T0295104

Hemodynamic Monitoring and Fluid Therapy during Surgery

Hemodynamic Monitoring and Fluid Therapy during Surgery

Edited by

Alexandre Joosten
University of California, Los Angeles

Maxime Cannesson
University of California, Los Angeles

Robert G. Hahn
Karolinska Institutet, Sweden

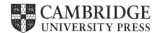

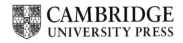

Shaftesbury Road, Cambridge CB2 8EA, United Kingdom

One Liberty Plaza, 20th Floor, New York, NY 10006, USA

477 Williamstown Road, Port Melbourne, VIC 3207, Australia

314–321, 3rd Floor, Plot 3, Splendor Forum, Jasola District Centre, New Delhi – 110025, India

103 Penang Road, #05–06/07, Visioncrest Commercial, Singapore 238467

Cambridge University Press is part of Cambridge University Press & Assessment,
a department of the University of Cambridge.

We share the University's mission to contribute to society through the pursuit of
education, learning and research at the highest international levels of excellence.

www.cambridge.org
Information on this title: www.cambridge.org/9781009226868

DOI: 10.1017/9781009226899

First published 2024

Printed in the United Kingdom by CPI Group Ltd. Croydon CR0 4YY

A catalogue record for this publication is available from the British Library

Library of Congress Cataloging-in-Publication Data
Names: Joosten, Alexandre, editor. | Cannesson, Maxime, editor. | Hahn, Robert G., editor.
Title: Hemodynamic monitoring and fluid therapy during surgery / edited by Alexandre Joosten, Maxime Cannesson,
Robert Hahn.
Other titles: Clinical fluid therapy in the perioperative setting. 2nd edition.
Description: Cambridge, United Kingdom ; New York, NY : Cambridge University Press, 2024. | Combined revised
volume of two successful texts: Clinical fluid therapy in the perioperative setting, 2nd edition; and Perioperative
hemodynamic monitoring and goal directed therapy. | Includes bibliographical references and index.
Identifiers: LCCN 2023044211 | ISBN 9781009226868 (hardback) | ISBN 9781009226899 (ebook)
Subjects: MESH: Hemodynamic Monitoring – methods | Fluid Therapy – methods | Monitoring, Intraoperative |
Intraoperative Care – methods | Intraoperative Period
Classification: LCC RC670.5.H45 | NLM WG 141.5.H3 | DDC 616.1/0754–dc23/eng/20231207
LC record available at https://lccn.loc.gov/2023044211

ISBN 978-1-009-22686-8 Hardback

Contents

Contributors

Metesh N. Acharya
Department of Cardiac Surgery, Glenfield Hospital, Leicester, UK

Brenton Alexander
Department of Anesthesiology, University of California, San Diego, CA, US

Achmet Ali
Department of Anesthesiology and Reanimation, Istanbul University, Istanbul, Turkey

Emre Sertaç Bingül
Department of Anesthesiology and Reanimation, Istanbul University, Istanbul, Turkey

Birgitte Brandstrup
Department of Surgery, Holbæk Hospital, Copenhagen University Hospitals, Copenhagen, Denmark

Jack E. Brooker
Anesthesiology Institute, Cleveland Clinic, Cleveland, OH, US

Pedro Cabrales
Department of Bioengineering, University of California, San Diego, CA, US

Lorenzo Calabrò
Humanitas Clinical and Research Center – IRCCS, Rozzano (Milan), Italy

Maxime Cannesson
Department of Anesthesiology and Intensive Care, Paris-Saclay University Hospitals, Paris-Saclay University, Paul-Brousse Hospital, Assistance Publique –

Hôpitaux de Paris, Villejuif, France, and Department of Anesthesiology and Perioperative Medicine, University of California, Los Angeles, CA, US

Maurizio Cecconi
Humanitas Clinical and Research Center – IRCCS, Rozzano (Milan), Italy, and Department of Biomedical Sciences, Humanitas University, Pieve Emanuele, MI, Italy

Sean Coeckelenbergh
Department of Anesthesiology and Intensive Care, Paris-Saclay University Hospital Group, Paris-Saclay University, Paul-Brousse Hospital, Assistance Publique – Hôpitaux de Paris, Villejuif, France, and Outcomes Research Consortium, Cleveland, OH, US

Diego Orbegozo Cortes
Department of Intensive Care, Erasme University Hospital, Free University of Brussels, Brussels, Belgium

Maxime Coutrot
Department of Anesthesiology and Critical Care and Burn Unit, St-Louis Hospital, Paris, France

Jérôme E. Dauvergne
Laënnec Hospital, University Hospital Center, Nantes, France

Daniel de Backer
Department of Intensive Care, Erasme University Hospital, Free University of Brussels, Brussels, Belgium

I.N. de Keijzer
Department of Anesthesiology, University Medical Center Groningen, University of Groningen, Groningen, The Netherlands

Benjamin Deniau
Department of Anesthesiology and Critical Care and Burn Unit, St-Louis Hospital, Paris, France

Nils W. Dennhardt
Department of Anaesthesiology and Intensive Care Medicine, Hannover Medical School, Hannover, Germany

François Depret
Department of Anesthesiology and Critical Care and Burn Unit, St-Louis Hospital, Paris, France

Emmanuel Dudoignon
Department of Anesthesiology and Critical Care and Burn Unit, St-Louis Hospital, Paris, France

Jacques Duranteau
Department of Anesthesiology and Intensive Care, Paris-Saclay University Hospitals, Paris-Saclay University, Paul-Brousse Hospital, Assistance Publique – Hôpitaux de Paris, Villejuif, France, and Department of Anesthesia and Surgical Intensive Care, Bicêtre University Hospital Assistance Publique – Hôpitaux de Paris, Paris-Saclay University Hospital Group, Kremlin-Bicêtre, France

Paul W.G. Elbers
Department of Intensive Care Medicine, Amsterdam UMC, Vrije Universiteit, Amsterdam, The Netherlands

Robert G. Hahn
Karolinska Institutet at Danderyds Hospital (KIDS), Stockholm, Sweden

Anatole Harrois
Department of Anesthesia and Surgical Intensive Care, Bicêtre University Hospital, Assistance Publique – Hôpitaux de Paris, Paris-Saclay University Hospital Group, Le Kremlin Bicêtre, France

Marcos Intaglietta
Department of Bioengineering, University of California, Diego, CA, US

Alexandre Joosten
Department of Anesthesiology and Perioperative Medicine, David Geffen School of Medicine, University of California, Los Angeles, CA, US

Indu Kapoor
Department of Neuroanaesthesiology and Critical Care, All India Institute of Medical Sciences, New Delhi, India

Hiromi Kato
Department of Anesthesiology and Intensive Care, Paris-Saclay University Hospitals, Paris-Saclay University, Paul-Brousse Hospital, Assistance Publique – Hôpitaux de Paris, Villejuif, France

Amanda M. Kleiman
Department of Anesthesiology, University of Virginia, Charlottesville, VA, US

Karim Lakhal
Laënnec Hospital, University Hospital Center, Nantes, France

Matthieu Legrand
Department of Anesthesia and Perioperative Medicine, Division of Critical Care Medicine, University of California, San Francisco, CA, US

Giulia Lionetti
Humanitas Clinical and Research Center – IRCCS, Rozzano (Milan), Italy

Charu Mahajan
Department of Neuroanaesthesiology and
Critical Care, All India Institute of Medical
Sciences, New Delhi, India

Kamal Maheshwari
Anesthesiology Institute, Cleveland Clinic,
Cleveland, OH, US

Giovanni Mariscalco
Department of Cardiac Surgery, Glenfield
Hospital, University of Leicester,
Leicester, UK

Judith Martini
Department of Anesthesia and Intensive
Care Medicine, Innsbruck Medical
University, Innsbruck, Austria

D. Massari
Department of Anesthesiology,
University Medical Center Groningen,
University of Groningen, Groningen,
The Netherlands

Antonio Messina
Humanitas Clinical and Research Center –
IRCCS, Rozzano (Milan), Italy, and
Department of Biomedical Sciences,
Humanitas University, Pieve Emanuele,
MI, Italy

Frédéric Michard
MiCo, Vallamand, Switzerland

Salima Naili
Department of Anesthesiology and
Intensive Care, Paris-Saclay University
Hospitals, Paris-Saclay University, Paul-
Brousse Hospital, Assistance Publique –
Hôpitaux de Paris, Villejuif, France

Chelsea A. Patry
Department of Anesthesiology,
University of Virginia, Charlottesville,
VA, US

Michael R. Pinsky
Department of Critical Care Medicine,
University of Pittsburgh, Pittsburgh, PA, US

Hemanshu Prabhakar
Department of Neuroanaesthesiology and
Critical Care, All India Institute of Medical
Sciences, New Delhi, India

Saqib H. Qureshi
Trent Cardiac Centre, University Hospital
of Nottingham, Nottingham, UK

Niels Van Regenmortel
Department of Intensive Care Medicine,
Ziekenhuis Netwerk Antwerpen Campus
Stuivenberg, Antwerp, Belgium, and
Department of Intensive Care Medicine,
Antwerp University Hospital, Antwerp,
Belgium

Joseph Rinehart
Outcomes Research Consortium,
Cleveland, OH, US, and Department of
Anesthesiology & Perioperative Care,
University of California, Irvine, US

Wouter Rosseels
Department of Intensive Care Medicine,
Ziekenhuis Netwerk Antwerpen Campus
Stuivenberg, Antwerp, Belgium

T.W.L. Scheeren
Critical Care, EMEACLA, Edwards
Lifesciences Services GmbH, Munich,
Germany

Mert Şentürk
Department of Anesthesiology and
Reanimation, Istanbul University, Istanbul,
Turkey

Robert Sümpelmann
Department of Anaesthesiology and Intensive
Care Medicine, Hannover Medical School,
Hannover, Germany

Zerrin Sungur
Department of Anesthesiology and
Reanimation, Istanbul University, Istanbul,
Turkey

Eryn R. Thiele
Department of Anesthesiology, University
of Virginia, Charlottesville, VA, US

Amy G. Tsai
Department of Bioengineering, University
of California, San Diego, CA, US

J.J. Vos
Department of Anesthesiology, University
Medical Center Groningen, University of
Groningen, Groningen, The Netherlands

Susan M. Walters
Department of Anesthesiology,
University of Virginia, Charlottesville,
VA, US

Laurence Weinberg
Department of Anaesthesia, Austin
Hospital, Melbourne, Australia, and
Department of Critical Care, University of
Melbourne, Australia

Marie Werner
Department of Anesthesia and Surgical
Intensive Care, Bicêtre University Hospital,
Assistance Publique – Hôpitaux de Paris,
Paris-Saclay University Hospital Group, Le
Kremlin-Bicêtre Villejuif, France

Foreword

Surgical interventions were documented for trauma already in prehistoric times, but the development of effective anesthetic agents in the mid-1800s, and later of muscle relaxants, paved the way for increasingly complex surgeries to be performed. As these interventions became more difficult, invasive, and thus longer, the need to maintain hemodynamic homeostasis and ensure adequate tissue oxygen delivery gained importance.

The word "hemodynamic" is derived from the Greek words *haima*, meaning blood, and *dunamis*, meaning power, and thus reflects the force involved in moving the circulation around the body. The word "monitoring" is derived from the Latin verb *monere*, meaning to warn or remind. "Hemodynamic monitoring" therefore essentially involves the use of methods to indicate the status of the blood circulation and to alert the clinician to any abnormalities. The very earliest form of hemodynamic monitoring was measurement of the pulse to estimate heart rate. In 1828, blood pressure was measured for the first time in humans and the sphygmomanometer was developed in the 1880s. A major advance in monitoring, and in our understanding of more complex hemodynamic interactions, came with the development of the Swan–Ganz catheter in the 1970s, enabling multiple variables to be measured simultaneously. More recent technological advances have seen a move toward increasingly non-invasive monitoring, notably for cardiac output assessment. Open-loop and closed-loop devices are also becoming available, which can assess hemodynamic status and offer advice or alerts regarding appropriate treatment (open-loop) or automatically provide treatment (closed-loop). And with the rapid advances currently taking place in artificial (or "augmented") intelligence, automatization of fluid therapy guided by continuous hemodynamic monitoring is likely to become a standard fixture in our operating rooms.

Indeed, among the multiple interventions used during surgery, fluid administration is one of the most frequent. Perioperative hypovolemia *and* fluid overload both impact negatively on patient outcomes, and appropriate administration of enough, but not too much, intravenous fluid is crucial to limit complications and ensure adequate tissue perfusion. Nevertheless, despite the widespread use of intravenous fluids questions still remain regarding the optimal approach to fluid administration, and there is wide variability in approaches to perioperative fluid management.

There are relatively few books specifically related to the combined notion of hemodynamic monitoring and fluid administration in the surgical patient, so this volume fills an important gap and provides a valuable up-to-date guide for all involved in the care of surgical patients. *Hemodynamic Monitoring and Fluid Therapy during Surgery*, a combined and updated version of two previous volumes, *Perioperative Hemodynamic Monitoring and Goal Directed Therapy: From Theory to Practice*[1] and *Clinical Fluid Therapy in the Perioperative Setting*,[2] is divided into four parts, providing comprehensive coverage of important aspects of hemodynamic monitoring and fluid therapy in chapters written by

---

[1] Cannesson M, Pearse R (Eds). (2014). *Perioperative Hemodynamic Monitoring and Goal Directed Therapy: From Theory to Practice*. Cambridge: Cambridge University Press. doi: 10.1017/CBO9781107257115

[2] Hahn RG (Ed). (2016). *Clinical Fluid Therapy in the Perioperative Setting* (2nd ed.). Cambridge: Cambridge University Press. doi: 10.1017/CBO9781316401972

an international panel of experts in their field. Part 1 sets the scene in terms of current concepts and aspects of hemodynamic monitoring. In Part 2, basic physiology of body volume distributions, fluid administration, and acid–base balance are revisited along with discussion of different fluid types. Part 3 focuses on the practicalities and complications of perioperative fluid infusion, including measures of fluid responsiveness and the role of goal-directed hemodynamic therapy. Several chapters in this section are then dedicated to specific types of surgery, trauma patients, and the pediatric population. Finally, Part 4 provides a vision of how the field is likely to advance in the future as new technology is employed to improve monitoring and provide more personalized patient care.

Despite the ever-increasing amounts of online material, books such as this, which gather together in one place chapters on related aspects of a specific topic written by known experts, are still valuable in providing an accurate and reliable source of information. The editors and authors are to be congratulated on this comprehensive volume, which covers the underlying physiology, available tools, current approaches, and a view of the future, to help improve knowledge about the appropriate use and application of hemodynamic monitoring to guide perioperative fluid therapy.

Jean-Louis Vincent MD PhD
Professor of Intensive Care Medicine (Université Libre de Bruxelles)
Consultant Intensivist, Dept of Intensive Care, Erasme University Hospital,
Brussels, Belgium

Preface

Over the past two decades, Cambridge University Press has published several books focused on perioperative hemodynamic care. Our present work incorporates and updates two of these texts. The first, *Clinical Fluid Therapy in the Perioperative Setting*, provided a means to understand fluid therapy and apply it to various perioperative situations. The second, *Perioperative Hemodynamic Monitoring and Goal Directed Therapy: From Theory to Practice*, established the importance of setting targets using monitors to improve perioperative vasopressor and fluid therapies. Our aims in the present work are similar to its predecessors: to convey a physiological foundation that will allow readers to transition with ease towards contemporary applications of perioperative hemodynamic therapy while simultaneously providing the knowledge required for advances in clinical hemodynamic research.

These messages are fundamental because hemodynamic monitoring and therapy have now become an integral part of perioperative care. Almost every patient who undergoes anesthesia receives intravenous fluids and many also require vasopressors. Every patient has blood pressure and heart rate monitoring, and higher risk patients benefit from continuous cardiac output monitoring. Physicians, nurses, patients, and even their families are thus faced with information and complex therapies that can be lifesaving. However, improper use can also be devastating and lead to severe iatrogenic morbidity. Today in perioperative medicine, it is indispensable to know the details of hemodynamics not only to give our patients the best quality of care but also to identify the limitations of these therapies and the potential of improvement through research.

Our work stems from a strong collaboration of world-renowned experts in the field of hemodynamics. We would like to wholeheartedly thank them for their contributions to both the updated and new chapters that will undoubtedly provide cutting-edge information for both clinicians and researchers. Although we provide detailed information on specialized topics, this text also provides a solid foundation for residents in anesthesia and critical care medicine as well as medical students who have a special focus on perioperative medicine.

Alexandre Joosten, Sean Coeckelenbergh, Robert Hahn and Maxime Cannesson

Chapter

1

Overview of the Circulation

Michael R. Pinsky

Introduction

Maintaining cardiovascular stability and reserve is fundamental to minimizing complications, morbidity and mortality in surgical patients and those otherwise critically ill. Titration of therapies aimed at supporting the cardiovascular system, respiratory gas exchange and internal homeostasis form the basis for acute care management. Diagnostic approaches, such as therapeutic trials and functional hemodynamic monitoring, or therapies, such as pre-optimization and other goal-directed therapies, are based on data derived from hemodynamic monitoring. Intraoperative clinical trial data documenting hemodynamic monitoring–defined resuscitation efforts that improve patient-centered outcomes were recently described.[1] Thus, the analysis of the cardiovascular status of patients and their response to therapies is tightly linked to physiological monitoring. Invasive hemodynamic monitoring includes arterial, central venous, and pulmonary arterial catheterization, transesophageal echo or ultrasound monitoring, non-invasive pulse oximetry, heart rate, blood pressure and arterial pressure waveform analysis. Similarly, using invasive monitoring one can measure O_2 saturation of central venous or mixed venous (within the pulmonary artery) blood (central venous oxygen saturation, $ScvO_2$, and venous oxygen saturation, SvO_2, respectively). Although specific combinations of hemodynamic variables often reflect certain disease states and their intrinsic physiological adaptive responses, there may be considerable overlap of hemodynamic data sets among markedly different pathological states that often may require different therapies. This diagnostic confusion can be minimized by examining the specific hemodynamic responses of the host to a specific therapy, often referred to as a therapeutic trial. For example, both severe sepsis and acute heart failure in the un-resuscitated patient will present with hypotension, a low cardiac output and SvO_2 and pulmonary artery occlusion pressure (Ppao). However, most patients in septic shock will be fluid responsive, increasing their cardiac output and SvO_2, whereas patients with acute heart failure will tend to increase both Ppao and blood pressure with less of an increase in cardiac output and SvO_2. Why these differences occur is a function of baseline cardiac function and reserve, vascular tone and reactivity, blood flow distribution and the effective circulating blood volume. To a large extent the information needed to identify which of these processes or groups of processes are driving a given pathological state requires hemodynamic monitoring targeted on the specific pathological processes most likely to be operational. Although the cardiovascular system is a tightly integrated system with close inherent and reflex feedback controls at multiple levels, one can artificially separate out the determinants of cardiovascular homeostasis into those that primarily are determined by: 1) ventricular pump function, 2) arterial vasomotor tone and blood flow distribution and 3) effective circulating blood volume and venous return. Although these processes are discussed further in several of the subsequent chapters in this volume, an overview of these processes is useful to place this massive system within context.

Ventricular Pump Function

Our fundamental understanding of cardiac myocyte contractile performance was initially defined by the pioneering work of Frank and Starling in the 1890s. Subsequently, we have come to realize that systolic and diastolic function can be linked or separated but carry a common determinant in adequate energy stores and delivery, calcium trafficking and structural changes in response to ischemia and either pressure or volume overload. Although most studies of ventricular function revolve around left ventricular (LV) function, right ventricular (RV) function is now getting well-deserved attention as a primary determinant of cardiovascular function. Still, understanding LV physiology is essential to diagnosing and managing critically ill patients. The two ventricles have different roles in sustaining cardiovascular homeostasis. The left ventricle's only role is to sustain a high central arterial pressure by ejecting a reasonable amount of its end-diastolic volume into the aorta with each heart beat without requiring high filling pressures or resulting in cardiac muscle ischemia. The maintenance of a high central arterial pressure allows the circulation to autoregulate blood flow amongst tissue beds relative to their different and often highly varying metabolic demands. The right ventricle's roles are to effectively transfer most of the varying venous return flow into the pulmonary arterial circuit with each beat without causing right atrial pressure (Pra) to increase, thus sustaining a maximal pressure gradient for venous return. Accordingly, LV failure is manifest by increased filling pressure and a low systolic pressure and profound pressure-dependent stroke volumes, whereas RV failure is defined by RV dilation, increased Pra, venous status and low cardiac outputs.

Frank, a German physiologist, noted that unlike skeletal muscle strips, when cardiac muscle strips were stretched above their resting length this increased their force of contraction. Starling reasoned that since the LV cavity approximated a sphere, increases in LV end-diastolic volume (EDV) should proportionally increase LV myocardial fiber stretch. Thus, he modified Frank's observations to say that force of LV contraction was related to LV EDV. According to this rule, increasing LV EDV when LV function is normal will increase LV stroke volume, and for a constant heart rate, cardiac output will increase as well. If LV pump function is impaired, then for the same increase in LV EDV stroke volume will increase much less (Fig. 1.1). This concept is central to most diagnostic and therapeutic protocols used to assess cardiac function.[2] The immediate treatment of acute cardiovascular insufficiency and arterial hypotension is to increase intravascular volume with the goal of increasing LV stroke volume via the Frank–Starling mechanism. If LV stroke volume increases, then the subject is said to be "preload-responsive," and the presumptive diagnosis of hypovolemia is made. The relation between LV EDV and either stroke volume or cardiac output is referred to as the Frank–Starling relationship. Still, focusing on the Frank–Starling mechanism to augment cardiac output when treating patients with presumed hypovolemia and preserved ventricular pump function is misleading and potentially dangerous. The Frank–Starling mechanism is primarily in place to match the varying outputs of the right and left ventricles over relatively short time intervals (e.g., 5–10 seconds) as venous return to the right ventricle varies with ventilation and subsequently varies to the left ventricle two to three beats later. In essence, it is an intrinsic process keeping the outputs of the two

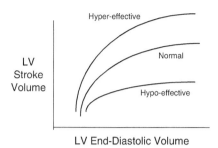

Figure 1.1 Graphic representation of the Frank–Starling relationship defining left ventricular (LV) function showing the relation between LV end-diastolic volume and stroke volume for normal, hyper- and hypo-functioning ventricles.

ventricles similar to prevent either pulmonary vascular congestion/edema or intrathoracic hypovolemia developing as either venous return or LV afterload are varied.

Importantly, it is difficult to document a sustained increase in LV EDV in an otherwise healthy subject following volume loading or exercise. Amazingly, with exercise or artificially increased venous return due to opening an arterio-venous fistula or rapid volume infusion, one sees a transient increase in both LV EDV and stroke volume. But after about 20 seconds, LV EDV returns to baseline values, although stroke volume remains elevated. The interpretation of these data must be that intrinsic contractility has increased. Indeed, this phenomenon, referred to as the Anrep effect or homeometric autoregulation, can be demonstrated in isolated perfused hearts, showing that it is intrinsic to the myocardium. [3] Presumably, increased myocardial wall stress increases local calcium flux by phosphorylation of the calcium channels, causing increased contractility. In fact, we can define patients as having systolic heart failure if they can only increase their LV stroke volume through the Starling mechanism.

However, with either the Frank–Starling or Anrep mechanisms in play, we still model the left ventricle as a pump, the work done is to create a stroke volume under pressure. The mechanical correlate of volumes moved under pressure is work, or stroke work. LV stroke volume will vary inversely with outflow pressure (arterial pressure) for a constant LV EDV and LV contractility. To account for this important influence, LV stroke work, rather than stroke volume, is often used to assess LV functional status. If stroke work is less for the same LV EDV, then LV contractility is also said to be less under this condition as well (Fig. 1.2). The measure of LV function used to assess cardiovascular status is highly dependent on the question being asked. If the clinician is wishing to assess the adequacy of LV output to meet the metabolic demands of the body, the cardiac output is most important, because it reflects blood flow. On the other hand, if the clinician wishes to understand the level of myocardial contractile reserve, independent of the level of blood flow, then the change in LV stroke work relative to the change in LV EDV is a better index.

Unfortunately, the Frank–Starling relationship is only a superficial description of the mechanical quality of ventricular ejection. The actual mechanical properties of the contracting ventricle are better characterized by the rate of increase in myocardial wall stiffness or elastance over systole, described as time-varying elastance.[4] Graphically, this distinction is better illustrated by displaying LV performance as a hydraulic pump plotting the relation between LV pressure and volume during the cardiac cycle.

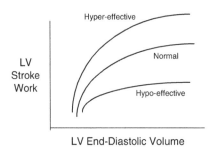

Figure 1.2 Same relation as shown in Figure 1.1, except left ventricular (LV) stroke work is substituted for stroke volume.

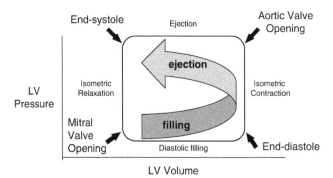

Figure 1.3 Stylized representation of the left ventricular (LV) pressure–volume relation over a complete cardiac cycle, referred to as the LV pressure–volume loop. Note that filling, contraction, emptying and relaxation proceed in a counterclockwise fashion.

The Left Ventricular Pressure–Volume Loop: When displayed as the changes in LV pressure and volume during a cardiac cycle, time is not seen (Fig. 1.3). Traditionally, LV volume is shown on the x-axis and LV pressure on the y-axis. Filling occurs during diastole when LV chamber pressure decreases to less than left atrial pressure. The slope of the passive LV distention is diastolic compliance. Right before the end of diastolic filling, the atria contract, rapidly increasing LV pressure at end-diastole. This results in a higher EDV but a lower overall filling pressure over diastole because LV end-diastolic pressure only increases rapidly at the end of diastole. Accordingly, myocardial blood flow is less impeded into the subendocardial regions during diastole than would otherwise be the case if LV filling pressure were always elevated across all diastolic pressure values. At end-diastole, defined by the electro-mechanical coupling of contraction, there exists the minimal LV pressure/volume ratio. This point is often used to assess diastolic compliance but is influenced the absolute volume restraint imposed by the pericardium, lungs and right ventricle. Thus, measures of LV end-diastolic pressure to LV EDV often vary widely without any actual changes in LV diastolic compliance. LV EDV is often used synonymously with LV preload as applied to the Frank–Starling relationship. However, LV preload by the Frank–Starling relationship is LV myocardial wall stress. If LV diastolic compliance changes from one beat to the next, as can easily occur with acute RV overload or hyperinflation, then for the same LV myocardial fiber stress LV EDV will be less. Thus, the bedside clinician is often left with the confusing situation of seeing increasing LV end-diastolic pressures without an increase in LV stroke volume and inferring that LV contractility is depressed. Although contractility may well be depressed, it is more likely in a non-cardiac patient that the decreased LV stroke volume reflects RV overload or hyperinflation. This process by which increased RV EDV or

RV end-diastolic pressures limit LV filling is referred to as ventricular interdependence and occurs commonly in both health and disease, making estimates of LV function by plotting the Frank–Starling curve using Ppao and LV stroke volume or stroke work inaccurate at best and often misleading.

With systolic contraction, LV intra-cavitary pressure rises, causing a passive closing of the mitral valve, changing the shape of the LV from an ellipsoid into a sphere as LV intra-cavitary pressure rapidly rises. The increased LV systolic intra-cavitary pressure caused by myofibril contraction results from three inter-related mechanisms. First, the myofibrils contract, shortening their individual fibers' long axis. This causes the circumference of fibrils to shorten along their myofibril orientation. Myofibrils are oriented in three ways: longitudinal, horizontal and spiral, relative to the long axis of the ventricle. Longitudinal myofibril contraction shortens the long axis from apex to base, causing the mitral annulus to migrate toward the base. Thus, mitral annual velocity measures reflect LV contraction. Horizontal myofibril contraction makes the cross-sectional circumference smaller. Finally, spiral myofiber contraction twists the chamber in a fashion analogous to the wringing of a washcloth. Second, myofibril contraction also results in thickening of the myofibrils at right angles at their longitudinal orientation. This thickening in a shortening circumference further increases the tension within the ventricle. Myofibril thickening primarily compresses the horizontal diameter of the LV chamber, whereas shortening primarily shortens the long axis and twists the heart. Third, the coordination of myofibril contraction allowing first the closure of the mitral and tricuspid values by the papillary muscles and then a generalized ventricular wall contractions requires an integrated His–Purkinjean conduction system that transfers atrio-ventricular nodal activation into myofibril activation. However, alterations in contraction synchrony caused by arrhythmias and regional contractile impairments induced by ischemia can profoundly impair LV contraction effects, rapidly leading to LV failure. All these processes combine to allow a single contraction to generate enough wall tension with a minimal amount of cellular energy requirement to cause effective LV ejection many times a minute for many years without the need for hypertrophy or the development of ischemia.

Once LV intra-cavitary pressure exceeds aortic pressure, the aortic valve passively opens, and ejection begins with continued LV contraction but now decreasing LV volume with no measurable resistance created by the aortic value. In normal subjects, the point where ejection occurs represents the maximal LV wall stress. By the law of Laplace, wall stress is the product of radius of curvature and developed pressure. Thus, diastolic arterial pressure being the pressure at which the aortic value opens during ejection is a major determinant of LV wall stress. LV wall stress is LV afterload and is often referred to inaccurately as LV ejection pressure. This concept is important because any therapy that selectively decreases diastolic arterial pressure will reduce LV afterload more than therapies that selectively decrease systolic arterial pressure. Similarly, if a vasodilator therapy, for example, induced both vasodilation and increased LV stroke volume, then diastolic arterial pressure will decrease, but systolic arterial pressure may either remain constant or increase. If the clinician were specifically targeting systolic arterial pressure as LV afterload, then they would incorrectly presume that the vasodilator therapy paradoxically increased afterload. This presumption potentially could lead to an incorrect decision to either increase vasodilator therapy further, which may induce coronary ischemia by further decreasing coronary perfusion pressure, or stop vasodilator therapy altogether despite the fact that such patients who increase their arterial pulse pressure in response to vasodilator therapy are actually showing a positive response to this treatment.

Importantly, for the LV pressure–volume loop, we see that LV ejection occurs as LV volume decreases and both LV pressure and aortic pressure rise. As LV ejection continues transferring blood into the thoracic aorta, the aorta distends. becoming stiffer. Thus, arterial pressure rises more toward the end of ejection even though the actual amount and rate of volume being ejected at the end is much less than in the beginning. Accordingly, most of the increase in arterial pressure occurs when the LV volume is already small. Interestingly, LV afterload is approximated by the product of the LV radius of curvature and the LV pressure; although LV pressure rises during ejection, the radius of curvature decreases. Thus, in otherwise normal subjects the product of LV radius of curvature and ejection pressure decreases during ejection. For example, assuming an ejection fraction of 60% and a normal LV EDV, then the LV radius of curvature should decrease by >300% from end-diastole to end-systole, while LV ejection pressure only increases by 20–40% from the opening of the aortic value (diastolic arterial pressure to systolic arterial pressure). Thus, LV wall stress should decrease by more than half from the start to the end of ejection. That the left ventricle unloads itself during ejection has important clinical implications. First, systolic hypertension is reasonably well tolerated on a short-term basis without much increase in myocardial O_2 demand (MVO_2). Diastolic hypertension, however, immediately increases MVO_2 and stimulates the development of LV hypertrophy. If the left ventricle is dilated and at end-ejection still has a large volume, then systolic pressure will be a major contributor to both LV wall stress and MVO_2. Under dilated cardiomyopathy conditions, a reduction of LV afterload only occurs if the LV cavity gets much smaller during ejection. So in dilated heart failure states, ejection only minimally decreases LV volumes, and systolic arterial pressure becomes the determinant of LV afterlaod. Accordingly, such patients are very sensitive to changes in systolic arterial pressure and specific decreases in systolic arterial pressure should decrease LV end-systolic volume and MVO_2.

Interestingly, LV end-ejection occurs at a pressure–volume ratio that appears to be only minimally altered by ejection history but highly influenced by end-ejection pressure and intrinsic contractility. If arterial resistance is high, then LV end-systolic pressure and end-systolic volume (ESV) increase, whereas if arterial resistance is low, both decrease. However, both end-systolic pressure and volume do so along an end-systolic elastance line, called the end-systolic pressure–volume relationship (ESPVR) that is independent of the actual pressure or volume. Importantly, the ESPVR slope varies in proportion to changes in contractility: increasing with increased contractility and decreasing with decreased contractility.[3] Thus, one can say that LV ESV then is a function of both afterload and contractility. As such increases in afterload will increase ESV whereas decreases in afterload will decrease ESV, the slope of the ESPVR, however, remains unchanged.

Once end-ejection has occurred, the left ventricle actively relaxes. Diastolic relaxation, or lusitropy, is the energy-dependent part of the cardiac cycle, causes LV intra-cavitary pressure to decrease faster than would be predicted by passive relaxation alone (i.e., sucking action occurs) and is impaired by myocardial ischemia. Thus, impaired active diastolic relaxation is the earliest manifestation of myocardial ischemia. Once LV intra-cavitary pressure decreases below aortic pressure, the aortic valve passively closes, allowing LV pressure to continue to decrease as aortic pressure remains elevated, creating a coronary artery pressure gradient needed to support LV coronary flow during diastole. Since coronary artery blood flow occurs primarily in diastole, when LV wall stress is low whereas perfusion pressure is high, any process that impairs diastolic relaxation will decrease coronary blood flow.

Expanding the ESPVR to Encompass All of Systole: Time-Varying Elastance: The entire LV contractile process can be understood better from the perspective not of a single pressure–volume loop, but from the pressure–volume domain of contraction across many potential LV pressure–volume loops that might be created for the same level of contractility but by varying preload and afterload. Within this analysis, one may describe increasing LV stiffness as an increasing slope of a theoretical LV pressure–volume domain as one point in time post-initiation of LV contraction, identical to the LV ESPVR but at earlier points during systole. Thus, as time progresses from the start of contraction to end-ejection the left ventricle becomes progressively stiffer, such that the slope of the unique LV elastance curves for each time post the start of contraction will become progressively greater until they merge with the ESPVR curve. Since stiffness is also referred to an elastance, this time-dependent increase in stiffness is referred to as time-varying elastance (Et). In essence, time-varying elastance describes the progressive stiffening of the left ventricle through systole and then its relaxation in diastole within the pressure–volume domain.[3] Time-varying elastance can be calculated as a plot of the slopes of the isochronic (similar point in time relative to the start of contraction) LV pressure–volume relations during ejection as the end-diastolic volume is rapidly varied (Fig. 1.4). The slopes of these sequential pressure–volume lines reflect the obligatory LV pressure–volume domain that must be followed during systole. Importantly, Et defines the LV systolic function. The slope of the ESPVR can then be defined as end-systolic elastance (E_{es}) and is usually calculated from the regression line of the ESPVR data pairs of repetitive LV pressure–volume loops.

Although this discussion may seem esoteric, it has important direct clinical applications and explains many of the previously unexplained physiological determinants of LV systolic function. Recall that the Frank–Starling relationship maintains that as LV EDV increases, LV stroke work also increases. Indeed, any ejection phase index, like stroke volume, velocity of circumferential fiber shortening, ejection fraction and LV pressure change (dP) over a period of time (dt), dP/dt, will all show an increase with increasing LV EDV. But why? Time varying elastance explains all these phenotypic outputs as epi-phenomena of time varying elastance. Note that as systole progresses, Et also increases. Since E_{es} is greater than end-diastolic elastance, any increase in LV EDV will create a lesser increase in ESV, if LV ejection pressure does not also increase significantly. Since the Et is always increasing up to

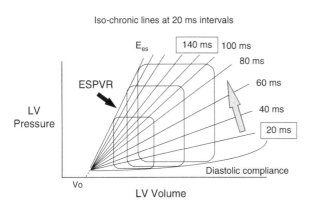

Figure 1.4 Stylized representation of three left ventricular (LV) pressure–volume loops at differing volumes showing how diastolic compliance, end-systolic elastance and the isochronic (same point in time following the start of systole) time-varying elastance are calculated. The estimated zero LV pressure residual volume of the heart is called V_0. E_{es}, end-systolic elastance; ESPVR, end-systolic pressure–volume relationship.

E_{es}, the resultant stroke volume, stroke work, LV dP/dt and velocity of circumferential fiber shortening must also increase for a given diastolic compliance and E_{es}. When does this not happen? When does increasing LV EDV not increase stroke volume or other ejection phase indices? This occurs when LV contractile function is depressed or LV diastolic compliance reduced so much that the slopes of the diastolic compliance and ESPVR become equal.

Applying Cardiac Physiology at the Bedside: The preload-dependent nature of LV perform-ance is a primary characteristic of normal ventricular function. Demonstrating that LV EDV is above some minimal value, despite cardiac output and stroke work both being depressed, and with increases in LV EDV further, neither cardiac output nor LV stroke work increase is a fundamental attribute of the phenotype of systolic heart failure. Regrettably, the opposite is not true. Documenting that LV EDV is reduced in the setting of hemodynamic instability does not identify hypovolemia because reduced LV EDV is also seen commonly in conditions associated with diastolic dysfunction, such as tamponade, cor pulmonale, hyperinflation and pulmonary hypertension. These conditions are common in the critically ill, making finding a reduced LV EDV not synonymous with volume responsiveness. These points are addressed further in the chapter on functional hemodynamic monitoring.

Right Ventricular Function: The *Forgotten Ventricle:* Traditionally, cardiovascular chapters would now switch to discussing the peripheral circulation, which is appropriate if the major aspects of ventricular pump function had already been covered. Regrettably, they have not. The right ventricle behaves in a very different manner when presented with increased volume (preload) or ejection pressure (afterload).

Under normal conditions, it is extremely difficult to document that RV filling pressure changes during RV filling. When RV filling pressure, defined as Pra minus pericardial pressure, was directly measured in patients undergoing open chest operations as RV volume was varied by acute volume loading, RV filling pressure is insignificantly altered.[5] Although Pra increases with volume loading, pericardial pressure also increases, such that RV filling pressure, defined as right atrial pressure minus pericardial pressure, remains unchanged. Similar data are seen when RV volumes are reduced by the application of positive end-expiratory pressure (PEEP) in post-operative cardiac patients.[6] Thus, under normal conditions, RV diastolic compliance is very high and most of the increase in Pra seen during volume loading reflects pericardial compliance and cardiac fossa stiffness. If RV wall stress is not increased during filling, then RV myofibril length remains constant. Presumably, conformational changes in the RV more than wall stretch are responsible for RV enlargement.[7] Accordingly, changes in Pra do not follow changes in RV end-diastolic volume, as has recently been validated to define why measures of right atrial pressure, or central venous pressure, cannot predict either intravascular volume status or RV preload.[8] When cardiac contractility is reduced and intravascular volume is expanded, RV filling pressure does increase as a result of either decreased RV diastolic compliance, increased pericardial compliance, increased end-diastolic volume or a combination of all three. RV over-distention has important clinical consequences. As RV EDV increases, the absolute volume remaining in the cardiac fossa decreases, making LV diastolic compliance less, by a process referred to as ventricular interdependence.[7] Lung expansion if causing hyperin-flation compresses the heart within the cardiac fossa in a fashion analogous to pericardial tamponade, but in this setting, it is the expanding lungs that increase intrathoracic pressure (ITP), and not pericardial restraint, limiting ventricular filling.[6]

As will be described further below, venous return, the primary determinant of cardiac output,[9] is maintained near maximal levels at rest [10] because RV filling occurs with minimal changes in filling pressure. This is because Pra is the back pressure to venous return. Accordingly, the closer Pra remains to zero relative to atmospheric pressure, the maximal is the pressure gradient for systemic venous blood flow.[11] For this mechanism to operate efficiently, RV output must equal venous return, otherwise sustained increases in venous blood flow would overdistend the RV, increasing Pra. Fortunately, under normal conditions of spontaneous ventilation this is not a problem because most of the increase in venous return is in phase with inspiration, when ITP decreases, such that Pra when measured relative to atmosphere also decreases. Likewise, the pulmonary arterial inflow circuit is highly compliant and can accept large increases in RV stroke volume without changing pressure. Thus, any transient increase in venous return within limits is proportionally delivered to the pulmonary circuit without forcing the RV to increase its force of contraction or myocardial oxygen demand.

This normal adaptive system will rapidly become dysfunctional if RV diastolic compliance decreases or if Pra increases independent of changes in RV EDV. Clinical examples of states where this usually occurs include acute RV dilation or cor pulmonale (pulmonary embolism, hyperinflation and RV infarction), which induce profound decreases in cardiac output not responsive to fluid resuscitation. Dissociation between Pra and RV EDV also occurs during either cardiac tamponade or positive-pressure ventilation. Thus, positive-pressure ventilation impairs circulatory adaptive processes normally occurring during spontaneous ventilation. Since the primary effect of ventilation on cardiovascular function in normal subjects is to alter RV preload via altering venous blood flow, the detrimental effect of positive pressure ventilation on cardiac output can be minimized by either fluid resuscitation to increase venous return or by keeping PEEP and tidal volumes as small as possible. Finally, over-resuscitation causes transient acute right heart failure, and though often underappreciated, it probably occurs more often than not with aggressive resuscitation scenarios not targeted as limited resuscitation to only preload responsive subjects. Excessive fluid resuscitation either by too much infused or too rapid an infusion rate will cause Pra to rise. Thus, a rising Pra of >2 mmHg during a fluid bolus maneuver is a stopping rule to limit fluid infusion. Such patients need to be reassessed as to the status of their right ventricle and their level of fluid responsiveness. Fluid responsiveness will be discussed below.

Arterial Pressure and Blood Flow Distribution

Arterial pressure is a primary determinant of organ perfusion. The other factor determining organ blood flow is intra-organ vascular resistance. Importantly, organ perfusion is independent of cardiac output. Cardiac output is only important within this context to maintain an adequate organ perfusion pressure, allowing autoregulation of organ blood flow by the organs themselves. Thus, hypotension blunts autoregulation of blood flow and directly reduces organ blood flow. Systemic hypotension is synonymous with cardiovascular instability. Since a fundamental goal of hemodynamic monitoring is to identify cardiovascular instability,[12] documenting systemic hypotension is essential in defining profound circulatory shock. Operationally, mean arterial pressure (MAP) is presumed to be the input pressure to the organs. However, LV perfusion occurs primarily during diastole and brain and intra-abdominal organs also see intra-cranial and intra-abdominal pressures as their back pressures to flow, respectively. Thus, actual organ perfusion pressure may be quite different amongst vital organs for the same MAP.

If MAP is the primary pressure defining organ perfusion, can a patient be in circulatory shock and not be hypotensive? The answer is yes. Normal homeostatic mechanisms functioning via carotid body baroreceptors vary arterial peripheral vascular tone through sympathetic nerves to maintain MAP relatively constant despite varying cardiac output. This profoundly conserved cardiovascular sympathetic reflex process is done to maintain cerebral and coronary blood flow at the expense of the remainder of the body. In an otherwise healthy subject, this reflex response can totally mask global hypoperfusion. For example, in the postoperative period, if occult hemorrhage causes progressive hypovolemia, then the initial findings are usually hypertension and tachycardia, not hypotension, as the increased sympathetic drive caused marked peripheral vasoconstriction. Clearly, baroreceptor response can only work effectively in the long term if the low cardiac output is not sustained; otherwise, marked end-organ hypoperfusion will manifest as decreased urine output, ileus and cold cyanotic extremities. Thus, MAP is a remarkably stable measure and relatively insensitive as a marker of cardiovascular instability or organ blood flow. Indirect measures of sympathetic tone, such as heart rate, respiratory rate and peripheral capillary filling and peripheral cyanosis, reflect better estimates of cardiovascular status than does MAP. Still, hypotension is a medical emergency because its presence defines that tissue hypoperfusion must exist and that normal homeostatic defense processes are inadequate.

MAP monitoring is still essential in the assessment and management of hemodynamically unstable subjects for several reasons. Measures that specifically increase MAP should also increase organ perfusion pressure if critical closing pressure does not also increase equally. In healthy subjects, vasopressors increase tone at all levels so organ blood flow usually remains constant despite increasing MAP. Vasoconstrictor therapies may increase vasomotor tone more in non-vital peripheral organs but almost always will maintain flow to the cerebral and coronary beds because their arteries have little or no alpha-adrenergic receptors, whereas the gut, kidneys, muscles and skin demonstrate a marked reduction in blood flow in response to marked sympathetic stimulation. Accordingly, short-term survival of the host is closely linked to MAP through the maintenance of cerebral and coronary blood flows. If profound hypotension persists for even a brief period of time, irreversible cerebral and cardiac damage can occur. Thus, the initial priority in resuscitation of a hypotensive patient is to restore MAP above a level that will ensure coronary and cerebral perfusion, usually >65 mmHg, and then to restore cardiac output once MAP is stabilized to restore vital organ blood flow.

The primary method of increasing vascular tone is to infuse vasopressor agents, like norepinephrine. Regrettably, vasopressor support in the absence of fluid resuscitation may improve transiently both global blood flow and MAP but worsen local non-vital blood flow and hasten tissue ischemia. Thus, initial resuscitative efforts should always include a volume expansion component and fluid challenge to identify preload-responsive shock states, prior to relying solely on vasopressors to support the unstable patient.

Arterial pressure is created by the ejection of LV stroke volume into the aorta, causing it to distend. Since LV ejection is rapid, absolute arterial blood volume increases with each systole and then decreases slowly during diastole as the arterial blood runoff into the organs continues. Since neither arterial pressure nor blood flow is ever constant during life, it is fundamentally difficult to assess arterial vasomotor tone from mean values of arterial pressure and cardiac output. Simplistically, one can estimate MAP and plot the relation between changes in MAP and changes in cardiac output over time. The inverse slope of this relationship, with flow on the *y*-axis, defines arterial tone (Fig. 1.5). With increased arterial vascular tone, a greater increase in arterial pressure is needed to cause the same increase in blood flow as would be the case if tone were less. Importantly, the zero-flow pressure intercept intersects the *x*-axis at a pressure significantly higher than Pra. In otherwise healthy individuals, this zero-flow intercept pressure is approximately 40–50 mmHg. This is because zero-flow pressure is the actual back pressure to arterial blood flow and reflects the mean-weighted (lumped parameter) critical closing pressure of the arterial circuit below which arterial vasomotor tone causes the arterioles to collapse. For the system as a whole, if arterial tone were to markedly increase, as is the case in severe heart failure, the zero-flow pressure will also increase. In vasodilatory state, like sepsis, zero-flow pressures usually decrease. Thus, for the same MAP, actual organ perfusion pressure can vary widely depending on overall vasomotor tone. Regrettably, the measure of an individual organ's critical closing pressures is impractical in clinical practice. Thus, clinicians use MAP as the primary pressure driver for organ blood flow. The other implication of this reality is that the artificial calculation of systemic vascular resistance as the ratio of the difference between MAP and Pra to cardiac output grossly overestimates vasomotor tone and places an inappropriately important value on the role Pra plays in defining arterial tone.[13]

Another way to analyze arterial tone is to assess the dynamic changes in arterial pressure and flow during ejection, as quantified by measures of aortic input impedance. Although this approach may seem daunting, if dynamic changes in arterial pulse pressure and stroke volume can be simultaneously recorded, as is often the case with the use of minimally invasive hemodynamic monitoring techniques, then both arterial elastance and the ratio of the pulse pressure variation to stroke volume variation, referred to as dynamic arterial elastance, can be estimated. Arterial elastance for a constant heart rate can be calculated as the ratio of 0.9 times the systolic arterial pressure to stroke volume, whereas the pulse pressure variation to stroke volume variation will reflect central arterial stiffness. The greater this dynamic arterial elastance is, the greater will be the variance of pulse pressure relative to stroke volume. Since these changes in pulse pressure and stroke volume are reported as percentage changes, dynamic arterial elastance is unitless. Normal subjects have a dynamic arterial elastance between 1.8 and 1.0, whereas a dynamic arterial elastance <0.8 reflects profound loss of arterial vasomotor tone.[14] If a patient is on vasopressor support and has an acceptable MAP and their dynamic arterial elastance is >1.0, then most can be

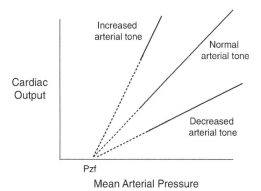

Figure 1.5 Relation between mean cardiac output and mean arterial pressure as cardiac output is varied over a normal physiological range for a normal, increased and decreased arterial vasomotor tone state. The zero cardiac output–mean arterial pressure intercept reflects arterial pressure at zero flow (Pzf) and is the effective back pressure to arterial blood flow.

safely weaned to a lower level of vasopressor support without causing systemic hypotension. This allows for the more rapid and highly personalized titration of vasopressors to vaso-plegic patients.

Blood Volume and Mean Systemic Pressure

Although ventricular pump function and arterial tone are extremely important in defining blood flow distribution once the blood is delivered to the heart, it is axiomatic that the heart can only pump the blood that it receives. In fact, up to the end of severe heart failure the heart pumps nearly 100% of the blood it receives back into the circulation. Clearly, as ventricular pump function decreases, increased filling pressures for the left ventricle can cause pulmonary edema and increased filling pressure for the right ventricle can cause peripheral edema. Indeed, it is only at the worst stages of cardiogenic shock that cardiac output decreases. Furthermore, when vascular pressures are measured along the route of blood flow from the heart, through the aorta into the arteries, arterioles, capillaries, venules and veins, one sees that most of the intravascular pressure generated by the ejecting heart is held constant down to the level of the small arteries and then drops quickly over the next 0.5 cm of vessel length as the circuit passes through the small arteries, arterioles, into the capillaries. This vascular waterfall occurs at a pressure measured as the zero flow pressure (Fig. 1.5) described above. That pressure drops beyond these vascular loci means that systemic capillaries are spared from seeing high hydrostatic pressures that would otherwise promote edema formation. However, the low capillary pressure demands that the resistance to venous return from the capillaries to the right side of the heart must remain very low or the pressure gradient for venous return will be inadequate to sustain flow. The maintenance of a low capillary and venous resistance is due to the markedly increased cross-sectional area of the capillaries relative to arterioles and the large diameters of the veins.

The blood flow back to the heart from the circulation is venous return and is the primary determinant of cardiac output.[11] Since the pressure in the periphery draining the organs is much lower than arterial pressure, the resistance to venous return is much lower than arterial resistance and flow much more dependent on small changes in downstream pressure. Guyton described this interaction over 50 years ago as the venous return curve (Fig. 1.6) wherein cardiac output or venous return is plotted on the y-axis against Pra on the x-axis. The summed weighted average systemic pressure in all the vascular reservoirs is referred to as mean systemic pressure (Pms) and is the subject of its own chapter later in this volume. Under steady-state conditions, Pms is a function of blood flow distribution amongst all the vascular reservoirs, their stressed and unstressed volumes and venomotor tone. Since venomotor tone and unstressed volume can be rapidly changed by increasing intra-abdominal pressure, muscle contraction, transferring blood flow from regions with high to low unstressed volumes and vice versa or changes in sympathetic tone, Pms is a highly dynamic variable under normal conditions. However, during rest, general anesthesia and critical illness wherein little changes in metabolic demand or blood flow distribution usually occur, Pms remains relatively constant over minutes, whereas Pra changes dynamically over the ventilatory cycle as changes in intrathoracic pressure artificially alter Pra relative to atmosphere. Spontaneous inspiration causes Pra to decrease, while positive pressure inspiration increases Pra. Thus, the blood flow back to the right ventricle can vary considerably throughout the ventilatory cycle. As mentioned above, one of the primary reasons for the Frank–Starling mechanism is to balance LV output to this changing RV output over a few heart beats. Still, sustained and rapid increases in Pra will markedly decrease venous return, inducing hypovolemic shock. This is the mechanism for cardiovascular collapse from an acute massive pulmonary embolism. The immediate pulmonary vascular obstruction blocks RV ejection, rapidly increasing Pra and stopping blood flow. By examining the venous return curve shown in Figure 1.6, this effect can be clearly understood. The normal Pra of healthy individuals is zero to 2 mmHg. This low Pra ensures a maximal venous return with minimal peripheral edema. If an acute obstruction of >50% of the pulmonary vascular were to occur, as is often the case with massive pulmonary embolism, then RV ejection will be markedly impeded, resulting in rapid RV dilation, intraventricular septal shift into the left ventricle, decreasing LV diastolic compliance, and a sudden and sustained increase in Pra, decreasing the pressure gradient for venous return. Thus, the underfilled left ventricle cannot adjust, and unless the pulmonary vascular obstruction is eliminated, profound circulatory shock and death ensue. Importantly, increasing venous return for fluid resuscitation alone will only cause further RV dilation, compromising LV function further. The immediate rescue treatment of this condition is to give systemic vasopressors to maintain coronary perfusion and Pms while instituting thrombolytic therapy to lyse the intravascular clot.

The determinants of venous return are Pms, Pra and the resistance to venous return. Although we discussed Pra and Pms and will discuss Pms in greater detail in a later, the resistance to venous return is often dismissed. This is a mistake. Since the pressure gradient for venous return is low and all of cardiac output must be defined by venous return, the small changes in the resistance to venous return will have profound effects on venous return for the same Pra and Pms. Importantly, venous resistance is not due to changes in downstream venomotor tone as seen in the arterial circuit, but due to changes in the total cross-sectional area of vascular and outflow resistance. Since the splanchnic circulation drains through a second organ, the liver, before returning to the heart, splanchnic blood flow carries with it twice the venous resistance of systemic vascular beds. Similarly, increasing sympathetic tone decreases unstressed volume, increasing Pms for the same blood volume, but also decreases the number of parallel venous conduits draining that organ by arterial constriction. This causes Pms to increase and increases the resistance to venous return. The results of vasopressor therapy on cardiac output are thus hard to predict beforehand unless one knows baseline contractile reserve, circulating blood volume and vasomotor tone. Increasing intra-abdominal pressure by gas insufflation for laparoscopic

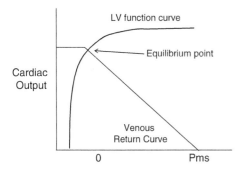

Figure 1.6 Relation between cardiac output and right atrial pressure when right atrial pressure (Pra) is independently varied defines two separate curves. The LV function curve also displayed in Figure 1.1, but with cardiac output and not stroke volume as the flow unit; and the venous return curve. The intersection of the two curves defines steady-state cardiac output and is referred to as the equilibrium point. The zero cardiac output Pra intercept of the venous return curve is mean systemic pressure (Pms); the slope of the cardiac output to Pra line is inversely proportional to the resistance to venous return.

surgery or proning a patient for surgery can also increase Pms and the resistance to venous return.[15] However, if vasopressor therapy while increasing MAP also increases cardiac output, then LV contractile reserve and circulating blood volume are adequate, whereas if the same increase in MAP causes cardiac output (CO) to decrease, then LV contractile reserve is limited. Accordingly, knowing the response to vasopressor therapy on cardiac output also allows the bedside clinician to know the patient's underlying cardiovascular reserve.

Cardiac Output, Oxygen Delivery and Oxygen Consumption

A central goal of normal homeostasis is to continually maintain delivery of oxygenated blood and nutrients to the metabolically active tissues in amounts adequate to sustain normal function overall and tissue viability in the short run without wasting energy or overstressing the cardiovascular circuit. The O_2 carrying capacity of the blood is the product of hemoglobin times O_2 saturation times cardiac output. If one assumes an adequate O_2 carrying capacity, then O_2 delivery to the tissues is dependent on cardiac output and blood flow distribution. Clearly, cardiac output and O_2 delivery may vary independently if arterial O_2 tension, hemoglobin levels or hemoglobin affinity for O_2 vary rapidly, as may occur during hemorrhage or rapid resuscitation with or without red blood cell infusions. Given this limitation, however, it is useful to consider the two together because cardiac output is relatively easy to measure, and in stress states, cardiac output and O_2 delivery share common determinants. Recall, however, that normal homeostasis allows for local metabolic demand to determine local blood flow and thus local O_2 delivery. Thus, loss of the ability to auto-regulate blood flow distribution relative to regional metabolic demands will also result in regional tissue hypoperfusion and tissue ischemia even if cardiac output and O_2 delivery are in a range that would otherwise ensure adequate tissue O_2 delivery. This is the scenario present in systemic hypotension wherein local vasodilation in response to increased metabolic demand does not equate with increased flow. The clinical example of this is severe sepsis wherein cardiac output is in either a normal or an elevated range and mixed venous O_2 saturation (SvO$_2$) is increased but clear evidence of tissue ischemia co-exists (e.g., lactic acidosis and organ dysfunction).

Since metabolic demand is ever changing even in the critically ill patient on mechanical ventilation and sedation, cardiac output usually co-varies with O_2 uptake.[16] O_2 supply and O_2 demand must co-vary as a normal and expected aspect of homeostasis. In cardiovascular insufficiency states, such as cardiogenic shock or hypovolemic shock, cardiac output is often limited and cannot increase in response to increasing metabolic demand. Under these conditions, O_2 consumption tends to remain constant despite minimal increases in cardiac output by increasing O_2 extraction. Different organs have different abilities to extract O_2 at low levels and still maintain function. Muscular activity effectively extracts O_2 from the blood because of the setup of the microcirculatory flow patterns and the large concentration of mitochondria in these tissues. Thus, sustained muscular activity is often associated with a marked decreased SvO$_2$ despite a normal circulatory system. Trained athletes can push their SvO$_2$ to very low levels during exercise. Muscular activities, such as moving in bed, physical therapy, being turned, "fighting the ventilator" and breathing spontaneously, can double resting O_2 consumption.[12,17] In the patient with an intact and functioning cardiopulmonary apparatus, this will translate into an increase in both cardiac output and O_2 consumption.

There is no level of cardiac output that is "normal," but there are thresholds of O_2 delivery below which normal metabolism can no longer occur.[18] Taking global measures first, if SvO_2 is less than 50%, then some vascular beds somewhere are at the brink of dysoxia because tissue O_2 extraction becomes inefficient at maintaining O_2 flux when end-capillary blood has little O_2 to unload.[10] Regrettably, the converse is not always true. A higher level of SvO_2 does not ensure adequate end-capillary O_2 levels because SvO_2 reflects the mix of all venous blood. Thus, some areas with low extraction may mix with areas of lesser extraction to create a "normal" SvO_2 of >70% despite the coexistence of tissue ischemia. Thus, measures of SvO_2 are useful only in defining the risk for ischemia and, by extension, circulatory insufficiency and not in excluding the presence of tissue ischemia. Measures of veno-arterial CO_2 differences reflect better adequacy of organ blood flow. Values of PCO_2 differences between venous and arterial blood gas of >6 mmHg suggest hypoperfusion, hypermetabolism or both.

Relevant to sustaining tissue blood flow, resuscitation from traumatic and septic shock is often at associated with immediate restoration of organ system function. Persistent coma, ileus and low urine output are commonly observed. End-organ function usually returns within hours to days. But measures of microcirculatory flow demonstrate that during resuscitation from circulatory shock, clear dissociations occur between macro-circulatory measures, like MAP, cardiac output and O_2 delivery and capillary blood flow and parenchymal cellular function. The causes of this commonly observed discordance are at present unknown but probably related to inherent down-regulation of the cellular metabolic function as a primordial defense mechanism against cellular death. This process and how to assess and reverse it once cardiovascular stability has been reinstated are currently areas of ongoing research.

References

1. Pinsky MR, Cecconi M, Chew MS, et al. Effective hemodynamic monitoring. *Crit Care*. 2022;**26**(1):294.

2. Ross J Jr, Peterson KL. On the assessment of cardiac inotropic state. *Circulation*. 1973;**47**(3):435–8.

3. Rosenblueth A, Alanis J, Lopez E, Rubio R. The adaptation of ventricular muscle to different circulatory conditions. *Arch Int Physiol Biochim*. 1959;**67**(3):358–73.

4. Suga H, Sagawa K. Instantaneous pressure-volume relationships and their ratio in the excised, supported canine left ventricle. *Circ Res*.1974;**35**(1):117–26.

5. Tyberg JV, Taichman GC, Smith ER, et al. The relationship between pericardial pressure and right atrial pressure: an intraoperative study. *Circulation*. 1986;**73**(3):428–32.

6. Pinsky MR, Desmet JM, Vincent JL. Effect of positive end-expiratory pressure on right ventricular function in humans. *Am Rev Respir Dis*. 1992;**146**(3):681–7.

7. Kingma I, Smiseth OA, Frais MA, Smith ER, Tyberg JV. Left ventricular external constraint: relationship between pericardial, pleural and esophageal pressures during positive end-expiratory pressure and volume loading in dogs. *Ann Biomed Eng*. 1987;**15**(3–4):331–46.

8. Marik PE, Cavallazzi R. Does the central venous pressure predict fluid responsiveness? An updated meta-analysis and a plea for some common sense. *Crit Care Med*. 2013;**41**(7):1774–81.

9. Goldberg HS, Rabson J. Control of cardiac output by systemic vessels. Circulatory adjustments to acute and chronic respiratory failure and the effect of therapeutic interventions. *Am J Cardiol*. 1981;**47**(3):696–702.

10. Scharf SM, Brown R, Saunders N, Green LH. Effects of normal and loaded

spontaneous inspiration on cardiovascular function. *J Appl Physiol Respir Environ Exerc Physiol*. 1979;**47**(3):582–90.

11. Guyton AC, Lindsey AW, Abernathy B, Richardson T. Venous return at various right atrial pressures and the normal venous return curve. *Am J Physiol*. 1957;**189**(3):609–15.

12. Wiedemann HP, Matthay MA, Matthay RA. Cardiovascular-pulmonary monitoring in the intensive care unit (part 1). *Chest*. 1984;**85**(4):537–49.

13. Geerts BF, Maas JJ, Aarts LP, Pinsky MR, Jansen JR. Partitioning the resistances along the vascular tree: effects of dobutamine and hypovolemia in piglets with an intact circulation. *J Clin Monit Comput* .2010;**24**(5):377–84.

14. Monge García MI, Gil Cano A, Gracia Romero M. Dynamic arterial elastance to predict arterial pressure response to volume loading in preload-dependent patients. *Crit Care*. 2011;**15**(1):R15.

15. Pinsky MR. Cardiovascular effects of prone positioning in acute respiratory distress syndrome patients: the circulation does not take it lying down. *Crit Care Med*. 2021;**49**(5):869–73.

16. Mohsenifar Z, Goldbach P, Tashkin DP, Campisi DJ. Relationship between O2 delivery and O2 consumption in the adult respiratory distress syndrome. *Chest*. 1983;**84**(3):267–71.

17. Annat G, Viale JP, Percival C, Froment M, Motin J. Oxygen delivery and uptake in the adult respiratory distress syndrome. Lack of relationship when measured independently in patients with normal blood lactate concentrations. *Am Rev Respir Dis*. 1986;**133**(6):999–1001.

18. Pinsky MR. The meaning of cardiac output. *Intensive Care Med*. 1990;**16**(7):415–17.

Invasive Hemodynamic Monitoring

Antonio Messina, Giulia Lionetti and Maurizio Cecconi

Introduction

Hemodynamic monitoring refers to continuous measurement of a hemodynamic variable. Cardiac output (CO) monitoring enables the clinician to guide hemodynamic management and improve oxygen delivery (DO_2). It began 50 years ago with the pulmonary artery catheter (PAC) and has evolved to the latest minimally invasive and non-invasive devices. The choice regarding the most appropriate form of hemodynamic monitoring in different settings should take into account several parameters. The performance of the system is certainly a key point, in terms of trueness (systematic error assessed by the closeness of agreement between the average of an infinite number of replicate measurements and the true or reference value), precision (how close two or more measurements are to each other, regardless of whether those measurements are accurate or not), accuracy (how close to the actual or real value the measurement is) and reliability to track a directional change of a measure (the ability to detect a significant change with high sensitivity and specificity).[1] However, the availability of a tool and the adoption of shared and validated therapeutic protocols and pathways based on the parameters obtained by the monitoring are also important.

The use of these monitors to optimize CO and tissue perfusion may positively influence the outcome for patients in the perioperative setting. Implementing this strategy successfully is dependent on correct interpretation of the information produced so that the appropriate interventions can be administered at the appropriate time.

This chapter will analyze the role of hemodynamic monitoring in the perioperative setting, describe some of the most commonly used invasive devices and discuss how to use the information obtained from them in clinical practice.

Evidence for Hemodynamic Monitoring and Optimization in the Perioperative Period

Postoperative complications occur in a significant proportion of patients undergoing surgery,[2–4] leading to mortality of about 4% in Europe [5] and having a significant impact on long-term morbidity and, in turn, on health and financial systems.[6,7] Several aspects including preoperative frailty, intraoperative management and events and postoperative care may influence the risk of developing postoperative complications.

Patients who achieve a higher CO, oxygen delivery and oxygen consumption after high-risk surgery have long been observed to have a greater chance of survival.[8,9] This led to the concept of an "oxygen debt" that accumulates within patients who were unable to mount a sufficient cardiorespiratory response to meet the increased metabolic demands that occur during and after surgery. In an important study, the use of fluid and inotrope administration to achieve supranormal hemodynamic targets, guided by the PAC, resulted in a decrease in mortality and morbidity in a cohort of high-risk surgical patients.[8] Other investigators subsequently studied goal-directed therapy (GDT), which is based on the purpose of balancing the increased oxygen demand during surgery, by the use of flow-based hemodynamic parameters, to achieve specific hemodynamic endpoints,[10,11] in the perioperative period and demonstrated similar results.[12,13] Unsurprisingly, using invasive monitoring was associated with increased resource utilization and complications.[14] Subsequent development of less-invasive technologies allowed the safe implementation of hemodynamic optimization to be applied to a wider surgical population.

The use of GDT to improve patient outcome has been repeatedly reproduced in a variety of clinical settings.[15–17] Recently published meta-analyses [10,18–20] and a Cochrane review [21] in perioperative patients have demonstrated that GDT reduces postoperative morbidity, length of hospital stay and mortality. In particular, mortality was reduced in patients undergoing high-risk surgery, and morbidity was reduced in all patient groups. [10,18] The most successful GDT protocols involved optimization of DO_2 or CO, and this was most effectively achieved if inotropes in addition to fluid therapy were used to meet these targets in the highest-risk group of patients.[10,18]

More recently, however, a number of studies have found no benefit in using GDT. [22,23] It is likely that after the introduction of initiatives that improve the overall standard of perioperative care, such as Enhanced Recovery After Surgery (ERAS), a single change in management has less of a demonstrable impact than it once did. The recent OPTIMISE trial [24] also failed to demonstrate an improvement in outcome when using GDT; however, in a sub-analysis in which the first 10 patients managed at each center were removed, the reduction in postoperative complications became significant. This suggests that optimization bundles are likely to require a period of familiarization before they are used to their full potential. Timing is also likely to be important: when GDT was used later after surgery (within 48 hours of intensive care unit [ICU] admission), it was not found to improve outcome and was even shown to harm some patients.[25]

Finally, it is important to consider the potential beneficial role of the GDT in the context of the most effective perioperative fluid management for each single patient. In this context, it is crucial to underline that in adopting a GDT approach, perioperative fluid balance is the effect of the individual response to fluid administration being titrated on the hemodynamic response to each fluid bolus. The ERAS pathways to support early recovery among patients undergoing major surgery recommend a restrictive approach aiming for the perioperative "zero-balance."[26] However, a recent large, randomized-controlled trial (RCT) performed by Myles et al. challenged this concept, and showed that a median intravenous-fluid intake of 3.7 liters as compared with 6.1 liters did not affect the rate of disability-free survival at 1 year, being also associated with higher rates of acute kidney injury, surgical-site infection and renal-replacement therapy.[27] As consequence, it is now suggested a moderately positive fluid balance of 1 to 2 liters at the end of surgery.[28]

In summary, it should be emphasized that a CO monitor is most effective in improving patient care if it is used to facilitate a validated hemodynamic optimization protocol. Used together correctly, hemodynamic monitoring and appropriate therapy have the potential to reduce mortality in high-risk patients and morbidity in moderate- to high-risk patients. It is important to remember that any monitor can be useful to improve outcome only if applied to the right population, at the right time and with the right strategy. The overall perioperative fluid balance is still a debated issue, with a recent large RCT suggesting a potential advantage in adopting a liberal fluid strategy. A recent metanalysis showed a trend toward the reduction of postoperative complications when a GDT is used in patients receiving large amounts of perioperative fluids.[20] Thus, rather than choosing between a fixed-volume regimen and a goal-directed concept, an alternative approach could be to combine the two strategies.

Assessing a Cardiac Output Monitor

Apart from safety and efficacy considerations, there are likely to be institutional and financial factors that may influence the choice of a particular CO monitor. The clinician must be aware of the limitations of a device with particular reference to the accuracy, the precision and the ability to track changes in physiology in the specific patient population used.

Despite limitations in clinical use, the PAC has become the gold standard by which most CO monitoring devices are assessed. The most frequently used statistical method for comparing the accuracy of two CO monitoring devices is the Bland–Altman method. Critchley and Critchley defined an acceptable percentage error of less than 30% for a clinical CO device.[29] However, comparison studies are not homogeneous, the statistical methods used for analysis have been questioned and acceptable performance limits remain debatable.[30]

The Role of Echocardiography

Trans-thoracic echocardiography (TTE) and trans-esophageal echocardiography (TEE) provide an immediate point-of-care assessment of fluid status, myocardial function, cardiac structure and response to treatment. Many hemodynamic measurements are possible, including measures of right heart function, and basic echocardiographic skills to perform a comprehensive exam have now been established by the European Society of Intensive Care Medicine.[31] Moreover, the use of echocardiography to manage the shocked patient is recommended by an expert panel in recent guidelines.[32] TTE use in the surgical setting as either continuous monitor or point-of-care tool remains impractical for the technical obstacles related to the position of the patients and the availability of appropriate views.

TEE has been adopted as imaging modality in a wide range of surgical settings including the cardiac operating theatre during cardiac operations, where its role has been well established in guiding and changing perioperative management.[33] The literature does not provide robust evidence regarding the clinical efficacy of TEE-guided protocols in non-cardiac settings, and the applications of perioperative TEE for non-cardiac surgery are often restricted for diagnosis and management of life-threatening disorders. Moreover, the availability of TEE equipment and trained personnel may limit the widespread implementation of perioperative monitoring. The lack of evidence supporting a therapeutic impact during high-risk non-cardiac surgery may be due to the combination of limited availability of TEE tools and anesthesiologist ability to interpret electrocardiograms.

TEE is overall considered a safe technique, however, it carries the risk of complications that range from mild to potentially life-threatening. The physical insertion and manipulation of the TEE probe in the intraoperative setting can cause a variety of gastric, esophageal and oropharyngeal complications. The overall rate of TEE-related complications reported in the literature ranges from 0.2% to 1.4%.

Very recently, a large retrospective cohort study (872 936 patients undergoing cardiac valve or aortic surgery between 2011 and 2019) compared clinical outcomes among patients undergoing cardiac valve or proximal aortic surgery with versus without intraoperative TEE and found that intraoperative TEE use was associated with lower 30-day mortality, a lower incidence of stroke or 30-day mortality and a lower incidence of cardiac reoperation or 30-day mortality. Despite the fact that the observational, non-randomized design of this study cannot confirm a causal link between TEE and improved clinical outcomes, it is likely that intraoperative TEE is conferring some degree of benefit for overall patient management.[34]

Intra-Pulmonary Thermodilution: The Pulmonary Artery Catheter

The PAC was introduced in the 1970s and was the first clinical hemodynamic monitor. Initially used for patients with cardiac dysfunction, it rapidly became the standard of care for perioperative monitoring in high-risk patients for the subsequent 20 years and has been extensively investigated in this context.

The PAC is a balloon-tipped catheter that is available in a range of lengths and sizes for adults and children. In addition to the balloon, there are three lumina, two of which terminate in the right atrium and one that terminates distal to the balloon. A thermistor wire is 4 cm from the tip, proximal to the balloon, and measures blood temperature used in the calculation of cardiac output.

Originally, an intermittent value for CO was produced using manual thermodilution, requiring a 10 ml bolus of cold fluid to be rapidly injected into a proximal port of the PAC at the end of expiration. The temperature of blood in the pulmonary artery is plotted against time, and the area under the curve is calculated (see Fig. 2.1) to produce CO. The addition of a heating element that automatically semi-continuously warms the blood in the pulmonary

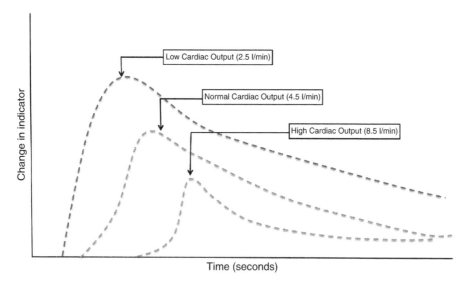

Figure 2.1 Change in an arbitrary indicator plotted against time in patients with normal and low cardiac output states. A high cardiac output state results in a greater dispersal of indicator, resulting in a lower peak concentration and a prolonged washout curve. Flow is inversely proportional to the rate of indicator change, and cardiac output is inversely proportional to the area under the curve.

artery allows more continuous CO monitoring and is the basis of the Vigilance^{TM} system. The mean CO is calculated over several minutes to improve the accuracy, resulting in a delay in the display of any acute changes.

Complications

The rate of complications when using the PAC may be inversely related to user experience. Complications related to insertion are observed in 6% of cases. Cardiac arrhythmias also occur frequently (12.5%) but are usually transient (including atrial and ventricular ectopic beats, ventricular tachycardia and right bundle branch block). Rare complications include catheter malposition or knotting, valve trauma and pulmonary arterial rupture. Late complications are infrequent if the catheter is removed within 72 hours and include infection, thrombosis and pulmonary infarction.[35]

Limitations

Reliable results depend on correct catheter position, injection technique and thermistor accuracy. The presence of intra-cardiac shunts, tricuspid or mitral valve regurgitation and mitral valve stenosis affects accuracy. High ventilator pressures may also result in falsely high CO readings. Furthermore, the avoidance of complications and the successful interpretation of the PAC data are user-dependent.

Validation

Outcome studies are conflicting. As discussed previously, when the PAC was used to guide therapy in high-risk surgical patients, a mortality and morbidity benefit was found by several investigators.[8,12,13] However, subsequent studies have demonstrated potential harm by using the PAC and increased resource utilization.[14,36,37] Some studies found that despite guiding therapy, no outcome benefit could be demonstrated.[36–38] In addition, the insertion and subsequent interpretation is heavily user-dependent, and operator experience is likely to be important. A Cochrane review concluded that PACs did not alter hospital length of stay, mortality or cost.[35] Importantly, complications occurring as a result of catheter insertion did not result in harm or death.[35,36]

Summary of the PAC

PAC use may still be beneficial in a select group of patients as discussed above and only if the operator and the institution have experience in the insertion, interpretation and subsequent care of these catheters. In this context, it is still an important monitoring tool and provides unique clinical information not easily obtained from other modalities. Overall, the PAC has seen a decline in its usage, justified by arguments concerning costs and invasiveness without robust data showing an improvement in patient outcomes.

Arterial Waveform Analysis

These devices use an arterial pressure trace to continuously calculate the CO. Compared with the PAC, they are less invasive and require less expertise to insert, maintain and interpret. Continuous stroke volume (SV) analysis allows the prediction of fluid responsiveness (discussed in other chapters), an advantage over intermittent measurements provided by the PAC.

To calculate flow from the pressure trace, the device must calculate the overall vascular impedance, based on the measurement or prediction of vascular resistance and compliance. This may be achieved by using a calibrated technique or by using an uncalibrated technique based on normograph data.

Calibrated Devices Using Pulse-Contour Analysis or Pulse-Power Analysis

A calibrated device will use an intermittent transpulmonary dilution technique (Table 2.1). An indicator injected into venous blood will dissipate through cardiac and pulmonary blood volumes before reaching the systemic circulation where it is measured. The change in indicator is plotted against time, and the area under the curve is calculated by the modified Stuart–Hamilton equation as for the PAC. Once calibrated, the device will utilize pulse-contour or pulse-power analysis to provide continuous SV and CO data.

PiCCO^{TM} (Pulsion Medical Systems, Munich, Germany)

The PiCCO^{TM} Family of Devices (PiCCOplus^{TM} and PiCCO02^{TM})

The PiCCO system [39] requires a calibration of three separate injections of 15 and 30 ml of a cold solution (ideally 0.9% saline, as both lipid and dextrose compounds can damage the sensors) within a 5-minute period. Calibration is considered appropriate when the variation of the obtained results is less then 20% and should also be repeated every 8 hours or following changes in the patient's hemodynamic setting (i.e., inotropes or vasopressor changes, fluid loss). A proprietary thermistor-tipped catheter, which detects the change in temperature, is inserted into the femoral or axillary artery. After calibration, the cardiac output is calculated from the area under curve analysis, using the Stewart–Hamilton equation, considering the temperature changes as an indicator:

$$PiCCO = Cal \times HR \int \left(\frac{p(t)}{SVR} + \frac{C(p) \times dp}{dt} \right)$$

- Cal: patient-specific calibration factor determined with thermodilution
- HR: heart rate
- $p(t)$/SVR [systemic vascular resistance]: area under curve
- $C(p)$: compliance
- dp/dt: shape of pressure curve

Apart from cardiac output, PiCCO can derive a number of static values of preload or fluid distribution:

ITTV: intrathoracic thermal volume

PTV: pulmonary thermal volume

GEDV: global end-diastolic volume

EVLW: extra-vascular lung water

SVV: stroke volume variation

Table 2.1 Algorithm characteristic of stroke volume measurement – uncalibrated pulse contour analysis systems

Device	Manufacturer	Algorithm characteristics
FloTrac™	Vigileo, Edwards Lifesciences, Irvine, CA, USA	The FloWTrac™ algorithm uses the standard of 2 000 arterial waveform points sampled each 20 s at 100 Hz. The stroke volume (SV) is estimated by the following equation: $SV = SD_{AP} \times \mu$. SD_{AP} = Standard deviation of data points that reflects pulse pressure. μ = Conversion factor depends on arterial compliance, mean arterial pressure, waveform characteristics. Vascular compliance is calculated considering patient's biometric value and waveform characteristics assessed by skewness (degree of asymmetry) and kurtosis (degree of peakedness) of the individual arterial pressure waveform.
LiDCORapid™	LiDCO Ltd, London, UK	The LiDCORapid™ uses the PulseCo™ algorithm. In the LiDCOPlus™ system, the nominal SV is calibrated using a lithium dilution technique to generate a true SV, whereas the LiDCORapid uses of a nomogram-based estimate (scaling factor) that incorporates patient age, height and weight to calibrate the nominal stroke volume.
Pulsio Flex™	Pulsion Medical Systems, Irving, TX, USA	Pulsio Flex™ measures cardiac output using the same pulse contour algorithm employed by the PiCCO™ system (transpulmonary thermodilution; Stewart–Hamilton principle). The device can be also calibrated using a cardiac output measurement derived from an external source. Autocalibration algorithm for vascular resistance and compliance estimation.
MostCare™	Vygon Health, Padua, Italy	MostCare is powered by the pressure recording analytical method (PRAM) and estimates SV and CO on a beat-by-beat basis by analyzing the whole cardiac cycle and area under the pressure wave (P/t) with a sampling rate of 1 000 points (P/t) per second. To optimize SV measurement, MostCare identifies specific parts over the pressure trace, especially the "points of instability," at which the reflected waves traveling from the periphery to the heart may affect the signal (backward-traveling waves).

The VolumeView™ Set EV1000™ Platform (Edwards Lifesciences, Irvine, CA, USA)

The VolumeView™ using the EV1000™ platform software is calibrated with cold-bolus thermodilution (as above) and uses pulse-contour analysis to measure similar values to the PiCCO™ system. A proprietary thermistor-tipped femoral arterial cannula is also required, and an optional PreSep™ catheter for continuous central venous oxygenation monitoring is available. The unique feature is the software package, which presents the hemodynamic data with a graphical interface facilitating interpretation by the operator.

The LiDCO™ System (LiDCO Ltd, Cambridge, UK)

LiDCO™ uses lithium as the indicator to calculate CO with the trans-pulmonary bolus technique.[40] The peripheral arterial catheter is connected to a proprietary lithium-sensitive electrode that creates a voltage proportional to the lithium concentration in the blood. The LiDCO system measures the stroke volume by means of Pulse Power analysis. The algorithm assumes net power change is equal to net flow change and calibration creates a correction factor for vascular compliance. Pulse-power analysis (rather than the pulse-contour) is subsequently used for continuous flow monitoring. This method is based on the principle that change in the blood pressure about the mean is directly related to the SV. A root mean square method is applied to the arterial pressure signal and the obtained "nominal SV" is adapted to the "actual SV" by means of a chemical calibration factor. In fact, the lithium is injected as indicator through central venous catheter and variation in its concentration is detected by a specialized probe attached to an arterial catheter.

By using a Stewart–Hamilton modified equation, cardiac output is calculated as below:

$$CO = \frac{LiCl \times 60}{Area \times (Cl - PCV)}$$

- LiCl: lithium chloride in mmol
- Area: AUC
- PCV: packed cell volume

Validation of Calibrated Devices

PiCCO™ in particular has been extensively validated in animal studies and in a variety of clinical conditions.[41] The use of GEDV to guide fluid administration in a cardiac ICU reduced duration of vasopressor and inotrope dependency, mechanical ventilation, and length of stay.[42,43] The EV1000/VolumeView™ monitor has demonstrated accuracy and reliability equal to that of PiCCO™, and superior accuracy in measurement of the GEDV.[43]

The LiDCO™ device has also been validated in numerous clinical situations, including in patients with impaired ventricular function after cardiac surgery and undergoing liver transplantation, with a wide variety of COs.[44,45] When used to facilitate GDT in postoperative patients to target a supranormal DO_2, a reduced rate of complications and length of hospital stay were demonstrated,[46] and this is used routinely in the author's institution.

Limitations

All pulse-contour devices, calibrated or not, depend on a good-quality arterial pressure trace. Severe arrhythmias and the use of intra-aortic balloon pump augmentation will result in unreliable data. A proprietary central arterial catheter and central venous access are required to calibrate the device, increasing the invasive nature of the technique. Owing to changes in the vascular resistance, recalibration is required frequently if there is an obvious clinical change. Moreover, the reliability of the pulse-contour analysis devices is remarkably affected by mechanical problems in the arterial wave signal transmission or resonance/ underdamping phenomena.[47]

Summary of Calibrated Devices

These devices provide accuracy comparable to the PAC with the obvious benefits of being less invasive and less user-dependent, and allowing assessment of dynamic indices. The limitations include reliance on a good-quality arterial pressure trace and the need for recurrent calibrations over time. Each device has been validated for use in perioperative clinical practice when used in conjunction with evidence-based optimization protocols, and they have found widespread clinical acceptance.

Uncalibrated Devices Using Pulse-Contour Analysis

Devices without the need for external calibration are a more recent development to meet a need for a user-independent system to display trend data (Table 2.1). This allows the assessment of dynamic indices to predict fluid responsiveness and protocol-guided optimization. Most devices use algorithms to calculate flow, which rely on databases containing information from laboratory or comparative studies. One newer system (MostCare^{TM}, Vytech) does not require calibration, as it analyzes the arterial waveform to calculate the vascular impedance.

Vigileo/FloTrac System^{TM} (Edward Life Sciences, Irvine, CA, USA)

This device requires a proprietary transducer to be connected to a standard arterial catheter. Demographic data (age, height, sex, weight) are manually supplied to calculate the predicted vascular impedance. The arterial trace is sampled at 100 Hz over a 20 second period and compliance and resistance are estimated. The arterial pressure waveform is continually analyzed for changes, and SV, CO, stroke volume variation (SVV) and pulse pressure variation (PPV) are displayed.

Pulsioflex^{TM} (Pulsion Medical Systems, Irving, TX, USA)

This system uses the same algorithm as the calibrated PiCCO^{TM} devices without in vitro calibration, instead relying on normograph data and biometric information. The basic module will monitor SV, CO, SVV, PPV and a contractility measurement. For greater accuracy, CO data for calibration can be supplied manually, for example from an esophageal Doppler device. The monitor is expandable, and modules can be added that allow bolus thermodilution calibration and continuous venous oxygen saturation (SvO$_2$) monitoring.

LiDCOrapid™ (LiDCO Ltd, Cambridge, UK)

This uncalibrated system by LiDCO™ calculates the correction factor for SVR. Using normograph data produced by the manufacturer, aortic blood volume is calculated based on age, height, weight, and body surface area. Newer models also allow the escalation of monitoring with transpulmonary dilution calibration, if required.

MostCare™ System (Vytech, Padua, Italy)

The MostCare™ system is the latest evolution of CO monitor that does not require in vitro or external calibration using a pressure recording analytical method (PRAM) to calculate vascular impedance. The SV is estimated as the ratio between the area under the systolic component of the curve and the systemic vascular impedance by analyzing the profile of the "points of instability" of the arterial waveform shape. The high sample rate of 1 000 Hz is able to identify these points, which are generated by the mechanical interaction between forward and backward pressure waves, and to define the specific profile of each arterial waveform, which is analyzed by MostCare® for the calculation of the vascular impedance. Arterial pressures (systolic, diastolic, mean and dicrotic) and the pulse pressure variation are directly measured from arterial pressure waveform, while SVV is calculated by analyzing the changes in SV overtime. Finally, the MostCare® estimates the performance of the cardiovascular system by considering the value of the cardiac cycle efficiency (CCE), which is calculated as follows:

$$CCE = W_{sys}/W_{beat} \times K_{(t)}.$$

where W_{sys} and W_{beat} are the systolic and complete beat power functions and $K_{(t)}$ is the ratio between the expected and measured mean arterial pressure. CCE varies from -1 to $+1$, with negative values corresponding to unfavorable energetic conditions and positive values related to beneficial energetic conditions.

Validation of Uncalibrated Devices

A number of studies have been performed comparing the accuracy of the three pulse-contour systems described above.

The accuracy of the Vigileo/FloTrac™ device has been questioned despite several incremental updates. The first iteration showed poor agreement with PAC- derived values, and later generations remain unacceptably inaccurate, with published error rates of 40% in non-cardiac patients.[48] Detection of cardiac output changes due to fluid bolus administration and vasopressor therapy [49] was also unreliable. It has, however, been used successfully in protocols for fluid administration in general surgical patients [50] and orthopedic patients.[51]

The uncalibrated LiDCO™ and PiCCO™ devices produce acceptably accurate results when compared with the PAC and are more able to track physiological changes than the FloTrac™ in a number of clinical situations.[52] The PiCCO™ device is able to accurately track the changes in the CO during fluid and vasopressor administration,[53] and both these devices have been successfully used to guide intravenous fluid therapy using GDT based on SV optimization and SVV in the perioperative period.

In different categories of ICU and surgical patients, PRAM performed well when compared with the PAC [54–56] and echocardiography.[56, 57] In addition, it appears to be accurate in patients with low CO states, receiving inotropes or intra-aortic balloon pump augmentation. This has been recently used in elective laparotomy surgery, showing a good accuracy in measuring SV changes.[58] Robust data regarding the reliability in hemodynamically unstable critically ill patients are still lacking.

Summary of Uncalibrated Devices

These devices are useful for the perioperative patient, as they are minimally invasive, do not require calibration and are not user dependent. The use of these devices in conjunction with evidence-based GDT protocols has been shown to reduce complications following surgery. However, convenience is traded for accuracy, and it is likely that in a hemodynamically compromised patient, an alternative monitoring device may be more appropriate.

Conclusion

Cardiac output monitoring in the perioperative period is now safely available to a greater number of patients owing to the improved risk–benefit profile of modern devices. These devices allow the judicious use of intravenous fluid therapy to optimize oxygen delivery and avoid hypervolemia. When used in conjunction with an evidence-based GDT protocol, it may improve the outcome of patients in the perioperative period. Adequate patient selection to identify moderate- to high-risk cases is probably one of the most important parts of these strategies.[10]

Each monitor has limitations that need to be considered by the clinician relying on the data provided. It is likely that the use of a particular monitor is less important than the implementation of a validated optimization protocol for the majority of patients. The monitoring tool may be escalated to a more invasive, accurate device and used in conjunction with echocardiography to manage the shocked perioperative patient.

References

1. Squara P, Cecconi M, Rhodes A, Singer M, Chiche JD. Tracking changes in cardiac output: methodological considerations for the validation of monitoring devices. *Intensive Care Med.* 2009 Oct;35(10):1801–8. PubMed PMID: 19593546. Epub 2009/07/14. eng.

2. Jhanji S, Thomas B, Ely A, Watson D, Hinds CJ, Pearse RM. Mortality and utilisation of critical care resources amongst high-risk surgical patients in a large NHS trust. *Anaesthesia.* 2008 Jul;63(7):695–700. PubMed PMID: 18489613. Epub 2008/05/21.

3. Thompson JS, Baxter BT, Allison JG, et al. Temporal patterns of postoperative complications. *Arch Surg.* 2003 Jun;138(6):596–602; discussion-3. PubMed PMID: 12799329. Epub 2003/06/12.

4. Tevis SE, Kennedy GD. Postoperative complications and implications on patient-centered outcomes. *J Surg Res.* 2013 May 1;181(1):106–13. PubMed PMID: 23465392. PMCID: PMC3637983. Epub 2013/03/08.

5. Pearse RM, Moreno RP, Bauer P, et al. Mortality after surgery in Europe: a 7 day cohort study. *Lancet.* 2012 Sep 22;380(9847):1059–65. PubMed PMID: 22998715. PMCID: PMC3493988. Epub 2012/09/25.

6. Khuri SF, Henderson WG, DePalma RG, et al. Determinants of long-term survival after major surgery and the adverse effect of postoperative complications. *Ann Surg.* 2005 Sep;242(3):326–41; discussion 41–3. PubMed PMID: 16135919. PMCID: PMC1357741. Epub 2005/09/02.

7. Healy MA, Mullard AJ, Campbell DA Jr., Dimick JB. Hospital and payer costs associated with surgical complications. *JAMA Surg.* 2016 Sep 1;**151**(9):823–30. PubMed PMID: 27168356. Epub 2016/ 05/12.

8. Shoemaker WC, Appel PL, Kram HB, Waxman K, Lee TS. Prospective trial of supranormal values of survivors as therapeutic goals in high-risk surgical patients. *Chest.* 1988 Dec;**94**(6):1176–86. PubMed PMID: 3191758. eng.

9. Ackland GL, Iqbal S, Paredes LG, et al. Individualised oxygen delivery targeted haemodynamic therapy in high-risk surgical patients: a multicentre, randomised, double-blind, controlled, mechanistic trial. *Lancet Respir Med.* 2015 Jan;**3**(1):33–41. PubMed PMID: 25523407. Epub 20141216. eng.

10. Cecconi M, Corredor C, Arulkumaran N, et al. Clinical review: goal-directed therapy-what is the evidence in surgical patients? The effect on different risk groups. *Crit Care.* 2013 Mar 05;**17**(2):209. PubMed PMID: 23672779. PMCID: 3679445.

11. Kaufmann T, Saugel B, Scheeren TWL. Perioperative goal-directed therapy – what is the evidence? *Best Pract Res Clin Anaesthesiol.* 2019 Jun;**33**(2):179–87. PubMed PMID: 31582097. Epub 2019/ 10/05.

12. Boyd O, Grounds RM, Bennett ED. A randomized clinical trial of the effect of deliberate perioperative increase of oxygen delivery on mortality in high-risk surgical patients. *JAMA.* 1993 Dec 8;**270**(22):2699–707. PubMed PMID: 7907668. eng.

13. Lobo SM, Salgado PF, Castillo VG, et al. Effects of maximizing oxygen delivery on morbidity and mortality in high-risk surgical patients. *Crit Care Med.* 2000 Oct;**28**(10):3396–404. PubMed PMID: 11057792. eng.

14. Connors AF Jr., Speroff T, Dawson NV, et al. The effectiveness of right heart catheterization in the initial care of critically ill patients. SUPPORT Investigators. *JAMA.* 1996 Sep 18;**276**(11):889–97. PubMed PMID: 8782638. eng.

15. Pölönen P, Ruokonen E, Hippeläinen M, Pöyhönen M, Takala J. A prospective, randomized study of goal-oriented hemodynamic therapy in cardiac surgical patients. *Anesth Analg.* 2000 May;**90**(5):1052–9. PubMed PMID: 10781452. eng.

16. Wakeling HG, McFall MR, Jenkins CS, et al. Intraoperative oesophageal Doppler guided fluid management shortens postoperative hospital stay after major bowel surgery. *Br J Anaesth.* 2005 Nov;**95**(5):634–42. PubMed PMID: 16155038. Epub 2005/09/13. eng.

17. Sinclair S, James S, Singer M. Intraoperative intravascular volume optimisation and length of hospital stay after repair of proximal femoral fracture: randomised controlled trial. *BMJ.* 1997 Oct 11;**315**(7113):909–12. PubMed PMID: 9361539. PMCID: 2127619.

18. Hamilton MA, Cecconi M, Rhodes A. A systematic review and meta-analysis on the use of preemptive hemodynamic intervention to improve postoperative outcomes in moderate and high-risk surgical patients. *Anesth Analg.* 2011 Jun;**112**(6):1392–402. PubMed PMID: 20966436. Epub 2010/10/23. eng.

19. Kern JW, Shoemaker WC. Meta-analysis of hemodynamic optimization in high-risk patients. *Crit Care Med.* 2002 Aug;**30**(8):1686–92. PubMed PMID: 12163777. eng.

20. Messina A, Robba C, Calabrò L, et al. Association between perioperative fluid administration and postoperative outcomes: a 20-year systematic review and a meta-analysis of randomized goal-directed trials in major visceral/ noncardiac surgery. *Crit Care.* 2021 Feb 1;**25**(1):43. PubMed PMID: 33522953. PMCID: Pmc7849093. Epub 2021/02/ 02. eng.

21. Grocott MP, Dushianthan A, Hamilton MA, et al. Perioperative increase in global blood flow to explicit defined goals and outcomes after surgery: a Cochrane Systematic Review.

Br J Anaesth. 2013 Oct;**111**(4):535–48. PubMed PMID: 23661403. Epub 20130509. eng.

22. Srinivasa S, Taylor MH, Singh PP, et al. Randomized clinical trial of goal-directed fluid therapy within an enhanced recovery protocol for elective colectomy. *Br J Surg.* 2013 Jan;**100**(1):66–74. PubMed PMID: 23132508.

23. McKenny M, Conroy P, Wong A, et al. A randomised prospective trial of intra-operative oesophageal Doppler-guided fluid administration in major gynaecological surgery. *Anaesthesia.* 2013 Dec;**68**(12):1224–31. PubMed PMID: 24116747. Epub 2013/10/15. eng.

24. Pearse RM, Harrison DA, MacDonald N, et al. Effect of a perioperative, cardiac output-guided hemodynamic therapy algorithm on outcomes following major gastrointestinal surgery: a randomized clinical trial and systematic review. *JAMA.* 2014 Jun 4;**311**(21):2181–90. PubMed PMID: 24842135. Epub 2014/05/21. eng.

25. Hayes MA, Timmins AC, Yau EH, et al. Elevation of systemic oxygen delivery in the treatment of critically ill patients. *N Engl J Med.* 1994 Jun 16;**330**(24):1717–22. PubMed PMID: 7993413. eng.

26. Gustafsson UO, Scott MJ, Schwenk W, et al. Guidelines for perioperative care in elective colonic surgery: Enhanced Recovery After Surgery (ERAS((R))) Society recommendations. *World J Surg.* 2013 Feb;**37**(2):259–84. PubMed PMID: 23052794. Epub 2012/10/12.

27. Myles PS, Bellomo R, Corcoran T, et al. Restrictive versus liberal fluid therapy for major abdominal surgery. *N Engl J Med.* 2018 Jun 14;**378**(24):2263–74. PubMed PMID: 29742967. Epub 2018/05/11. eng.

28. Miller TE, Myles PS. Perioperative fluid therapy for major surgery. *Anesthesiology.* 2019 May;**130**(5):825–32. PubMed PMID: 30789364. Epub 2019/02/23.

29. Critchley LA, Critchley JA. A meta-analysis of studies using bias and precision statistics to compare cardiac output measurement techniques. *J Clin Monit Comput.* 1999 Feb;**15**(2):85–91. PubMed PMID: 12578081.

30. Cecconi M, Rhodes A, Poloniecki J, Della Rocca G, Grounds RM. Bench-to-bedside review: the importance of the precision of the reference technique in method comparison studies–with specific reference to the measurement of cardiac output. *Crit Care.* 2009;**13**(1):201. PubMed PMID: 19183431. PMCID: PMC2688094. Epub 20090113. eng.

31. Robba C, Wong A, Poole D, et al. Basic ultrasound head-to-toe skills for intensivists in the general and neuro intensive care unit population: consensus and expert recommendations of the European Society of Intensive Care Medicine. *Intensive Care Med.* 2021 Dec;**47**(12):1347–67. PubMed PMID: 34787687. PMCID: PMC8596353. Epub 2021/11/18.

32. Cecconi M, De Backer D, Antonelli M, et al. Consensus on circulatory shock and hemodynamic monitoring. Task force of the European Society of Intensive Care Medicine. *Intensive Care Med.* 2014 Dec;**40**(12):1795–815. PubMed PMID: 25392034. PMCID: 4239778.

33. Fanshawe M, Ellis C, Habib S, Konstadt SN, Reich DL. A retrospective analysis of the costs and benefits related to alterations in cardiac surgery from routine intraoperative transesophageal echocardiography. *Anesth Analg.* 2002 Oct;**95**(4):824–7, table of contents. PubMed PMID: 12351252. eng.

34. MacKay EJ, Zhang B, Augoustides JG, Groeneveld PW, Desai ND. Association of Intraoperative Transesophageal Echocardiography and Clinical Outcomes After Open Cardiac Valve or Proximal Aortic Surgery. *JAMA Netw Open.* 2022 Feb 1;**5**(2):e2147820. PubMed PMID: 35138396. PMCID: PMC8829659. Epub 2022/02/10.

35. Rajaram SS, Desai NK, Kalra A, et al. Pulmonary artery catheters for adult patients in intensive care. *Cochrane Database Syst Rev.* 2013;**2**:CD003408. PubMed PMID: 23450539. Epub 2013/03/02. eng.

36. Harvey S, Harrison DA, Singer M, et al. Assessment of the clinical effectiveness of pulmonary artery catheters in management of patients in intensive care (PAC-Man): a randomised controlled trial. *Lancet.* 2005 Aug 6–12;**366**(9484):472–7. PubMed PMID: 16084255. eng.

37. Sandham JD, Hull RD, Brant RF, et al. A randomized, controlled trial of the use of pulmonary-artery catheters in high-risk surgical patients. *N Engl J Med.* 2003 Jan 2;**348**(1):5–14. PubMed PMID: 12510037. Epub 2003/01/03. eng.

38. Wheeler AP, Bernard GR, Thompson BT, et al. Pulmonary-artery versus central venous catheter to guide treatment of acute lung injury. *N Engl J Med.* 2006 May 25;**354** (21):2213–24. PubMed PMID: 16714768. Epub 2006/05/23. eng.

39. Litton E, Morgan M. The PiCCO monitor: a review. *Anaesth Intensive Care.* 2012 May;**40**(3):393–409. PubMed PMID: 22577904. Epub 2012/05/15. eng.

40. Pearse RM, Ikram K, Barry J. Equipment review: an appraisal of the LiDCO plus method of measuring cardiac output. *Crit Care.* 2004 Jun;**8**(3):190–5. PubMed PMID: 15153237. PMCID: 468899.

41. Goedje O, Hoeke K, Lichtwarck-Aschoff M, et al. Continuous cardiac output by femoral arterial thermodilution calibrated pulse contour analysis: comparison with pulmonary arterial thermodilution. *Crit Care Med.* 1999 Nov;**27**(11):2407–12. PubMed PMID: 10579256. eng.

42. Goepfert MS, Reuter DA, Akyol D, et al. Goal-directed fluid management reduces vasopressor and catecholamine use in cardiac surgery patients. *Intensive Care Med.* 2007 Jan;**33**(1):96–103. PubMed PMID: 17119923. Epub 20061121. eng.

43. Kiefer N, Hofer CK, Marx G, et al. Clinical validation of a new thermodilution system for the assessment of cardiac output and volumetric parameters. *Crit Care.* 2012 May 30;**16**(3):R98. PubMed PMID: 22647561. PMCID: PMC3580647. Epub 20120530. eng.

44. Mora B, Ince I, Birkenberg B, et al. Validation of cardiac output measurement with the LiDCO™ pulse contour system in patients with impaired left ventricular function after cardiac surgery. *Anaesthesia.* 2011 Aug;**66**(8):675–81. PubMed PMID: 21564044. Epub 20110513. eng.

45. Costa MG, Della Rocca G, Chiarandini P, et al. Continuous and intermittent cardiac output measurement in hyperdynamic conditions: pulmonary artery catheter vs. lithium dilution technique. *Intensive Care Med.* 2008 Feb;**34**(2):257–63. PubMed PMID: 17922106. Epub 20071006. eng.

46. Pearse R, Dawson D, Fawcett J, et al. Early goal-directed therapy after major surgery reduces complications and duration of hospital stay. A randomised, controlled trial [ISRCTN38797445]. *Crit Care.* 2005;**9** (6):R687–93. PubMed PMID: 16356219. PMCID: PMC1414018. Epub 2005/12/17. eng.

47. Vincent JL, Rhodes A, Perel A, et al. Clinical review: Update on hemodynamic monitoring–a consensus of 16. *Crit Care.* 2011 Aug 18;**15**(4):229. PubMed PMID: 21884645. PMCID: 3387592.

48. Østergaard M, Nielsen J, Nygaard E. Pulse contour cardiac output: an evaluation of the FloTrac method. *Eur J Anaesthesiol.* 2009 Jun;**26**(6):484–9. PubMed PMID: 19436173. eng.

49. Phan TD, Kluger R, Wan C, Wong D, Padayachee A. A comparison of three minimally invasive cardiac output devices with thermodilution in elective cardiac surgery. *Anaesth Intensive Care.* 2011 Nov;**39**(6):1014–21. PubMed PMID: 22165352. eng.

50. Senn A, Button D, Zollinger A, Hofer CK. Assessment of cardiac output changes using a modified FloTrac/Vigileo algorithm in cardiac surgery patients. *Crit Care.* 2009;**13**(2):R32. PubMed PMID: 19261180. PMCID: PMC2689464. Epub 20090304. eng.

51. Cecconi M, Fasano N, Langiano N, et al. Goal-directed haemodynamic therapy during elective total hip arthroplasty under regional anaesthesia. *Crit Care.* 2011;**15**(3):

R132. PubMed PMID: 21624138. PMCID: 3218998.

52. Hadian M, Kim HK, Severyn DA, Pinsky MR. Cross-comparison of cardiac output trending accuracy of LiDCO, PiCCO, FloTrac and pulmonary artery catheters. *Crit Care*. 2010;**14**(6):R212. PubMed PMID: 21092290. Epub 2010/11/26. eng.

53. Monnet X, Anguel N, Naudin B, et al. Arterial pressure-based cardiac output in septic patients: different accuracy of pulse contour and uncalibrated pressure waveform devices. *Crit Care*. 2010;**14**(3): R109. PubMed PMID: 20537159. PMCID: PMC2911755. Epub 20100610. eng.

54. Romano SM, Pistolesi M. Assessment of cardiac output from systemic arterial pressure in humans. *Crit Care Med*. 2002 Aug;**30**(8):1834–41. PubMed PMID: 12163802. eng.

55. Giomarelli P, Biagioli B, Scolletta S. Cardiac output monitoring by pressure recording analytical method in cardiac surgery. *Eur J Cardiothorac Surg*. 2004

Sep;**26**(3):515–20. PubMed PMID: 15302045. eng.

56. Calamandrei M, Mirabile L, Muschetta S, et al. Assessment of cardiac output in children: a comparison between the pressure recording analytical method and Doppler echocardiography. *Pediatr Crit Care Med*. 2008 May;**9**(3):310–2. PubMed PMID: 18446106. eng.

57. Scolletta S, Franchi F, Romagnoli S, et al. Comparison between doppler-echocardiography and uncalibrated pulse contour method for cardiac output measurement: a multicenter observational study. *Crit Care Med*. 2016 Jul;**44**(7):1370–9. PubMed PMID: 27097293.

58. Messina A, Lionetti G, Foti L, et al. Mini fluid challenge and end-expiratory occlusion test to assess fluid responsiveness in the operating room (MANEUVER study): a multicentre cohort study. *Eur J Anaesthesiol*. 2021 Apr 1;**38** (4):422–31. PubMed PMID: 33399372. Epub 2021/01/06.

Non-Invasive Blood Pressure Monitoring

Karim Lakhal and Jérôme E. Dauvergne

Introduction

In acute care settings, protracted and/or profound arterial hypotension is associated with a higher risk of mortality, myocardial ischemia, stroke and acute kidney injury.[1–3] Arterial hypertension is also potentially harmful.[1,2] After major surgery, organ dysfunction can be limited by ensuring that blood pressure (BP) deviates only slightly from its usual level.[4] This underscores the importance of a proper measurement of BP. To that end, three options are often available: the arterial catheter, the automatic upper arm cuff and, more and more frequently, the automatic finger cuff. The paradox of the automatic upper arm cuff is that its performance is almost as decried as its use is frequent. The automatic finger cuff is appealing because it combines an advantage of the arterial catheter (the "beat-to-beat" measurement) with an advantage of the upper arm cuff (the non-invasiveness). Studies addressing the performance of these non-invasive techniques are manifold, some with an enthusiastic conclusion and others with a somewhat discouraging one. This chapter aims to describe the recent advances in this field, mainly in adult patients, while reminding the reader some basic principles. Figure 3.1 summarizes the key messages.

Automatic Upper Arm Cuff

Principles of the Technique

The technique, based on principles discovered in the late nineteenth century, is called oscillometry. It is only since the 1970s that automatic devices have been marketed on a large scale. Briefly, cuff inflation above the systolic BP (SBP) occludes the brachial artery. The gradual deflation of the cuff progressively restores blood flow, permitting the oscillometer to detect pulse wave–induced oscillations of the arterial wall. External compression of the artery by the cuff reduces vessel transmural pressure, which promotes its oscillations. When the magnitude of the oscillations is maximal, the pressure in the cuff is the mean BP (MBP).[5] The systolic and diastolic BP (DBP) are then derived from the envelope of all oscillations that were recorded during cuff deflation. Manufacturer-specific algorithms that are used to that end are usually kept secret.[5] This secrecy is a matter of concern.[6] Indeed, it is challenging to know, for one given device, whether the embedded software takes into account the various parameters that can affect BP measurement: stiffness of the artery, thickness of the tissue that is interposed between the artery and the cuff, cardiac arrhythmia, or artefacts linked to the patient's movements or to the vibrations related to patient transport (intra- or out-of-hospital). It is also difficult to know whether there was

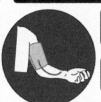

Automatic upper arm cuff

- MBP measurement can be true and precise in acute care settings.
- Performance varies from device model to model.
- SBP is often displayed with a significant error.

- Reliable identification of patients responding to therapy.
- Remarkable ability to detect hypo- and hypertension
  If MBP displayed > 70 mm Hg, hypotension (actual MBP<65 mmHg) is very unlikely)

Beliefs to be (likely) abandoned

- "The upper arm cuff systematically (over-) underestimates BP"
  The direction of the measurement error is often unpredictable!

- "This technique is unreliable during the infusion of a vasopressive drug"
  - Vasopressive drugs: impact on the measurement error is uncertain.
  - Caution 1: the intermittent nature of the measurement may delay the detection of hypo- or hypertension related to infusion issues.
  - Caution 2: in the event of an infusion through a peripheral vein of the upper limb, the upper arm cuff is preferably placed at the opposite upper limb.

Cardiac arrhythmia

Consider the average of 3 consecutive measurements.

Obese patients

Place the cuff at the wrist (especially if the upper arm is large and conically shaped).

Contra-indication for placing the cuff at the upper limb

Keep in mind that placing the cuff at the lower leg is associated with a higher degree of measurement error.

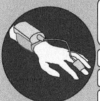

Automatic finger cuff

- Measurement error does not fulfil the requirements of the current international standard.
  However, more appropriate assessments are needed for acute care settings.
- Lower measurement error for MBP than SBP or DBP.

Beat-to-beat BP monitoring : earlier detection of hypo-/hypertension.

Trending ability of uncertain performance.

Beware of the limitations of photoplethysmography (vasoconstriction).

The impact of obesity/finger edema and/or cardiac arrhythmia is uncertain.

Displays a reliable estimate of respiratory changes in pulse pressure.

Displays an estimate of cardiac output (not interchangeable with more reliable techniques).

Figure 3.1 Key messages. DBP, diastolic blood pressure; MBP, mean blood pressure; SBP, systolic blood pressure. A black and white version of this figure will appear in some formats. For the color version, please refer to the plate section.

a significant improvement in measurement trueness and precision over the different evolutions of a given oscillometer model. As MBP is the only component of BP that is directly measured, it is likely that the trueness and precision of its measurement varies less between oscillometer models/versions than that of SBP and DBP.

Choosing the correct cuff size is important to prevent over- or underestimation of BP.[7] Recommendations for cuff length and width exist.[8] The easiest way to choose the adequate cuff size is to thoroughly follow the manufacturer's instructions, using the information printed on the inner side of the cuff.

Measurement Error with the Upper Arm Cuff

A non-invasive BP measurement is compared with a simultaneous invasive reference measurement. The measurement error, for this pair of measurements, is easily calculated by subtraction. In the available studies, from several pairs of measurements, in different patients and at different BP levels, the authors averaged all the measurements errors to calculate the measurement bias. It is an estimate of the systematic measurement error that reflects the trueness of measurement with an instrument.[9] The standard deviation of observed measurement errors was used to estimate the random measurement error that reflects the measurement precision. Trueness and precision of measurement are more appropriate metrological terms than the often misused term "accuracy," which only applies to a single pair of measurements.[9] As trueness and precision should ideally refer to the assessment of replicate measurements in the same patient in steady-state conditions, and as most of the available studies did not fulfil this prerequisite, we acknowledge that the use of these terms in the present chapter is still semantically improper.[9]

According to the current international standard ISO 81060–2:2018, a BP measuring instrument has acceptable trueness and precision if the measurement bias and its standard deviation do not exceed 5 mmHg and 8 mmHg, respectively.[10]

Some large retrospective studies, based on post-hoc analyses of databases, have reported that these ISO 81060–2:2018 criteria were not fulfilled with the automatic upper arm cuff. [11,12] However, in such retrospective studies, one could not guarantee that the cuff was correctly chosen and placed or that no patient movement interfered with the measurements. Likewise, how can we retrospectively ensure that the pressure transducer of the arterial line was placed at the appropriate level, that the zero was correctly set and that the BP waveform was neither under- nor overdamped?[13] It is noteworthy that several prospective studies in anaesthesia and critical care reported that some automatic upper arm cuff devices fulfil the ISO 81060–2:2018 standard.[14–16] This was true for MBP and even DBP, but exceptionally so for SBP. Hence, the measurement bias and the random error are better for MBP than for SBP. This is possibly related to the fact that MBP is directly measured, whereas SBP is only extrapolated. DBP is not directly measured either, but as DBP is the lowest of the three BP components, it may benefit from the fact that the tolerable measurement error (5 mmHg) is similar to that of SBP and is expressed as an absolute value rather than a relative error.

Of the three components of BP, MBP is the one that is measured with the lowest measurement error by the automatic upper arm cuff. Directly measured, MBP is less likely to vary from one model of oscillometer to another, although some models/versions perform better than others.[15,17,18] Furthermore, MBP is the perfusion pressure of most organs. Thus, first and foremost, it is the MBP value that one should pay attention to, although some devices only display it in small font and/or within brackets or even do not display it at all! Since even prospective studies have only inconsistently reported that measurements of MBP are true and precise (according to the ISO standard) with an automatic upper arm cuff, [19,20] it is difficult to make a definitive statement on this point. A meta-analysis of prospective studies will be available soon.[21]

Some beliefs like "the automatic upper arm cuff systematically overestimates (or under-estimates) BP" should be abandoned since the direction of the measurement error is unpredictable from one device to another and from one patient to another. Additionally, it may vary from one BP level to another.[11,12,14,17,19]

Lastly, it is noteworthy that the maximum error tolerated by the ISO 81060–2:2018 standard is independent of the BP level. However, a given non-invasive measurement error (10 mmHg) is likely to be much more acceptable at a very high level of BP (MBP=110 mmHg, for example) or very low level of BP (MBP=40 mmHg) than at a "borderline" BP level (MBP=68 mmHg). Particularly in anaesthesia and critical care, BP can reach extreme values. Thus, one could question whether the same maximum error should be tolerated at each BP level and whether it should indistinctly apply to SBP, MBP and DBP. In order to better tailor the maximum tolerated error, an error grid analysis has been proposed.[22] It classifies for SBP and MBP at each BP level the degree of risk in relation to the magnitude of the measurement error (nil, low, moderate, significant or life-threatening). This error grid is increasingly used [20,23] and may contribute, in future studies, to a better assessment of the performance of the automatic upper arm cuff in acute care settings.

Detection of Hypo- or Hypertension and of Response to Therapy

If a device is unable to measure BP with trueness and precision, it should at least be able to indicate whether the patient is hypotensive or hypertensive and whether he/she has responded to the treatment initiated. Indeed, this crucial information may be sufficient in many situations before invasive monitoring is considered, if necessary. The few available studies reported a remarkable ability to detect arterial hypotension (MBP < 65 mmHg) and hypertension (SBP > 140 mmHg): the corresponding areas under the receiver operating characteristics (ROC) curves were 0.89–0.98 [14,15,17,19] and 0.88–0.94,[15,17,24] that is, close to the maximum of 1. One take-home message could be the following: if the MBP displayed by the automatic cuff is at least 70 mmHg, it is very likely that the patient is not hypotensive, that is, the MBP would be at least 65 mmHg if measured invasively. Taken with the automatic upper arm cuff, an MBP of at least 70 mmHg seems to be a reasonable target during shock resuscitation in patients with no chronic hypertension.

The automatic upper arm cuff allows a reliable identification of patients who have responded to urgent therapy (e.g., 10% increase in MBP after fluid loading, initiation/change in vasopressive drug dosage): area under the ROC curve of 0.89–0.98.[14,15,17,19] In addition, when BP increase is used as a surrogate for cardiac output increase during a fluid challenge, BP measurements taken with an automatic upper arm cuff were reported to be as informative as invasive measurements.[25]

Automatic Upper Arm Cuff in Common Situations

Cardiac Arrhythmia

Cardiac arrhythmia entails anarchy in pulse wave (in both magnitude and frequency) and therefore in oscillations of the arterial wall. This anarchy may impact the reliability of the non-invasive measurements. Whether arrhythmia is taken into account by the algorithms embedded in each model of automatic upper arm cuff is poorly known. Furthermore, before being marketed, the device is validated in a population from which patients with cardiac arrhythmia were excluded, although such a device is often used in patients with arrhythmia. This is paradoxical. So, does cardiac arrhythmia distort the measurements taken with an automatic upper arm cuff? Studies that used the historical auscultatory method as a reference are not informative, since measurements taken with this technique can also be corrupted by arrhythmia.[8] A few studies have used invasive measurements as reference. With a given model of automatic upper arm cuff, MBP readings were not distorted by arrhythmia.[15] For some other models tested, averaging three consecutive BP measurements was necessary to mitigate the arrhythmia-associated high degree of random error. [17,26] Even in the presence of arrhythmia, one device (and possibly others, not investigated) was able to meet the criteria of the ISO 81060–2:2018 standard.[15]

Vasopressive Drugs, Arterial Hypotension

In several studies, the infusion of vasopressive drugs did not impede the fulfilment of the ISO 81060–2:2018 standard.[12,14,27] Hypotension does not seem to increase the non-invasive measurement error,[12,14,15,19] but some data encourage exercising caution on this point.[20] A meta-analysis would be welcome.[21] During extreme hypotension, the failure of the automatic cuff to display any BP value should be interpreted as an alert, especially when other signs of tissue hypoperfusion coexist.

Obesity

Even after a thorough selection of the cuff size, non-invasive measurements at the upper arm are often neither true nor precise in the obese patient.[23] As the interposition of fatty tissue reduces the signal-to-noise ratio, the body mass index is probably less crucial than the upper arm circumference. The shape of the upper arm is also an important factor, as we have all experienced difficulties in placing and maintaining the cuff when the upper arm is more conically than cylindrically shaped.[28] The automatic finger cuff is a possible alternative,[23,29] provided that it does not require calibration with an upper arm cuff.[30]

In morbidly obese patients, placing the automatic cuff at the forearm [23] – or at best, at the wrist [24] – has been reported to be an easy means to limit the measurement error observed when the cuff is placed at the upper arm.

Impossibility to Place the Cuff at the Upper Limb

Vascular access device, arteriovenous fistula, fracture, wound, burn and ongoing surgery on the upper limb are frequently encountered issues that justify placing the automatic cuff on the thigh, the calf or the ankle rather than the upper arm.[31] Nevertheless, this practice is associated with a higher measurement error.[14,32] In the absence of any more appropriate alternative, the automatic cuff placed at the lower limb at least allows the simple detection of hypotension or and the identification of response to urgent therapy (area under the ROC curve of 0.93 and 0.96, respectively).[14]

Continuous Blood Pressure Monitoring: The Automatic Finger Cuff

Measurements with the automatic upper arm cuff are non-invasive but intermittent. Too frequent cuff inflations may cause skin or nerve damage,[5] whereas too frequent measurements expose to a delayed detection of hypo- or hypertension and their morbid consequences. [1–4,33,34] To benefit from continuous and non-invasive monitoring, innovative devices have been marketed and promoted.[35] Are they the missing link in the armamentarium of BP monitoring?

Principles of the Technique

The automatic finger cuff device consists of a photoplethysmographic sensor and an inflatable cuff. The principle is called volume clamp:[5] the inflatable cuff aims at keeping constant the volume of blood contained in the finger, despite the inflow of blood from each pulse wave. This supposes instant changes in the counterpressure exerted by the inflatable cuff wrapped around the finger. Finger cuff pressure automatic adjustments at a high frequency (1 000 times/second) depends on the photoplethysmographic signal. The latter determines that the blood volume in the finger remains constant. The counterpressure exerted by the finger cuff – that is, the pressure in the finger cuff – is the digital BP. An algorithm embedded in the device allows a more proximal BP waveform (the one that would be obtained at the brachial artery) to be constructed. This requires periodic calibrations of the device, either via an oscillometric cuff measurement at the upper arm (in the case of the CNAP™ device, CNSystems) or directly at the finger cuff itself, via a proprietary algorithm (in the case of the ClearSight™ device, Edwards Lifesciences Corporation, previously branded as Nexfin™, an evolution of Finapress™).[5,35]

Measurement Error with the Automatic Finger Cuff

Interpreting the abundant literature addressing the performance of the automatic finger cuff is often challenging. Indeed, some studies reported that the measurement error is acceptable, while others reported that it is not.[5] Acceptability criteria may vary from one study to another, some authors arguing that the ISO 81060–2:2018 standard has not been developed for the continuous BP monitoring.[36] A meta-analysis of 24 studies among 1 164 patients in anaesthesia and critical care found that the automatic finger cuff monitoring of BP did not meet the ISO 81060–2:2018 standard because of a too high random measurement error. [37] Indeed, although the mean measurement error was acceptable (≤5 mmHg), a given non-invasive measurement over- or underestimated BP too often and too widely, as reflected by the excessive standard deviation of the measurement errors and therefore the too wide limits of agreement (which frame 95% of the measurement errors). This was true for each of the two main devices:[37]

- Clearsight™: for MBP, mean measurement error = 4.9 mmHg; 95% limits of agreement: – 11 to 21 mmHg.
- CNAP™: for MBP, mean error = 3.7 mmHg; 95% limits of agreement: –16 to 23 mmHg.

For SBP and DBP, the performance was poorer.[37] Thus, as for the oscillometric upper arm cuff, one should pay attention to MBP rather than SBP or DBP.

Rather than definitively concluding that finger cuff measurements are unreliable, it is noteworthy, as highlighted for the automatic upper arm cuff, that the maximum error tolerated by the ISO 81060–2:2018 standard applies indiscriminately to SBP, MBP or DBP and does not take into account the BP level. Therefore, the grid assessing the risk associated with each degree of error for each level of BP [22] is increasingly applied to the evaluation of the finger cuff device.[29,38,39] Another approach worth exploring is to determine a range of values of BP (or of another physiological parameter) for which the device under test can be considered interchangeable with the reference measurement.[40] These new approaches could permit a more specific evaluation of the performance of the automatic finger cuff in acute care settings. Finally, beyond trueness and precision of the measurement, knowing whether BP is above or below a critical level could be valuable information but very few studies have evaluated this performance.[41,42]

Trending Ability

When an innovative and minimally invasive device does not display true and precise measurements of the physiological parameter of interest, one expect the device to be at least able to assess variations of the parameter, that is, to have a reliable trending ability.[43] Measuring changes in BP implies that the device detects and accounts for changes in the properties of the arterial tree. These changes could be induced by fluid loading, initiation/modification of vasopressive drugs dosage, postural change or arterial clamping during surgery, for instance. Trending ability may therefore rely on a new calibration, ideally automatically, as soon as a change is detected or suspected.

The trending ability of the Clearsight™ and the CNAP™ devices has been poorly evaluated, and the methodology that was used was often perfectible. Indeed, detection of the direction of the BP variation (increase, decrease or stability) is the minimum expected, and the few studies that have included trending analysis have often only reported the concordance rate, reflecting the ability to detect the direction of BP variation.[43] The concordance rate ranged from poor to excellent.[23,29,38,41,44–56]

Beyond the sole direction of BP change, it is relevant to know whether the increase (or decrease) in BP displayed by the monitor is of a similar magnitude to the actual increase (or decrease) in BP. For example, if MBP has increased by 20 mmHg but the non-invasive device only displays an increase of 5 mmHg, its trending ability will be considered poor. To illustrate the ability of the device to provide the magnitude of the BP change, a graph using polar coordinates could be used, as well as other methods.[43,57] In the few studies that have used polar coordinate analysis of BP changes, a moderate to good performance has been reported.[46,50,52,53,55,58]

In summary, drawing a definitive conclusion about the trending ability of the Clearsight™ and CNAP™ devices is impossible. Indeed, beyond the limited amount of available evidence and studies' heterogeneous conclusions, methodological considerations call for caution. Firstly, as mentioned above, the trending ability analysis rarely included the detection of the magnitude of BP variations. Secondly, trending ability was often assessed during periods of BP relative stability: significant BP changes were infrequent, even in studies with an impressive initial number of measurements,[51,55] since small changes in BP were excluded from the analysis deemed to be random noise.[43] Finally, the detection of rapid or even abrupt changes in BP deserves further investigation. Thus, for the CNAP™ device, reliable detection of BP changes is highly uncertain with the finger cuff alone, as this detection seems to mostly rely on the recalibration (by oscillometric upper arm cuff), which only occurs intermittently, often 15 minutes apart.[55] In one study between two oscillometric cuff calibrations, the BP effects of a cardiovascular intervention were poorly detected by the CNAP™ device.[41] For the ClearSight™ device, the few available studies have limited size, and they reported that the detection of fluid challenge-induced changes in BP were poorly to correctly detected.[53,54] During the induction of anaesthesia and tracheal intubation, the CNAP™ and ClearSight™ devices provided a very early detection of a change in BP but not its magnitude.[52,59]

Other Data Provided by the Automatic Finger Cuff

Prediction of Arterial Hypotension

So far, emphasis has been on the early detection of hypotension in order to treat it quickly. Predicting its occurrence in order to initiate a so-called pre-emptive treatment is a more ambitious task. Via artificial intelligence, multiple physiological variables and their variations, imperceptible to the human eye, can be analyzed to that end. This tool is now available at the patient's bedside.[60] The hypotension prediction index, displayed by some Edwards Lifesciences monitors, ranges from 0 to 100 and reflects the probability of the occurrence of decrease in MBP below 65 mmHg within the next 15 minutes. Promising sensitivity and specificity have been reported.[60,61] This tool includes the easily identifiable events related to anaesthesia or surgery: induction and deepening of anaesthesia, arterial clamping/declamping, insufflation during laparoscopy, for instance.[62] The use of this early alert system was associated, in a preliminary study, with a lower rate of episodes of hypotension.[63] Initially developed from the invasive BP waveform, the hypotension prediction index is now proposed with the ClearSight™ system, and an encouraging predictive performance has been reported in preliminary studies in the operating room.[64–66]

Fluid Management

Mechanical ventilation-induced cyclic changes in BP waveform can be analyzed. Finger cuff devices provide the percentage change in pulse pressure (ΔPP) or in stroke volume (ΔSV). These indices have been proposed to predict the response to fluid loading [67] or to evaluate its effects.[68] In the operating theatre or in the intensive care unit,[69,70] several studies (but not all of them [71,72]) have reported that a non-invasive measurement of ΔPP can substitute for its invasive measurement.[73–77] The limitations to the use of ΔPP are well known (arrhythmia, inspiratory efforts, low tidal volume [78]) and naturally apply to its non-invasive measurement.

Cardiac Output Measurement

It is possible to determine the stroke volume (and thus cardiac output) rather reliably by the analysis of the invasive BP waveform, ideally after thermodilution calibration.[79] What about stroke volume determination from a non-invasive waveform and with no thermodilution calibration? Recent meta-analyses have reported that cardiac output measurement error by the Clearsight™ and CNAP™ devices was poor.[37,80,81] This was also true for the measurement of cardiac output changes.[81] A word of caution is necessary: in these works, baseline cardiac output was determined by thermodilution, an invasive method reserved for patients undergoing moderate- to high-risk surgery or resuscitation. Hence, the Clearsight™ and CNAP™ devices were tested in this population. However, these patients are neither the ones in whom the device algorithms were developed nor the ones for whom non-invasive cardiac output monitoring was intended.[80]

Limitations to the Use of the Finger Cuff

The cost of the device may be prohibitive for some invasive procedures, facilities or healthcare systems. For example, the finger cuff of the ClearSight™ system is for single patient use and costs €160 at our hospital. For the CNAP™ system, the finger cuff can be reused from one patient to another, but the monitor must be purchased. Medico-economic studies are needed in order to put the cost of the device into perspective with the possible savings allowed by the reduction in rate, depth and duration of hypotensive episodes and their morbid consequences.

Since the finger cuff embeds a photoplethysmograph, it is expected that finger vasoconstriction (induced by hypothermia, circulatory insufficiency and/or a vasopressive drug) would expose to BP measurement error or failure. Obesity and/or digital edema could decrease the signal-to-noise ratio and thus also contribute to measurement error.[38,82] The former also contributes to distort the calibration of the CNAP™ system with its upper arm cuff. Finally, the impact of cardiac arrhythmia on the various proprietary algorithms embedded in the monitors is poorly divulgated or investigated.[41,83] These limitations, which are more or less prevalent from one study population to another, contribute to the heterogeneity of the performances reported for these devices. For example, the incidence of measurement failure (failure to display a BP value) varied considerably between studies (0 to 17%).[41,70,72] A between-study heterogeneity in the reported trueness and precision is therefore expected as well as a better performance of these innovative devices in relatively "healthy" patients, that is, patients who are not critically ill and who do not undergo major surgery.[82]

Arterial Catheter, Automatic Upper Arm Cuff or Automatic Finger Cuff?

Non-Invasive or Invasive Monitoring?

The aim of this chapter is not to claim, for each specific situation, whether the use of the arterial catheter is strictly required or whether a non-invasive monitoring could be considered. This chapter rather aims at providing keys to guide individual decisions. BP monitoring is a field where individual or departmental practices, or even beliefs, considerably vary,[84] and opposing non-invasive and invasive monitoring often yields to endless debates.[85,86] Nevertheless, whatever the setting, it is remarkable that the technique that is used is, transiently or exclusively, non-invasive in the vast majority of cases:

- In minimal- to moderate-risk surgery, the arterial catheter is often perceived as too invasive and non-invasive monitoring is preferred.
- Even when invasive intra-operative BP monitoring is planned, during induction of anaesthesia and tracheal intubation, BP is commonly monitored only non-invasively, the arterial catheter being placed afterwards.
- During the surgical procedure, the arterial catheter allows the early detection of episodes of arterial hypotension;[87] however, it is withdrawn as soon as the patient is transferred to the ward. Monitoring then only relies on the automatic upper arm cuff, although arterial hypotension and hypertension occurring in the postoperative hours/days may negatively impact patients' outcomes.[2,34]
- During pre-hospital care, an arterial catheter is seldom inserted, even in severely ill patients. Non-invasive monitoring is used.
- When a critically ill patient is admitted to the hospital, inserting an arterial catheter is far from being a priority, especially as its insertion may be difficult/impossible in the event of

acute circulatory failure and therefore consuming precious time.[88] Establishing the diagnosis and prompting urgent therapies are the actual priorities: performing imaging procedures, before initiating antimicrobial therapy (after microbiological sampling), fluid loading, transfusion, vasoactive and inotropic drugs, transfer to the operating theatre and so forth. Thus, even in patients receiving vasopressive drugs and invasive mechanical ventilation, BP monitoring mostly relies on the automatic upper cuff.[31] It allows a sufficiently low measurement error with some devices or, at least, a reliable detection of hypo-, hypertension and response to treatment.[5] It therefore seems reasonable to consider the insertion of an arterial catheter only secondarily, that is, after the completion of the abovementioned urgent diagnostic and therapeutic measures and under optimal conditions (of BP level, asepsis, time allowed), if the patient's condition still requires it. Such a strategy is currently studied in France.[89]

- During the stay in the intensive care unit, one of the undeniable advantages of the arterial catheter is the ease of arterial blood sampling. The counterpart is that it may encourage blood samplings that are not strictly necessary, yielding avoidable extra costs and anemia.[90] In addition, using an arterial catheter exposes the patient to hematoma, arterial thrombosis, pseudo-aneurysm, infection, air embolism and nerve damage.[91] These complications are rare but their consequences are potentially life-threatening, especially in critically ill patients. It is also important to keep in mind that invasive monitoring does not prevent significant measurement errors.[13] Of note, no study has reported an association between the use of an arterial catheter and an improvement in the patients' outcomes. On the other hand, two observational studies reported the lack of association between survival and the use of an arterial catheter.[92,93] In a cohort of almost 11 000 patients receiving a vasopressive drug, arterial catheter use was even associated with a higher risk of death as compared with patients with no arterial catheter.[93]

Non-Invasive Monitoring: Intermittent or Continuous?

Are finger cuff BP measurements less accurate than measurements taken with an automatic upper arm cuff? Surprisingly, only a few studies have compared these two techniques using the invasive reference method. Except in obese patients,[24,49] the ClearSight™ [94] and CNAP™ [41] systems seem to be of similar performance as compared with the automatic upper arm cuff. Most importantly, the continuous nature of the monitoring with these innovative devices is likely to allow an earlier detection and therefore a lower duration and depth of hypotensive or hypertensive episodes as compared with intermittent monitoring.[3,95–97]

Rather than opposing intermittent and continuous non-invasive monitoring, why not combine them? Indeed, an early detection of hypo- or hypertension with the automatic finger cuff as an alert system and its confirmation with the automatic cuff would be an appealing approach, yet to be tested comprehensively.[98,99]

Future Directions

As continuous non-invasive monitoring represents a lead market, it is likely that endeavors will remain intense to continue to develop and refine innovative tools. Hence, besides the automatic finger cuff, there are other devices for non-invasive continuous BP monitoring.

They use other technological principles: arterial tonometry, analysis of the different components of the pulse wave or analysis of the pulse wave transit time.[5,35,100]

In a near future, there may be no need for any specific device for non-invasive monitoring of BP. Indeed, the signal obtained by a conventional pulse oximeter and analyzed via a patented algorithm can provide a reliable detection of significant changes in BP during anaesthesia induction.[101] Within the few minutes after initial calibration (with a conventional automatic oscillometric upper arm cuff, for instance), photoplethysmographic waveform analysis even allowed reliable measurements of BP.[101] This could be a remarkable application of the aforementioned combination of intermittent and continuous non-invasive monitoring. The pulse oximeter may even be replaced by a smartphone to measure BP. Indeed, after placing the fingertip on its camera sensor and its flashlight, a smartphone application analyses the captured optical signals in order to provide an estimation of BP after initial calibration with an automatic upper arm cuff.[102,103] Such advances are noteworthy as, even in low-income settings, smartphones are often available, whereas automatic devices specifically dedicated to BP monitoring may not. Those preliminary findings spur the conduction of studies aiming at determining whether such "minimally invasive–minimally expensive" monitoring is reliable and suitable for acute care settings.

References

1. Sessler DI, Bloomstone JA, Aronson S, et al. Perioperative Quality Initiative consensus statement on intraoperative blood pressure, risk and outcomes for elective surgery. *Br J Anaesth.* 2019 May;**122**(5):563–74.

2. McEvoy MD, Gupta R, Koepke EJ, et al. Perioperative Quality Initiative consensus statement on postoperative blood pressure, risk and outcomes for elective surgery. *Br J Anaesth.* 2019 May;**122** (5):575–86.

3. Maheshwari K, Khanna S, Bajracharya GR, et al. A randomized trial of continuous noninvasive blood pressure monitoring during noncardiac surgery. *Anesth Analg.* 2018 Aug;**127**(2):424–31.

4. Futier E, Lefrant JY, Guinot PG, et al. Effect of individualized vs standard blood pressure management strategies on postoperative organ dysfunction among high-risk patients undergoing major surgery: a randomized clinical trial. *JAMA.* 2017 Oct 10;**318** (14):1346–57.

5. Lakhal K, Ehrmann S, Boulain T. Noninvasive BP monitoring in the critically ill: time to abandon the arterial catheter? *Chest.* 2018 Apr;**153**(4):1023–39.

6. Jilek J. Electronic sphygmomanometers: the problems and some suggestions. *Biomed Instrum Technol.* 2003 Aug;**37**(4):231–3.

7. Bur A, Hirschl MM, Herkner H, et al. Accuracy of oscillometric blood pressure measurement according to the relation between cuff size and upper-arm circumference in critically ill patients. *Crit Care Med.* 2000 Feb;**28**(2):371–6.

8. Pickering TG, Hall JE, Appel LJ, et al. Recommendations for blood pressure measurement in humans and experimental animals: part 1: blood pressure measurement in humans: a statement for professionals from the Subcommittee of Professional and Public Education of the American Heart Association Council on High Blood Pressure Research. *Circulation.* 2005 Feb 8;**111** (5):697–716.

9. Squara P, Scheeren TWL, Aya HD, et al. Metrology part 1: definition of quality criteria. *J Clin Monit Comput.* 2021 Feb;**35** (1):17–25.

10. Stergiou GS, Alpert B, Mieke S, et al. A universal standard for the validation of blood pressure measuring devices: Association for the Advancement of

Medical Instrumentation/European Society of Hypertension/International Organization for Standardization (AAMI/ESH/ISO) collaboration statement. *Hypertension*. 2018 Mar;**71**(3):368–74.

11. Wax DB, Lin HM, Leibowitz AB. Invasive and concomitant noninvasive intraoperative blood pressure monitoring: observed differences in measurements and associated therapeutic interventions. *Anesthesiology*. 2011 Nov;**115**(5):973–8.

12. Lehman L wei H, Saeed M, et al. Methods of blood pressure measurement in the ICU. *Crit Care Med*. 2013 Jan;**41**(1):34–40.

13. Romagnoli S, Ricci Z, Quattrone D, et al. Accuracy of invasive arterial pressure monitoring in cardiovascular patients: an observational study. *Crit Care*. 2014 Nov 30;**18**(6):644.

14. Lakhal K, Macq C, Ehrmann S, Boulain T, Capdevila X. Noninvasive monitoring of blood pressure in the critically ill: reliability according to the cuff site (arm, thigh, or ankle). *Crit Care Med*. 2012 Apr;**40**(4):1207–13.

15. Lakhal K, Ehrmann S, Martin M, et al. Blood pressure monitoring during arrhythmia: agreement between automated brachial cuff and intra-arterial measurements. *Br J Anaesth*. 2015 Oct;**115**(4):540–9.

16. Xu J, Wu Y, Su H, et al. The value of a BP determination method using a novel non-invasive BP device against the invasive catheter measurement. *PLoS One*. 2014;**9**(6):e100287.

17. Lakhal K, Martin M, Ehrmann S, et al. Non-invasive blood pressure monitoring with an oscillometric brachial cuff: impact of arrhythmia. *J Clin Monit Comput*. 2018 Aug;**32**(4):707–15.

18. Bur A, Herkner H, Vlcek M, et al. Factors influencing the accuracy of oscillometric blood pressure measurement in critically ill patients. *Crit Care Med*. 2003 Mar;**31**(3):793–9.

19. Lakhal K, Ehrmann S, Runge I, et al. Tracking hypotension and dynamic changes in arterial blood pressure with

brachial cuff measurements. *Anesth Analg*. 2009 Aug;**109**(2):494–501.

20. Meidert AS, Dolch ME, Mühlbauer K, et al. Oscillometric versus invasive blood pressure measurement in patients with shock: a prospective observational study in the emergency department. *J Clin Monit Comput*. 2021 Apr;**35**(2):387–93.

21. Dauvergne JE, Lakhal K, Boulain T, Rozec B. Accuracy and precision of oscillometric automated cuff measurements of arterial blood pressure in the acute care setting: systematic review and meta-analysis of individual participant data from studies with invasive measurements serving as reference. [Internet]. National Institute for Health Research: PROSPERO (international prospective register of systematic reviews). 2021. Available from: www.crd.york.ac.uk/prospero/display_record.php?RecordID=233707

22. Saugel B, Grothe O, Nicklas JY. Error grid analysis for arterial pressure method comparison studies. *Anesth Analg*. 2018 Apr;**126**(4):1177–85.

23. Schumann R, Meidert AS, Bonney I, et al. Intraoperative blood pressure monitoring in obese patients. *Anesthesiology*. 2021 Feb 1;**134**(2):179–88.

24. Mostafa MMA, Hasanin AM, Alhamade F, et al. Accuracy and trending of non-invasive oscillometric blood pressure monitoring at the wrist in obese patients. *Anaesth Crit Care Pain Med*. 2020 Apr;**39**(2):221–7.

25. Lakhal K, Ehrmann S, Perrotin D, Wolff M, Boulain T. Fluid challenge: tracking changes in cardiac output with blood pressure monitoring (invasive or non-invasive). *Intensive Care Med*. 2013 Nov;**39**(11):1953–62.

26. Pagonas N, Schmidt S, Eysel J, et al. Impact of atrial fibrillation on the accuracy of oscillometric blood pressure monitoring. *Hypertension*. 2013 Sep;**62**(3):579–84.

27. Riley LE, Chen GJ, Latham HE. Comparison of noninvasive blood pressure monitoring with invasive arterial pressure monitoring in medical ICU patients with

septic shock. *Blood Press Monit.* 2017 Aug;**22**(4):202–7.

28. Eley VA, Christensen R, Guy L, Dodd B. Perioperative blood pressure monitoring in patients with obesity. *Anesth Analg.* 2019;**128**(3):484–91.

29. Rogge DE, Nicklas JY, Schön G, et al. Continuous noninvasive arterial pressure monitoring in obese patients during bariatric surgery: an evaluation of the vascular unloading technique (Clearsight system). *Anesth Analg.* 2019;**128**(3):477–83.

30. Lakhal K. Non-invasive measurements of blood pressure in obese patients: where should I place the cuff? *Anaesth Crit Care Pain Med.* 2020 Apr;**39**(2):193–4.

31. Chatterjee A, DePriest K, Blair R, Bowton D, Chin R. Results of a survey of blood pressure monitoring by intensivists in critically ill patients: a preliminary study. *Crit Care Med.* 2010 Dec;**38**(12):2335–8.

32. Siaron KB, Cortes MX, Stutzman SE, et al. Blood pressure measurements are site dependent in a cohort of patients with neurological illness. *Sci Rep.* 2020 Feb 25;**10**(1):3382.

33. Maheshwari K, Nathanson BH, Munson SH, et al. The relationship between ICU hypotension and in-hospital mortality and morbidity in septic patients. *Intensive Care Med.* 2018 Jun;**44**(6):857–67.

34. Sessler DI, Meyhoff CS, Zimmerman NM, et al. Period-dependent associations between hypotension during and for four days after noncardiac surgery and a composite of myocardial infarction and death: a substudy of the POISE-2 Trial. *Anesthesiology.* 2018 Feb;**128**(2):317–27.

35. Michard F, Sessler DI, Saugel B. Non-invasive arterial pressure monitoring revisited. *Intensive Care Med.* 2018 Dec;**44**(12):2213–15.

36. Lakhal K, Martin M, Ehrmann S, Boulain T. Noninvasive monitors of blood pressure in the critically ill: what are acceptable accuracy and precision? *Eur J Anaesthesiol.* 2015 May;**32**(5):367–8.

37. Saugel B, Hoppe P, Nicklas JY, et al. Continuous noninvasive pulse wave analysis using finger cuff technologies for arterial blood pressure and cardiac output monitoring in perioperative and intensive care medicine: a systematic review and meta-analysis. *Br J Anaesth.* 2020 Jul;**125**(1):25–37.

38. Eley V, Christensen R, Guy L, et al. ClearSight^{TM} finger cuff versus invasive arterial pressure measurement in patients with body mass index above 45 kg/m^2. *BMC Anesthesiol.* 2021 May 18;**21**(1):152.

39. Bugarini A, Young AJ, Griessenauer CJ, et al. Perioperative continuous noninvasive arterial pressure monitoring for neuroendovascular interventions: prospective study for evaluation of the vascular unloading technique. *World Neurosurg.* 2021 Sep;**153**:e195–203.

40. Lorne E, Diouf M, de Wilde RBP, Fischer MO. Assessment of interchangeability rate between 2 methods of measurements: an example with a cardiac output comparison study. *Medicine (Baltimore).* 2018 Feb;**97**(7):e9905.

41. Lakhal K, Martin M, Faiz S, et al. The CNAP^{TM} finger cuff for noninvasive beat-to-beat monitoring of arterial blood pressure: an evaluation in intensive care unit patients and a comparison with 2 intermittent devices. *Anesth Analg.* 2016;**123**(5):1126–35.

42. Wang Z, Chen G, Lu K, Zhu Y, Chen Y. Investigation of the accuracy of a noninvasive continuous blood pressure device in different age groups and its ability in detecting hypertension and hypotension: an observational study. *BMC Anesthesiol.* 2019 Dec 5;**19**(1):223.

43. Critchley LA, Lee A, Ho AMH. A critical review of the ability of continuous cardiac output monitors to measure trends in cardiac output. *Anesth Analg.* 2010 Nov;**111**(5):1180–92.

44. Lu SY, Dalia AA. Continuous noninvasive arterial pressure monitoring for transcatheter aortic valve replacement. *J Cardiothorac Vasc Anesth.* 2021 Jul;**35**(7):2026–33.

45. Mukai A, Suehiro K, Kimura A, et al. Effect of systemic vascular resistance on the

reliability of noninvasive hemodynamic monitoring in cardiac surgery. *J Cardiothorac Vasc Anesth.* 2021 Jun;**35**(6):1782–91.

46. Kanazawa H, Maeda T, Miyazaki E, et al. Accuracy and trending ability of blood pressure and cardiac index measured by ClearSight system in patients with reduced ejection fraction. *J Cardiothorac Vasc Anesth.* 2020 Dec;**34**(12):3293–9.

47. Noto A, Sanfilippo F, De Salvo G, et al. Noninvasive continuous arterial pressure monitoring with Clearsight during awake carotid endarterectomy: a prospective observational study. *Eur J Anaesthesiol.* 2019 Feb;**36**(2):144–52.

48. Rogge DE, Nicklas JY, Haas SA, Reuter DA, Saugel B. Continuous noninvasive arterial pressure monitoring using the vascular unloading technique (CNAP system) in obese patients during laparoscopic bariatric operations. *Anesth Analg.* 2018 Feb;**126**(2):454–63.

49. Berkelmans GFN, Kuipers S, Westerhof BE, Spoelstra-de Man AME, Smulders YM. Comparing volume-clamp method and intra-arterial blood pressure measurements in patients with atrial fibrillation admitted to the intensive or medium care unit. *J Clin Monit Comput.* 2018 Jun;**32**(3):439–46.

50. Ameloot K, Van De Vijver K, Van Regenmortel N, et al. Validation study of Nexfin® continuous non-invasive blood pressure monitoring in critically ill adult patients. *Minerva Anestesiol.* 2014 Dec;**80**(12):1294–301.

51. Broch O, Bein B, Gruenewald M, et al. A comparison of continuous non-invasive arterial pressure with invasive radial and femoral pressure in patients undergoing cardiac surgery. *Minerva Anestesiol.* 2013 Mar;**79**(3):248–56.

52. Weiss E, Gayat E, Dumans-Nizard V, Le Guen M, Fischler M. Use of the Nexfin^TM device to detect acute arterial pressure variations during anaesthesia induction. *Br J Anaesth.* 2014 Jul;**113**(1):52–60.

53. Hofhuizen C, Lansdorp B, van der Hoeven JG, Scheffer GJ, Lemson J. Validation of noninvasive pulse contour cardiac output using finger arterial pressure in cardiac surgery patients requiring fluid therapy. *J Crit Care.* 2014 Feb;**29**(1):161–5.

54. Schramm P, Tzanova I, Gööck T, et al. Noninvasive hemodynamic measurements during neurosurgical procedures in sitting position. *J Neurosurg Anesthesiol.* 2017 Jul;**29**(3):251–7.

55. Smolle KH, Schmid M, Prettenthaler H, Weger C. The accuracy of the CNAP® device compared with invasive radial artery measurements for providing continuous noninvasive arterial blood pressure readings at a medical intensive care unit: a method-comparison study. *Anesth Analg.* 2015 Dec;**121**(6):1508–16.

56. Biais M, Vidil L, Roullet S, et al. Continuous non-invasive arterial pressure measurement: evaluation of CNAP device during vascular surgery. *Ann Fr Anesth Reanim.* 2010 Aug;**29**(7–8):530–5.

57. Fischer MO, Lorne E. The trend interchangeability method. *Br J Anaesth.* 2016 Dec;**117**(6):826–8.

58. Balzer F, Habicher M, Sander M, et al. Comparison of the non-invasive Nexfin® monitor with conventional methods for the measurement of arterial blood pressure in moderate risk orthopaedic surgery patients. *J Int Med Res.* 2016 Aug;**44**(4):832–43.

59. Gayat E, Mongardon N, Tuil O, et al. CNAP(®) does not reliably detect minimal or maximal arterial blood pressures during induction of anaesthesia and tracheal intubation. *Acta Anaesthesiol Scand.* 2013 Apr;**57**(4):468–73.

60. Hatib F, Jian Z, Buddi S, et al. Machine-learning algorithm to predict hypotension based on high-fidelity arterial pressure waveform analysis. *Anesthesiology.* 2018 Oct;**129**(4):663–74.

61. Davies SJ, Vistisen ST, Jian Z, Hatib F, Scheeren TWL. Ability of an Arterial Waveform Analysis-Derived Hypotension Prediction Index to Predict Future Hypotensive Events in Surgical Patients. *Anesth Analg.* 2020 Feb;**130**(2):352–9.

62. Saugel B, Kouz K, Hoppe P, Maheshwari K, Scheeren TWL. Predicting hypotension in perioperative and intensive care medicine. *Best Pract Res Clin Anaesthesiol.* 2019 Jun;**33**(2):189–97.

63. Wijnberge M, Geerts BF, Hol L, et al. Effect of a machine learning–derived early warning system for intraoperative hypotension vs standard care on depth and duration of intraoperative hypotension during elective noncardiac surgery: the HYPE randomized clinical trial. *JAMA.* 2020 Mar 17;**323**(11):1052–60.

64. Frassanito L, Giuri PP, Vassalli F, et al. Hypotension Prediction Index with non-invasive continuous arterial pressure waveforms (ClearSight): clinical performance in gynaecologic oncologic surgery. *J Clin Monit Comput.* 2022 Oct;**36**(5):1325–2.

65. Frassanito L, Sonnino C, Piersanti A, et al. Performance of the Hypotension Prediction Index with noninvasive arterial pressure waveforms in awake cesarean delivery patients under spinal anesthesia. *Anesth Analg.* 2022 Mar 1;**134**(3):633–43.

66. Maheshwari K, Buddi S, Jian Z, et al. Performance of the Hypotension Prediction Index with non-invasive arterial pressure waveforms in non-cardiac surgical patients. *J Clin Monit Comput.* 2021 Feb;**35**(1):71–8.

67. Vallet B, Blanloeil Y, Cholley B, et al. [Guidelines for perioperative haemodynamic optimization. Société française d'anesthésie et de réanimation]. *Ann Fr Anesth Reanim.* 2013 Jun;**32**(6):454–62.

68. Lakhal K, Nay MA, Kamel T, et al. Change in end-tidal carbon dioxide outperforms other surrogates for change in cardiac output during fluid challenge. *Br J Anaesth.* 2017 Mar 1;**118**(3):355–62.

69. Lansdorp B, Ouweneel D, de Keijzer A, et al. Non-invasive measurement of pulse pressure variation and systolic pressure variation using a finger cuff corresponds with intra-arterial measurement. *Br J Anaesth.* 2011 Oct;**107**(4):540–5.

70. Monnet X, Dres M, Ferré A, et al. Prediction of fluid responsiveness by a continuous non-invasive assessment of arterial pressure in critically ill patients: comparison with four other dynamic indices. *Br J Anaesth.* 2012 Sep;**109**(3):330–8.

71. Fischer MO, Coucoravas J, Truong J, et al. Assessment of changes in cardiac index and fluid responsiveness: a comparison of Nexfin and transpulmonary thermodilution. *Acta Anaesthesiol Scand.* 2013 Jul;**57**(6):704–12.

72. Flick M, Schumann R, Hoppe P, et al. Non-invasive measurement of pulse pressure variation using a finger-cuff method in obese patients having laparoscopic bariatric surgery. *J Clin Monit Comput.* 2021 Dec;**35**(6):1341–7.

73. Renner J, Gruenewald M, Hill M, et al. Non-invasive assessment of fluid responsiveness using CNAP[TM] technology is interchangeable with invasive arterial measurements during major open abdominal surgery. *Br J Anaesth.* 2017 Jan;**118**(1):58–67.

74. Biais M, Stecken L, Ottolenghi L, et al. The ability of pulse pressure variations obtained with CNAP[TM] device to predict fluid responsiveness in the operating room. *Anesth Analg.* 2011 Sep;**113**(3):523–8.

75. Biais M, Stecken L, Martin A, et al. Automated, continuous and non-invasive assessment of pulse pressure variations using CNAP® system. *J Clin Monit Comput.* 2017 Aug;**31**(4):685–92.

76. Solus-Biguenet H, Fleyfel M, Tavernier B, et al. Non-invasive prediction of fluid responsiveness during major hepatic surgery. *Br J Anaesth.* 2006 Dec;**97**(6):808–16.

77. de Wilde RBP, de Wit F, Geerts BF, et al. Non-invasive continuous arterial pressure and pulse pressure variation measured with Nexfin(®) in patients following major upper abdominal surgery: a comparative study. *Anaesthesia.* 2016 Jul;**71**(7):788–97.

78. Lakhal K, Biais M. Pulse pressure respiratory variation to predict fluid responsiveness: from an enthusiastic to a rational view. *Anaesth Crit Care Pain Med.* 2015 Feb;**34**(1):9–10.

79. Jozwiak M, Monnet X, Teboul JL. Pressure waveform analysis. *Anesth Analg.* 2018 Jun;**126**(6):1930–3.

80. Joosten A, Desebbe O, Suehiro K, et al. Accuracy and precision of non-invasive cardiac output monitoring devices in perioperative medicine: a systematic review and meta-analysis†. *Br J Anaesth.* 2017 Mar 1;**118**(3):298–310.

81. Fischer MO, Joosten A, Desebbe O, et al. Interchangeability of cardiac output measurements between non-invasive photoplethysmography and bolus thermodilution: a systematic review and individual patient data meta-analysis. *Anaesth Crit Care Pain Med.* 2020 Feb;**39** (1):75–85.

82. Hohn A, Defosse JM, Becker S, et al. Non-invasive continuous arterial pressure monitoring with Nexfin does not sufficiently replace invasive measurements in critically ill patients. *Br J Anaesth.* 2013 Aug;**111**(2):178–84.

83. Ilies C, Grudev G, Hedderich J, et al. Comparison of a continuous noninvasive arterial pressure device with invasive measurements in cardiovascular postsurgical intensive care patients: a prospective observational study. *Eur J Anaesthesiol.* 2015 Jan;**32**(1):20–8.

84. Gershengorn HB, Garland A, Kramer A, et al. Variation of arterial and central venous catheter use in United States intensive care units. *Anesthesiology.* 2014 Mar;**120**(3):650–64.

85. Garland A. Arterial lines in the ICU: a call for rigorous controlled trials. *Chest.* 2014 Nov;**146**(5):1155–8.

86. Jiang Y, Liu J, Peng W, et al. Comparison of invasive blood pressure monitoring versus normal non-invasive blood pressure monitoring in ST-elevation myocardial infarction patients with percutaneous coronary intervention. *Injury.* 2022 Mar;**53** (3):1108–13.

87. Naylor AJ, Sessler DI, Maheshwari K, et al. Arterial catheters for early detection and treatment of hypotension during major noncardiac surgery: a randomized trial. *Anesth Analg.* 2020 Nov;**131**(5):1540–50.

88. Mouncey PR, Osborn TM, Power GS, et al. Trial of early, goal-directed resuscitation for septic shock. *N Engl J Med.* 2015 Apr 2;**372**(14):1301–11.

89. Muller G, Kamel T, Contou D, et al. Early versus differed arterial catheterisation in critically ill patients with acute circulatory failure: a multicentre, open-label, pragmatic, randomised, non-inferiority controlled trial: the EVERDAC protocol. *BMJ Open.* 2021 Sep 14;**11**(9):e044719.

90. Low LL, Harrington GR, Stoltzfus DP. The effect of arterial lines on blood-drawing practices and costs in intensive care units. *Chest.* 1995 Jul;**108**(1):216–9.

91. Scheer B, Perel A, Pfeiffer UJ. Clinical review: complications and risk factors of peripheral arterial catheters used for haemodynamic monitoring in anaesthesia and intensive care medicine. *Crit Care.* 2002 Jun;**6**(3):199–204.

92. Hsu DJ, Feng M, Kothari R, et al. The association between indwelling arterial catheters and mortality in hemodynamically stable patients with respiratory failure: a propensity score analysis. *Chest.* 2015 Dec;**148**(6):1470–6.

93. Gershengorn HB, Wunsch H, Scales DC, et a. Association between arterial catheter use and hospital mortality in intensive care units. *JAMA Intern Med.* 2014 Nov;**174** (11):1746–54.

94. Vos JJ, Poterman M, Mooyaart EAQ, et al. Comparison of continuous non-invasive finger arterial pressure monitoring with conventional intermittent automated arm arterial pressure measurement in patients under general anaesthesia. *Br J Anaesth.* 2014 Jul;**113**(1):67–74.

95. Meidert AS, Nold JS, Hornung R, et al. The impact of continuous non-invasive arterial blood pressure monitoring on blood pressure stability during general anaesthesia in orthopaedic patients: a randomised trial. *Eur J Anaesthesiol.* 2017 Nov;**34**(11):716–22.

96. Ilies C, Kiskalt H, Siedenhans D, et al. Detection of hypotension during Caesarean section with continuous non-invasive arterial pressure device or

intermittent oscillometric arterial pressure measurement. *Br J Anaesth*. 2012 Sep;**109**(3):413–19.

97. Wagner JY, Prantner JS, Meidert AS, et al. Noninvasive continuous versus intermittent arterial pressure monitoring: evaluation of the vascular unloading technique (CNAP device) in the emergency department. *Scand J Trauma Resusc Emerg Med*. 2014 Jan 29;**22**:8.

98. Chen G, Chung E, Meng L, et al. Impact of non invasive and beat-to-beat arterial pressure monitoring on intraoperative hemodynamic management. J Clin Monit Comput. 2012 Apr;**26**(2):133–40.

99. Müller G, Thierry Boulain, Ehrmann S, Karim Lakhal. Prospective, multi-center evaluation of the accuracy of non-invasive measurement of blood pressure using an arm, calf and finger cuff. [Internet]. 2021. Available from: https://clinicaltrials.gov/ct2/show/NCT04269382

100. Bilo G, Zorzi C, Ochoa Munera JE, et al. Validation of the Somnotouch-NIBP noninvasive continuous blood pressure

monitor according to the European Society of Hypertension International Protocol revision 2010. *Blood Press Monit*. 2015 Oct;**20**(5):291–4.

101. Ghamri Y, Proença M, Hofmann G, et al. Automated pulse oximeter waveform analysis to track changes in blood pressure during anesthesia induction: a proof-of-concept study. *Anesth Analg*. 2020 May;**130**(5):1222–33.

102. Desebbe O, El Hilali M, Kouz K, et al. Evaluation of a new smartphone optical blood pressure application (OptiBPTM) in the post-anesthesia care unit: a method comparison study against the non-invasive automatic oscillometric brachial cuff as the reference method. *J Clin Monit Comput*. 2022 Oct;**36**(5):1525–33.

103. Desebbe O, Tighenifi A, Jacobs A, et al. Evaluation of a novel mobile phone application for blood pressure monitoring: a proof of concept study. *J Clin Monit Comput*. 2022 Aug;**36**(4):1147–53.

Microcirculation and Mitochondrial Dysfunction

Daniel De Backer and Diego Orbegozo Cortes

Introduction

Organ dysfunction often occurs in the perioperative setting and in sepsis. Alterations in systemic hemodynamics may play a role, but even when these are within therapeutic goals, organ dysfunction may still occur. Microcirculatory alterations, a key determinant of tissue perfusion and of mitochondrial dysfunction, may play a role in the development of organ dysfunction. In this chapter, we discuss the evidence for alterations in microcirculatory and mitochondrial functions, and their relevance, in circulatory failure and in the perioperative setting.

Microcirculatory Alterations in Sepsis: Where Is the Evidence?

Multiple experimental studies have found that sepsis induces marked alterations in the microcirculation. Compared with normal conditions where there is a dense network of well-perfused capillaries, sepsis is associated with a decrease in capillary density. More importantly, intermittently perfused or not perfused capillaries are located in proximity to well-perfused capillaries, which results in shunt.[1–4] Importantly, this is a dynamic process, as the stop-flow capillaries may be perfused a few minutes later and vice versa. In addition, there is an increase in heterogeneity in microvascular perfusion between areas separated by a few microns. These alterations have been reported after administration of endotoxin or live bacteria and during bacterial peritonitis,[2,3,5] and have been observed in small [6,7] as well as in large animals.[3,4] In addition, all studied organs are affected, including the skin,[8] muscle,[6,7] eye,[9] tongue,[3] gut,[3,4] liver,[1] heart,[10] and the brain.[5] Hence, these changes seem to be ubiquitous and to have common pathophysiological mechanisms.

Technical limitations have long impaired the demonstration of microcirculatory alterations in patients. The development of new imaging techniques has enabled direct visualization of the human microcirculation with small handheld microscopes.[11,12] In patients with severe sepsis and septic shock, we observed a decrease in vascular density, together with an increased number of capillaries with stopped or intermittent flow.[13] Typical examples of normal and septic microcirculations are shown in Figures 4.1 and 4.2. These alterations are very similar to those occurring in experimental models of sepsis. Since this initial study, more than 30 studies have shown similar results.

This chapter was originally published in *Perioperative Hemodynamic Monitoring and Goal Directed Therapy*, ed. Maxime Cannesson and Rupert Pearse. Published by Cambridge University Press.

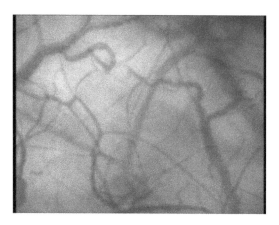

Figure 4.1 Sublingual microcirculation in normal conditions. Photograph of the sublingual microcirculation in a normal individual with septic shock using a sidestream dark field (SDF) imaging device. A black and white version of this figure will appear in some formats. For the color version, please refer to the plate section.

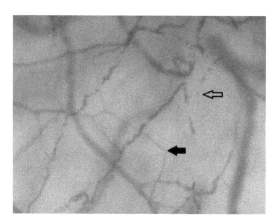

Figure 4.2 Sublingual microcirculation in sepsis. Photograph of the sublingual microcirculation in a patient with septic shock using a sidestream dark field (SDF) imaging device. The solid arrow shows a well-perfused capillary; the empty arrow identifies a stopped flow capillary. A black and white version of this figure will appear in some formats. For the color version, please refer to the plate section.

What Are the Consequences of These Alterations?

Tissue oxygenation is impaired as the diffusion distance for oxygen increases as a result of the decreased capillary density.[10] In addition, the heterogeneity in microvascular blood flow with perfused capillaries in close vicinity to non-perfused capillaries leads to alterations in oxygen extraction capabilities [4,14–17] and heterogeneity in tissue oxygenation.[18] Hence zones of tissue hypoxia may develop, even when total blood flow to the organ is preserved.[19]

Importantly, heterogeneity in perfusion leads to more severe alterations in tissue oxygenation than a homogeneous decrease in perfusion.[14,17] During episodes of hypo-perfusion, the heterogeneity of microvascular perfusion further increases in sepsis instead of being minimized as in normal conditions.[16]

These alterations play an important role in the development of organ dysfunction and are not just an indication of the severity of sepsis. Microvascular alterations can lead to cellular injury,[20] and reversal of these alterations is associated with improvement in lactate [21] and NADH [22] levels, suggesting that microvascular alterations directly impair tissue oxygenation. In addition, several trials have demonstrated an association between the severity of microvascular dysfunction and the development of organ dysfunction [23–25] and mortality.[13,19,24,26–30]

In 252 patients with septic shock, microvascular perfusion was an independent factor associated with survival.[31] Dividing the population into quartiles of proportions of perfused capillaries, mortality rates markedly increased with alterations in the microcirculation.[31] The proportion of perfused capillaries was the strongest predictor of outcome, but vascular density of perfused capillaries and heterogeneity index were also associated with outcome.[13,19,31] Similar results were reported in a multicentric study in the United States.[32] Of note, the velocity in perfused capillaries was not associated with outcome,[19] illustrating that the diffusive component of oxygen transport seems to be more important at the microcirculatory level than its convective component.

The evolution over time of these alterations also differed in patients with good or poor outcomes.[27,30] Microvascular perfusion rapidly improved in survivors, but remained disturbed in non-survivors, whether these patients died of acute circulatory failure or organ failure after resolution of shock.[27,30]

Mitochondrial Dysfunction: Where Is the Evidence?

Mitochondrial dysfunction is characterized by alteration in the mitochondrial electron transport chain by cytochromes I to IV. Several experimental models have reported decreased complex I, II, and/or complex IV activity.[33,34] In a long-term model of sepsis in rodents, mitochondrial dysfunction, mostly characterized by decreased complex I activity, was associated with organ dysfunction and mortality.[32] In late phases of sepsis, administration of exogenous cytochrome C corrected mitochondrial alterations and reversed myocardial depression.[35]

Several publications investigated skeletal muscle mitochondria in septic patients.[36–38] Complexes I and IV as well as citrate synthase activity were reduced in septic patients if the enzymatic activity was expressed per tissue weight, and again, no change was observed when normalized to citrate synthase activity.[36,37] Additionally, the muscle ATP content was decreased in septic patients. Brealey et al. [38] observed differences between surviving and non-surviving septic patients and controls: complex I activity decreased compared with controls and ATP content decreased compared with survivors of sepsis and controls. However, complex IV activity increased in non-survivors compared with controls. Overall, skeletal muscle mitochondria and tissue ATP content seem mainly to be reduced in patients who will later die of sepsis.

On the other hand, other studies have demonstrated normal or even increased mitochondrial function. In hearts demonstrating impairment in systolic and diastolic function at the early phase of sepsis, mitochondrial histology and function were normal.[39] In peripheral white blood cells obtained from patients with sepsis, mitochondrial respiratory function was increased, not decreased.[40] Oxidative phosphorylation and electron transfer were increased in patients with sepsis, suggesting integrity of cytochrome pathways.

In a systematic review, which included 76 trials, Jeger et al. [41] pointed out the different factors contributing to these different results. In addition to species and organ specificities, the methods used to investigate cellular respiration, in particular the way results were expressed, should be examined carefully. Results can be expressed per tissue weight, mitochondrial protein, or citrate synthase activity. As citrate synthase activity is down-regulated by ATP content, results of mitochondrial function expressed per citrate synthase activity should be looked at with caution. In addition, it appears to change throughout the course of sepsis. Mitochondrial function seems to be increased in early sepsis, but impaired in later stages [38,42] mitochondrial dysfunction is more severe in non-resuscitated than in resuscitated models,[43] and more severe in non-survivors than in survivors.[38]

Microcirculatory and Mitochondrial Dysfunction: A Different Relevance at Different Periods?

As alterations in systemic hemodynamics, microvascular perfusion, and mitochondrial function may all occur, it is quite difficult to determine which contributes most to the development of organ dysfunction.

Several factors suggest that the microcirculatory alterations are important at the early stages and act as a primary event leading to cellular dysfunction. First, microcirculatory alterations are co-localized with low PO_2, production of hypoxia-inducible factor,[10] or redox potential [22] in experimental conditions. Second, oxygen saturation at the capillary end of well-perfused capillaries is low, suggesting that the tissues are using the delivered oxygen.[15] Third, there is an inverse relationship between microvascular perfusion and tissue to arterial PCO_2 gradient, in the sublingual area and in the ileal mucosal area.[44,45] This gradient would be normal if flow was matching metabolism, as CO_2 production would be low because the primary alteration is the decrease in metabolism. Fourth, perfusion abnormalities precede alterations in organ function.[46] Fifth, improvement in the sublingual microcirculation in response to initial resuscitation procedures was associated with an improvement of organ function 24 hours later.[25] Finally, the decrease in lactate levels is proportional to the improvement of the microcirculation during dobutamine administration.[21] Hence, it seems that, at early stages, flow alterations seem to precede and maybe contribute to cellular alterations.

One may thus raise the following unifying theory: at initial stages, systemic hemodynamic alterations predominate. Once these are within targets (i.e., arterial pressure, cardiac index, and SvO_2), the contribution of microcirculatory alterations becomes predominant. After some time, cellular alterations dominate. This suggests that there is a time window opportunity for therapeutic interventions aiming at improving tissue perfusion. This view is supported by some experimental and clinical data. In animals with sepsis, delayed fluid resuscitation, compared with timely resuscitation, was associated with increased levels of inflammatory mediators and impairment of cytochrome function.[43] In patients with septic shock, Rivers et al. [47] reported that patients undergoing early goal-directed therapy had lower activation of inflammatory and apoptotic pathways.

Do These Alterations Also Occur in High-Risk Surgery?

Microcirculatory alterations also occur in the perioperative period.[48–50] In patients submitted to high-risk surgery, the severity of the alterations was associated with development of perioperative complications.[50] In patients submitted to cardiac surgery, the microvascular alterations culminated during the surgical procedure and the severity of these alterations correlated with peak levels of lactate and Sequential Organ Failure Assessment (SOFA) score in the perioperative period.[48] Various factors may influence the development of such microvascular alterations during high-risk surgery. First, hypovolemia (and preload-dependence) may promote the occurrence of microvascular alterations, but these usually easily reverse after correction of hypovolemia.[51] Second, ischemia-reperfusion injury and inflammatory processes related to the surgical procedure may alter the microcirculation. Finally, the impact of anesthesia should not be neglected, but this effect is not sustained and rapidly disappears in the postoperative period.[48]

Mitochondrial dysfunction occurs in organs submitted to clamping as a consequence of the ischemic process. Hearts submitted to cardioplegic arrest under cardiopulmonary bypass demonstrate a diffuse loss of mitochondrial cytochrome C, and in particular complex I, and a decrease in mitochondrial oxygen consumption.[52–54] Do we also observe similar alterations in remote organs? This issue has not yet been evaluated in humans.

Conclusions

Multiple experimental and clinical trials have shown that microcirculatory alterations occur in sepsis and that they may play a role in the development of organ dysfunction. Similar alterations occur in the perioperative period. In addition, mitochondrial dysfunction also occurs, especially in late stages of sepsis, and is associated with organ dysfunction. The relative contribution of both factors is difficult to determine at this stage.

It seems that temporal factors may play a role and that microcirculatory alterations prevail at early stages, once global hemodynamic variables are within target values, and that mitochondrial dysfunction dominates at later stages.

References

1. Croner RS, Hoerer E, Kulu Y, et al. Hepatic platelet and leukocyte adherence during endotoxemia. *Crit Care.* 2006;**10**:R15.

2. Secor D, Li F, Ellis CG, et al. Impaired microvascular perfusion in sepsis requires activated coagulation and P-selectin-mediated platelet adhesion in capillaries. *Intens Care Med.* 2010;**36**:1928–34.

3. Verdant CL, De Backer D, Bruhn A, et al. Evaluation of sublingual and gut mucosal microcirculation in sepsis: a quantitative analysis. *Crit Care Med.* 2009;**37**:2875–81.

4. Farquhar I, Martin CM, Lam C, et al. Decreased capillary density in vivo in bowel mucosa of rats with normotensive sepsis. *J Surg Res* 1996;**61**:190–6.

5. Taccone FS, Su F, Pierrakos C, et al. Cerebral microcirculation is impaired during sepsis: an experimental study. *Crit Care.* 2010;**14**:R140.

6. Hollenberg SM, Broussard M, Osman J, et al. Increased microvascular reactivity and improved mortality in septic mice lacking inducible nitric oxide synthase. *Circ Res.* 2000;**86**:774–8.

7. McKinnon RL, Lidington D, Tyml K. Ascorbate inhibits reduced arteriolar conducted vasoconstriction in septic mouse cremaster muscle. *Microcirculation.* 2007;**14**:697–707.

8. Ruiz C, Hernandez G, Godoy C, et al. Sublingual microcirculatory changes during high-volume hemofiltration in hyperdynamic septic shock patients. *Crit Care.* 2010;**14**:R170.

9. Pranskunas A, Pilvinis V, Dambrauskas Z, et al. Early course of microcirculatory perfusion in eye and digestive tract during hypodynamic sepsis. *Crit Care.* 2012;**16**:R83.

10. Bateman RM, Tokunaga C, Kareco T, et al. Myocardial hypoxia-inducible HIF-1α, VEGF and GLUT1 gene expression is associated with microvascular and ICAM-1 heterogeneity during endotoxemia. *Am J Physiol Heart Circ Physiol.* 2007;**293**:H448–56.

11. Groner W, Winkelman JW, Harris AG, et al. Orthogonal polarization spectral imaging: a new method for study of the microcirculation. *Nat Med.* 1999;**5**:1209–12.

12. Goedhart P, Khalilzada M, Bezemer R, et al. Sidestream Dark Field (SDF) imaging: a novel stroboscopic LED ring-based imaging modality for clinical assessment of the microcirculation. *Optics Express.* 2007;**15**:15101–14.

13. De Backer D, Creteur J, Preiser JC, et al. Microvascular blood flow is altered in patients with sepsis. *Am J Respir Crit Care Med.* 2002;**166**:98–104.

14. Goldman D, Bateman RM, Ellis CG. Effect of decreased O_2 supply on skeletal muscle oxygenation and O_2 consumption during sepsis: role of heterogeneous capillary spacing and blood flow. *Am J Physiol Heart Circ Physiol.* 2006;**290**:H2277–85.

15. Ellis CG, Bateman RM, Sharpe MD, et al. Effect of a maldistribution of microvascular blood flow on capillary O_2 extraction in sepsis. *Am J Physiol.* 2002;**282**:H156–64.

16. Humer MF, Phang PT, Friesen BP, et al. Heterogeneity of gut capillary transit times and impaired gut oxygen extraction in endotoxemic pigs. *J Appl Physiol,* 1996;**81**:895–904.

17. Walley KR. Heterogeneity of oxygen delivery impairs oxygen extraction by peripheral tissues: theory. *J Appl Physiol.* 1996;**81**:885–94.

18. Legrand M, Bezemer R, Kandil A, et al. The role of renal hypoperfusion in development of renal microcirculatory dysfunction in endotoxemic rats. *Intens Care Med.* 2011;**37**:1534–42.

19. Edul VS, Enrico C, Laviolle B, et al. Quantitative assessment of the microcirculation in healthy volunteers and in patients with septic shock. *Crit Care Med.* 2012;**40**:1443–8.

20. Eipel C, Bordel R, Nickels RM, et al. Impact of leukocytes and platelets in mediating hepatocyte apoptosis in a rat model of systemic endotoxemia. *Am J Physiol Gastrointest Liver Physiol.* 2004;**286**: G769–76.

21. De Backer D, Creteur J, Dubois MJ, et al. The effects of dobutamine on microcirculatory alterations in patients with septic shock are independent of its systemic effects. *Crit Care Med.* 2006;**34**:403–8.

22. Kao R, Xenocostas A, Rui T, et al. Erythropoietin improves skeletal muscle microcirculation and tissue bioenergetics in a mouse sepsis model. *Crit Care.* 2007;**11**:R58.

23. Doerschug KC, Delsing AS, Schmidt GA, et al. Impairments in microvascular reactivity are related to organ failure in human sepsis. *Am J Physiol Heart Circ Physiol.* 2007;**293**:H1065–71.

24. Shapiro NI, Arnold R, Sherwin R, et al. The association of near-infrared spectroscopy-derived tissue oxygenation measurements with sepsis syndromes, organ dysfunction and mortality in emergency department patients with sepsis. *Crit Care.* 2011;**15**:R223.

25. Trzeciak S, McCoy JV, Phillip DR, et al. Early increases in microcirculatory perfusion during protocol-directed resuscitation are associated with reduced multi-organ failure at 24 h in patients with sepsis. *Intens Care Med.* 2008;**34**:2210–17.

26. De Backer D, Creteur J, Dubois MJ, et al. Microvascular alterations in patients with acute severe heart failure and cardiogenic shock. *Am Heart J.* 2004;**147**:91–9.

27. Sakr Y, Dubois MJ, De Backer D, et al. Persistant microvasculatory alterations are associated with organ failure and death in patients with septic shock. *Crit Care Med.* 2004;**32**:1825–31.

28. Den Uil CA, Lagrand WK, van der Ent M, et al. Impaired microcirculation predicts poor outcome of patients with acute myocardial infarction complicated by cardiogenic shock. *Eur Heart J.* 2010;**31**:3032–9.

29. Creteur J, Carollo T, Soldati G, et al. The prognostic value of muscle StO(2) in septic patients. *Intens Care Med.* 2007;**33**:1549–56.

30. Top AP, Ince C, de Meij N, et al. Persistent low microcirculatory vessel density in nonsurvivors of sepsis in pediatric intensive care. *Crit Care Med.* 2011;**39**:8–13.

31. De Backer D, Donadello K, Sakr Y, et al. Microcirculatory alterations in patients with severe sepsis: impact of time of assessment and relationship with outcome. *Crit Care Med.* 2013;41:791–9.

32. Massey MJ, Hou PC, Filbin M, et al. Microcirculatory perfusion disturbances in septic shock: results from the ProCESS trial. *Crit Care.* 2018;22:308.

33. Brealey D, Karyampudi S, Jacques TS, et al. Mitochondrial dysfunction in a long-term rodent model of sepsis and organ failure. *Am J Physiol Regul Integr Comp Physiol.* .2004;286:R491–7.

34. Levy RJ, Piel DA, Acton PD, et al. Evidence of myocardial hibernation in the septic heart. *Crit Care Med.* 2005;33:2752–6.

35. Piel DA, Deutschman CS, Levy RJ. Exogenous cytochrome C restores myocardial cytochrome oxidase activity into the late phase of sepsis. *Shock.* 2008;29:612–16.

36. Fredriksson K, Tjader I, Keller P, et al. Dysregulation of mitochondrial dynamics and the muscle transcriptome in ICU patients suffering from sepsis induced multiple organ failure. *PLoS One.* 2008;3:e3686.

37. Fredriksson K, Hammarqvist F, Strigard K, et al. Derangements in mitochondrial metabolism in intercostal and leg muscle of critically ill patients with sepsis-induced multiple organ failure. *Am J Physiol Endocrinol Metab.* .2006;291:E1044–50.

38. Brealey D, Brand M, Hargreaves I, et al. Association between mitochondrial dysfunction and severity and outcome of septic shock. *Lancet.* 2002;360:219–23.

39. Smeding L, van der Laarse WJ, van Veelen TA, et al. Early myocardial dysfunction is not caused by mitochondrial abnormalities in a rat model of peritonitis. *J Surg Res.* 2012;176:178–84.

40. Sjovall F, Morota S, Persson J, et al. Patients with sepsis exhibit increased mitochondrial respiratory capacity in peripheral blood immune cells. *Crit Care.* 2013;17:R152.

41. Jeger V, Djafarzadeh S, Jakob SM, et al. Mitochondrial function in sepsis. *Eur J Clin. Invest* 2013;43:532–42.

42. Fredriksson K, Flaring U, Guillet C, et al. Muscle mitochondrial activity increases rapidly after an endotoxin challenge in human volunteers. *Acta Anaesthesiol Scand.* 2009;53:299–304.

43. Correa TD, Vuda M, Blaser AR, et al. Effect of treatment delay on disease severity and need for resuscitation in porcine fecal peritonitis. *Crit Care Med.* 2012;40:2841–9.

44. Creteur J, De Backer D, Sakr Y, et al. Sublingual capnometry tracks microcirculatory changes in septic patients. *Intens Care Med.* 2006;32:516–23.

45. Dubin A, Edul VS, Pozo MO, et al. Persistent villi hypoperfusion explains intramucosal acidosis in sheep endotoxemia. *Crit Care Med.* 2008;36:535–42.

46. Rosengarten B, Hecht M, Auch D, et al. Microcirculatory dysfunction in the brain precedes changes in evoked potentials in endotoxin-induced sepsis syndrome in rats. *Cerebrovasc Dis.* 2007;23:140–7.

47. Rivers EP, Kruse JA, Jacobsen G, et al. The influence of early hemodynamic optimization strategies on biomarker patterns of severe sepsis and septic shock. *Crit Care Med.* 2007;35:2016–2024.

48. Greenwood JC, Jang DH, Hallisey SD, et al. Severe impairment of microcirculatory perfused vessel density is associated with postoperative lactate and acute organ injury after cardiac surgery. *J Cardiothorac Vasc Anesth.* 2021;35:106–15

49. De Backer D, Dubois MJ, Schmartz D, et al. Microcirculatory alterations in cardiac surgery: effects of cardiopulmonary bypass and anesthesia. *Ann Thorac Surg.* 2009;88:1396–403.

50. Atasever B, Boer C, Goedhart P, et al. Distinct alterations in sublingual microcirculatory blood flow and hemoglobin oxygenation in on-pump and off-pump coronary artery bypass graft surgery. *J Cardiothorac Vasc Anesth.* 2010;25:784–90.

51. Bouattour K, Teboul J-L, Varin L, Vicaut E, Duranteau J. Preload dependence is associated with reduced sublingual microcirculation during major abdominal surgery. *Anesthesiology.* 2019;**130**:541–9.

52. Jhanji S, Lee C, Watson D, et al. Microvascular flow and tissue oxygenation after major abdominal surgery: association with post-operative complications. *Intens Care Med.* 2009;**35**:671–7.

53. Caldarone CA, Barner EW, Wang L, et al. Apoptosis-related mitochondrial dysfunction in the early postoperative neonatal lamb heart. *Ann Thorac Surg.* 2004;78:948–55.

54. Oka N, Wang L, Mi W, et al. Cyclosporine A prevents apoptosis-related mitochondrial dysfunction after neonatal cardioplegic arrest. *J Thorac Cardiovasc Surg.* 2008;135:123–30

Cerebral Oximetry

D. Massari, I.N. de Keijzer, J.J. Vos and T.W.L. Scheeren

Background

Most hemodynamic monitoring techniques provide direct or indirect information related to the systemic oxygen delivery or to the balance between oxygen delivery and consumption. Organs and tissues have different metabolic demands and thus different oxygen consumption. The human brain consumes on average 3.5 ml min^{-1} of oxygen per 100 g of tissue, which translates to ~50 ml min^{-1} of oxygen, that is, around 20% of the oxygen consumption of the entire human body.[1] In the perioperative period, it would be desirable to be able to monitor the adequacy of cerebral perfusion and oxygen delivery, since they can be compromised by several factors related to surgery and anesthesia, for example, hypotension or a reduced cardiac output. Cerebral oximetry is a simple and effective way to monitor (regional) cerebral oxygen saturation. This chapter presents the characteristics of cerebral oximetry and its clinical applications in the perioperative period.

Near Infrared Spectroscopy

Cerebral oximeters are monitoring devices based on near infrared spectroscopy (NIRS), and consist of a portable device connected to one or more adhesive sensors, each constituted by an electrode emitting near infrared light, and one or more electrodes receiving near infrared light reflected by the tissues.[2] Using algorithms based on the Lambert–Beer law – which relates the difference in transmitted and received light to the concentration of a substance (i.e., hemoglobin) in a solution – NIRS devices measure the amount of oxygenated and deoxygenated hemoglobin in the monitored tissue sample underneath the sensor, similarly to pulse oximeters. In fact, NIRS devices share some features with pulse oximeters, including the non-invasiveness, the portability, and the use of distinct wavelengths that interact with hemoglobin and are in part absorbed and in part reflected by this chromophore. In contrast with pulse oximetry, NIRS is based on wavelengths in the near infrared spectrum that are capable of penetrating tissues – including bone – to a greater extent, allowing the monitoring of the frontal lobes of the brain when the NIRS sensors are applied on the forehead. The depth of penetration is estimated to be around 1.5 to 2 cm – about one-third to one-half of the distance between the emitting and receiving electrodes of the sensor – hence the grey matter of the brain is within the range monitored with cerebral oximetry (Fig. 5.1). Additionally, unlike pulse oximeters, NIRS devices are not dependent on pulsatile blood flow or temperature, but instead monitor hemoglobin in small vessels (<100 µm in diameter) including arterioles, venules, and capillaries. It follows that NIRS devices provide a composite measure of arterial, venous, and capillary saturation: depending on the device, the venous contribution accounts for 70–80% of the signal, and the arterial contribution for

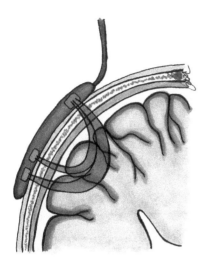

Figure 5.1 Representation of a near infrared spectroscopy sensor with one electrode emitting near infrared light and two electrodes detecting light reflected by the grey matter of the brain. A black and white version of this figure will appear in some formats. For the color version, please refer to the plate section.

20–30%.[3] This constitutes the first key feature of cerebral *oximetry*: it provides a measure of the balance between oxygen delivery and consumption in the cerebral microcirculation, that is, close to the site of oxygen consumption (mitochondria). The second key feature relies in the ability of cerebral oximetry to provide real-time monitoring, that allows detecting changes in cerebral oxygen saturation, maybe even before – or in the absence of – changes in macrohemodynamic variables monitored routinely (such as blood pressure or cardiac output). Several drawbacks of cerebral oxygen saturation must be noted. First, absolute cerebral oxygen saturation values obtained with different devices are not directly comparable and therefore not interchangeable.[4] The algorithms employed by different devices use fixed but slightly different values of arterial and venous contribution (arterial–venous ratio) for computing cerebral oxygen saturation. Additionally, such values are assumed constant, while it is known that the arterial–venous ratio varies both between individuals, and within the same individual under different physiological or pathological conditions (e.g., body position or hypoxia).[4] Hence, it has been suggested that cerebral oximeters are more reliable in monitoring trends or changes in cerebral oxygen saturation (from an individual baseline value) compared with monitoring absolute values of cerebral oxygen saturation.[4] Second, the NIRS signal can be contaminated from extracerebral tissues including bone and cutaneous tissue. This issue is in part overcome since most devices employ two detecting electrodes, one measuring superficial tissues and one measuring deeper tissues, with algorithms allowing discrimination between the two signals. Third, sensors for cerebral oximetry are commonly placed on the forehead and thus only the frontal lobes of the brain are monitored, and so desaturation(s) in other areas of the brain will probably go undetected.

Cardiac Surgery

Cerebral oximetry is commonly adopted in cardiac anesthesia, with the widest application in aortic arch procedures and pediatric congenital heart surgery. In this setting, patient- and surgery-related factors (e.g., cardiac structural abnormalities, carotid stenosis, and cardiopulmonary bypass itself, to name a few) pose the brain at high risk of hypoperfusion, leading to intraoperative and postoperative adverse events including postoperative cognitive decline or dysfunction, delirium, prolonged mechanical ventilation, stroke, and death.[5] In this context, the purpose of cerebral oximetry is to detect cerebral oxygen desaturations, in order to take direct corrective measures to promptly restore cerebral oxygen saturation and possibly avoid immediate and delayed complications. Before looking at clinical applications, the reader may ask how "cerebral oxygen desaturation" is defined. Since NIRS values are probably best interpreted as trending values, a commonly accepted definition is a ≥20% decrease from individual baseline cerebral oxygen saturation (generally established after induction of anesthesia with a stable fraction of inspired oxygen and stable vital signs).[3] Yet, *absolute* cerebral oxygen saturation values <50% are also commonly regarded as abnormal. Other definitions have been used (≥10–30% decreases from baseline, or absolute values <40–60%), but the mentioned thresholds are probably the most widely accepted.

In some case reports and observational studies, cerebral oximetry has been shown to help detect malpositioned vascular cannulas during cardiac surgery with cardiopulmonary bypass (causing a bilateral or unilateral decrease in cerebral oxygen saturation), and to help confirm effective selective antegrade cerebral perfusion or changing the position of the cannulas in patients undergoing aortic arch surgery.[6]

What has been investigated more extensively is the relationship between cerebral desaturation during cardiac surgery and neurological complications occurring in the post-operative period. It has been hypothesized that intraoperative cerebral desaturations are associated with the development of postoperative neurocognitive disorders and postoperative delirium.[7] A recent systematic review reported substantial variability in the findings of observational studies aiming to establish an association between intraoperative cerebral desaturations and postoperative neurologic complications (delirium, early and late neuro-cognitive disorders, and stroke).[8] Only one observational study supported an association between intraoperative cerebral desaturation and postoperative delirium, while three other studies did not. Similarly, the association with perioperative stroke is not certain, and the evidence is limited. A few more observational studies showed an association between cerebral desaturation and early postoperative cognitive disorders within 7 days after surgery. However, when only interventional trials were considered, the majority of them did not support cerebral oximetry and therapeutic actions aimed at correcting cerebral desaturations. Hence, these studies raise doubt about the causal relationship between cerebral desaturations and adverse neurological outcomes.[8] In 2020, a panel of experts issued a consensus statement about the role of cerebral oximetry in perioperative outcomes, in which the use of preoperative and intraoperative cerebral oximetry was recommended to identify cardiac surgery patients at risk of adverse outcomes.[9] The strength of the statement was weak, reflecting the variability in the results of the studies. In summary, while additional evidence is still needed to give a clear answer, it can be concluded that preoperative or intraoperative cerebral desaturations can at least be considered a risk factor for adverse postoperative neurological outcomes, probably reflecting a reduced cerebral reserve or cognitive frailty in patients undergoing cardiac surgery.[8] In accordance with this view, it was found that a low preoperative cerebral oxygen saturation is an independent predictor of postoperative delirium (cerebral oxygen saturation < 60%) [10] and mortality (cerebral oxygen saturation < 50%).[11]

Congenital heart surgery in neonates and infants poses additional challenges to the brain: the positioning of cardiopulmonary bypass cannulas and vascular clamps is extremely delicate, and the pathophysiology of the underlying congenital abnormality is often complex and can encompass intra- and extracardiac shunts and/or a cyanotic pathology. All these factors contribute to cerebral monitoring as an essential part of anesthetic care. In fact, in this population, cerebral hypoperfusion or desaturation can occur even when cardiac output is maintained – for example, in case of pulmonary overflow – or, on the opposite, cerebral oxygen saturation might be adequate even if peripheral oxygen saturation is low, as in cyanotic diseases.[12] Besides this role in "tracking" the effects of pathological circulations, there is also some evidence that cerebral oximetry can predict neurodevelopmental and neurocognitive outcomes after pediatric cardiac surgery, as well as major morbidity and mortality.[13,14] Yet, pediatric patients with congenital heart disease are a population with an unmatched complexity in terms of physiological derangements, making it intrinsically hard to prove the usefulness of cerebral oximetry in this context. Consequently, it is not yet possible to make strong recommendations about the use of cerebral oximetry for predicting or improving outcomes in pediatric cardiac anesthesia.

Among the applications of cerebral oximetry, the possibility of monitoring cerebral blood flow autoregulation is gaining popularity. Cerebral blood flow is kept constant across a wide range of values of cerebral perfusion pressure, and cerebral oximetry has been demonstrated to be an acceptable surrogate of cerebral blood flow. The cerebral oximetry index is an NIRS-derived variable that has been validated for cerebral blood flow autoregulation monitoring in patients undergoing cardiopulmonary bypass.[15] In brief, the cerebral oximetry index is obtained by calculating a continuous, moving Pearson correlation coefficient between the mean arterial pressure and cerebral oxygen saturation values: cerebral oximetry index values close to 0 indicate preserved blood flow autoregulation (no correlation between changes in mean arterial pressure and cerebral oxygen saturation), whereas values close to 1 indicate impaired autoregulation (correlation between changes in mean arterial pressure and cerebral oxygen saturation). Recent studies reported an association between an impaired cerebral autoregulation in the immediate postoperative period and postoperative delirium.[16,17] The importance of monitoring cerebral autoregulation relies on the fact that certain conditions (e.g., chronic hypertension) can shift the limits of cerebral autoregulation – which has been demonstrated to be highly variable [18] – to the right, making mean arterial pressures that were generally believed to be safe, potentially deleterious for cerebral perfusion in concerned individuals. Therefore, cerebral oximetry has the potential to allow personalization of mean arterial pressure targets, and its role in this field is undoubtedly expanding.

Non-Cardiac Surgery

Cerebral oximetry is less commonly adopted in non-cardiac surgery. However, evidence supporting the use of cerebral oximetry for improving perioperative care in different types of non-cardiac surgery is emerging. A few challenges that anesthesiologists may encounter during non-cardiac surgery are surgery-related alterations in cerebral blood flow during specific surgical procedures such as carotid endarterectomy or intracerebral thrombectomy. Other indications include lung surgery with one-lung ventilation, and operations performed in certain positioning of the patient such as beach-chair or steep Trendelenburg positions.

The use of cerebral oximetry to detect cerebral ischemia during carotid endarterectomy remains controversial. Cerebral oximetry and transcranial Doppler had similar accuracy to detect cerebral ischemia in one study,[19] whereas another found that transcranial Doppler was more accurate than NIRS.[20] One of the concerns using NIRS is that it has a high negative predictive value, but a low positive predictive value [21] and low specificity,[20,22] which could result in the placement of unnecessary shunts when solely cerebral oxygenation is used as an indicator for shunt placement.[23] Another concern is that as long as critical cerebral ischemia is not defined, interventions based on cerebral oximetry values cannot be justified.[24] In patients who underwent endovascular therapy for an acute ischemic stroke, a sustained increase in cerebral oxygenation was observed after recanalization in only 4.7%, yet the interhemispheric oxygenation difference, oxygenation variability, and area under 10% from baseline values were predictive of reperfusion and mortality.[25] A case study of three patients, of whom two had a successful recanalization, showed a rise in cerebral oxygenation in the infarcted side and a decrease in the interhemispheric saturation difference.[26] One important drawback is that NIRS sensors should be applied to the hypoperfused area in order to potentially capture cerebral ischemia and subsequent reperfusion. Therefore, future studies are needed to establish the value of cerebral oximetry in this specific population.

During surgery requiring one-lung ventilation, cerebral desaturations (<65% for more than 3 minutes) occurred in a large proportion (51.3%), and those patients suffered from impaired cognitive recovery directly after surgery and had an increased risk of delirium and a longer hospital stay.[27] The risk of impaired early cognitive recovery increased with a longer duration of cerebral desaturation (<60%).[28]

Surgeries performed in beach chair position (BCP) may pose challenges to hemo-dynamic management. In BCP, cardiac preload decreases due to venous pooling in the lower limbs, and cerebral perfusion pressure decreases due to the positioning of the head well above the level of the heart, and thus there is an increase in the risk of intraoperative cerebral hypoperfusion and adverse neurological events.[29] The majority of studies found a decrease in cerebral oxygen saturation after positioning in the BCP compared with values recorded after induction of anesthesia in the supine position,[30–32] or compared with the lateral decubitus position.[33–35] Additionally, a decrease in cerebral oxygen saturation was found in BCP compared with supine position only in anesthetized patients, but not in a control group of healthy awake volunteers, indicating that the combination of anesthesia and BCP results in a decrease in cerebral oxygen saturation. Of note, mean arterial pressure in anesthetized patients was kept above 70 mmHg, and did not differ in BCP compared with the supine position, while in healthy awake volunteers blood pressure spontaneously increased after positioning in BCP.[36] Yet, when NIRS-monitored patients were compared with a control group in which the anesthesiologist was blinded to NIRS values, no reduction of incidence of cerebral desaturation was found, and no decrease in postoperative cognitive function was observed in either group.[37] It is possible that intraoperative cerebral desaturation does not lead to adverse cognitive or neurological outcomes per se, but plays a role as a cofactor adding to other patient-related risk factors. Moreover, the incidence of poor neurological outcomes after surgery in BCP may be too low to be detected by relatively small studies. Finally, the absence of reduction of cerebral desaturations in patients managed according to cerebral NIRS values might be due to the reactive approach, rather than using a proactive approach to prevent desaturation from occurring, or to the fact that the intervention initiated after desaturation was inappropriate or ineffective.

At the other extreme of patient positioning during surgery, the steep Trendelenburg position – commonly used during robotic prostatectomy – poses the patient at risk of increased cerebral blood flow and volume due to congestion, resulting in elevated intracranial pressure. A gradual increase in cerebral oxygen saturation has been found during surgery in the steep Trendelenburg position, and the increase persisted after resuming the supine position.[38] Additionally, no difference in cerebral autoregulation was found when robotic prostatectomy in the steep Trendelenburg position was compared with radical prostatectomy in the supine position.[39]

The use of cerebral oximetry has been investigated in other clinical settings (e.g., abdominal, orthopedic, and spinal surgery) where the risk of cerebral desaturations is related less to the type of surgery or patient position per se, but more to factors related to the patient (comorbidities) or the intraoperative management. The evidence for the use of cerebral oximetry in patients undergoing abdominal surgery is conflicting. In a population of elderly patients, cerebral desaturations were found to be associated with postoperative cognitive decline and increased length of hospital stay.[40] The same authors found a higher mean cerebral oxygen saturation and a lower area under the curve below 75% of baseline values in a group that was monitored with cerebral oximetry compared with the group that was blinded for cerebral oximetry values.[41] However, in an elderly population of abdominal and orthopedic surgery patients ($n = 40$), cerebral desaturation occurred only twice and no association was found between cerebral desaturation and postoperative complications.[42] In studies only focusing on orthopedic surgery, the maximal drop in cerebral oxygen saturation was an independent predictor of postoperative cognitive dysfunction,[43] and perioperative cerebral oxygenation was lower in patients with postoperative cognitive dysfunction compared with patients without postoperative cognitive dysfunction.[44]

In patients undergoing spinal surgery, it was found that cerebral desaturation occurred, while other clinical signs, for example, mean arterial pressure, peripheral oxygen saturation, and end-tidal CO_2, remained constant.[45] A correlation was found between the duration of cerebral desaturation <60% and the development of postoperative cognitive dysfunction 7 days after surgery.[46] Additionally, a decrease in incidence of postoperative cognitive dysfunction at 7 and 30 days after surgery was demonstrated in patients monitored with NIRS compared with patients without NIRS monitoring.[47] On the contrary, another study described an association between muscular tissue oxygenation and postoperative complications, but found no association between cerebral desaturation and postoperative complications.[48]

In summary, cerebral oximetry is commonly used in cardiac surgery, and new fields of application in non-cardiac surgery are under investigation. Cerebral oximetry offers the chance to unveil cerebral desaturation and prompt actions attempting to correct it, keeping in mind that intraoperative cerebral desaturation is only one of several insults contributing to neurological complications after surgery. While the evidence for a role in impacting patient outcomes in cardiac surgery is still not entirely clear, cerebral oximetry can be considered as an adjunctive tool in the perioperative monitoring and hemodynamic management, provided that it is interpreted in the context of other physiological variables that may affect it.[9] In contrast, the usefulness of cerebral oximetry in non-cardiac surgery remains controversial, and there is insufficient evidence of its ability to help improving patient outcomes.[9]

Acknowledgements
We thank C. K. Niezen for providing Figure 5.1.

References

1. Clarke DD, Sokoloff L. Circulation and energy metabolism of the brain. In GJ Siegel, BW Agranoff, AW Albers, SK Fisher, MD Uhler, eds., *Basic Neurochemistry: Molecular, Cellular and Medical Aspects*, 6th ed. Philadelphia: Lippincott Williams & Wilkins; 1999: Chapter 31.

2. Scheeren TWL, Kuizenga MH, Maurer H, Struys MMRF, Heringlake M. Electroencephalography and brain oxygenation monitoring in the perioperative period. *Anesth Analg*. 2019 Feb;**128**(2):265–77.

3. Hogue CW, Levine A, Hudson A, Lewis C. Clinical applications of near-infrared spectroscopy monitoring in cardiovascular surgery. *Anesthesiology*. 2021 May 1;**134**(5):784–91.

4. Bickler PE, Feiner JR, Rollins MD. Factors affecting the performance of 5 cerebral oximeters during hypoxia in healthy volunteers. *Anesth Analg*. 2013 Oct;**117**(4):813–23.

5. Seese L, Sultan I, Gleason TG, et al. The Impact of major postoperative complications on long-term survival after cardiac surgery. *Ann Thorac Surg*. 2020 Jul;**110**(1):128–35.

6. Zheng F, Sheinberg R, Yee M-S, et al. Cerebral near-infrared spectroscopy monitoring and neurologic outcomes in adult cardiac surgery patients: a systematic review. *Anesth Analg*. 2013 Mar;**116**(3):663–76.

7. Yu Y, Zhang K, Zhang L, et al. Cerebral near-infrared spectroscopy (NIRS) for perioperative monitoring of brain oxygenation in children and adults. *Cochrane Database Syst Rev*. 2018 Jan 17;**1**: CD010947.

8. Semrau JS, Motamed M, Ross-White A, Boyd JG. Cerebral oximetry and preventing neurological complication post-cardiac surgery: a systematic review. *Eur J Cardiothorac Surg*. 2021 Jun 14;**59**(6):1144–54.

9. Thiele RH, Shaw AD, Bartels K, et al. American Society for Enhanced Recovery and Perioperative Quality Initiative Joint Consensus Statement on the Role of Neuromonitoring in Perioperative Outcomes: cerebral near-infrared spectroscopy. *Anesth Analg*. 2020 Nov;**131**(5):1444–55.

10. Soh S, Shim J-K, Song J-W, Choi N, Kwak Y-L. Preoperative transcranial Doppler and cerebral oximetry as predictors of delirium following valvular heart surgery: a case-control study. *J Clin Monit Comput*. 2020 Aug;**34**(4):715–23.

11. Heringlake M, Garbers C, Käbler J-H, et al. Preoperative cerebral oxygen saturation and clinical outcomes in cardiac surgery. *Anesthesiology*. 2011 Jan;**114**(1):58–69.

12. Frogel J, Kogan A, Augoustides JGT, et al. The value of cerebral oximetry monitoring in cardiac surgery: challenges and solutions in adult and pediatric practice. *J Cardiothorac Vasc Anesth*. 2019 Jun;**33**(6):1778–84.

13. Flechet M, Güiza F, Vlasselaers D, et al. Near-infrared cerebral oximetry to predict outcome after pediatric cardiac surgery: a prospective observational study. *Pediatr Crit Care Med*. 2018 May;**19**(5):433–41.

14. Kussman BD, Wypij D, Laussen PC, et al. Relationship of intraoperative cerebral oxygen saturation to neurodevelopmental outcome and brain magnetic resonance imaging at 1 year of age in infants undergoing biventricular repair. *Circulation*. 2010 Jul 20;**122**(3):245–54.

15. Brady K, Joshi B, Zweifel C, et al. Real-time continuous monitoring of cerebral blood flow autoregulation using near-infrared spectroscopy in patients undergoing cardiopulmonary bypass. *Stroke*. 2010 Sep;**41**(9):1951–6.

16. Chan B, Aneman A. A prospective, observational study of cerebrovascular autoregulation and its association with delirium following cardiac surgery. *Anaesthesia*. 2019 Jan;**74**(1):33–44.

17. Nakano M, Nomura Y, Whitman G, et al. Cerebral autoregulation in the operating

room and intensive care unit after cardiac surgery. *Br J Anaesth.* 2021 May;**126**(5):967–74.

18. Joshi B, Ono M, Brown C, et al. Predicting the limits of cerebral autoregulation during cardiopulmonary bypass. *Anesth Analg.* 2012 Mar;**114**(3):503–10.

19. Moritz S, Kasprzak P, Arlt M, Taeger K, Metz C. Accuracy of cerebral monitoring in detecting cerebral ischemia during carotid endarterectomy: a comparison of transcranial Doppler sonography, near-infrared spectroscopy, stump pressure, and somatosensory evoked potentials. *Anesthesiology.* 2007 Oct;**107**(4):563–9.

20. Grubhofer G, Plöchl W, Skolka M, et al. Comparing Doppler ultrasonography and cerebral oximetry as indicators for shunting in carotid endarterectomy. *Anesth Analg.* 2000 Dec;**91**(6):1339–44.

21. Samra SK, Dy EA, Welch K, et al. Evaluation of a cerebral oximeter as a monitor of cerebral ischemia during carotid endarterectomy. *Anesthesiology.* 2000 Oct;**93**(4):964–70.

22. Rigamonti A, Scandroglio M, Minicucci F, et al. A clinical evaluation of near-infrared cerebral oximetry in the awake patient to monitor cerebral perfusion during carotid endarterectomy. *J Clin Anesth.* 2005 Sep;**17**(6):426–30.

23. Friedell ML, Clark JM, Graham DA, Isley MR, Zhang X-F. Cerebral oximetry does not correlate with electroencephalography and somatosensory evoked potentials in determining the need for shunting during carotid endarterectomy. *J Vasc Surg.* 2008 Sep;**48**(3):601–6.

24. Beese U, Langer H, Lang W, Dinkel M. Comparison of near-infrared spectroscopy and somatosensory evoked potentials for the detection of cerebral ischemia during carotid endarterectomy. *Stroke.* 1998 Oct;**29**(10):2032–7.

25. Hametner C, Stanarcevic P, Stampfl S, et al. Noninvasive cerebral oximetry during endovascular therapy for acute ischemic stroke: an observational study. *J Cereb Blood Flow Metab.* 2015 Nov;**35**(11):1722–8.

26. Ritzenthaler T, Cho T-H, Luis D, Berthezene Y, Nighoghossian N. Usefulness of near-infrared spectroscopy in thrombectomy monitoring. *J Clin Monit Comput.* 2015 Oct;**29**(5):585–9.

27. Roberts ML, Lin H-M, Tinuoye E, et al. The association of cerebral desaturation during one-lung ventilation and postoperative recovery: a prospective observational cohort study. *J Cardiothorac Vasc Anesth.* 2021 Feb;**35**(2):542–50.

28. Tang L, Kazan R, Taddei R, et al. Reduced cerebral oxygen saturation during thoracic surgery predicts early postoperative cognitive dysfunction. *Br J Anaesth.* 2012 Apr;**108**(4):623–9.

29. Murphy GS, Greenberg SB, Szokol JW. Safety of beach chair position shoulder surgery: a review of the current literature. *Anesth Analg.* 2019 Jul;**129**(1):101–18.

30. Picton P, Dering A, Alexander A, et al. influence of ventilation strategies and anesthetic techniques on regional cerebral oximetry in the beach chair position: a prospective interventional study with a randomized comparison of two anesthetics. *Anesthesiology.* 2015 Oct;**123**(4):765–74.

31. Moerman AT, De Hert SG, Jacobs TF, De Wilde LF, Wouters PF. Cerebral oxygen desaturation during beach chair position. *Eur J Anaesthesiol.* 2012 Feb;**29**(2):82–7.

32. Jeong H, Jeong S, Lim HJ, Lee J, Yoo KY. Cerebral oxygen saturation measured by near-infrared spectroscopy and jugular venous bulb oxygen saturation during arthroscopic shoulder surgery in beach chair position under sevoflurane-nitrous oxide or propofol-remifentanil anesthesia. *Anesthesiology.* 2012 May;**116**(5):1047–56.

33. Laflam A, Joshi B, Brady K, et al. Shoulder surgery in the beach chair position is associated with diminished cerebral autoregulation but no differences in postoperative cognition or brain injury biomarker levels compared with supine

positioning: the anesthesia patient safety foundation beach chair study. *Anesth Analg.* 2015 Jan;**120**(1):176–85.

34. Meex I, Vundelinckx J, Buyse K, et al. Cerebral tissue oxygen saturation values in volunteers and patients in the lateral decubitus and beach chair positions: a prospective observational study. *Can J Anaesth.* 2016 May;**63**(5):537–43.

35. Murphy GS, Szokol JW, Marymont JH, et al. Cerebral oxygen desaturation events assessed by near-infrared spectroscopy during shoulder arthroscopy in the beach chair and lateral decubitus positions. *Anesth Analg.* 2010 Aug;**111**(2):496–505.

36. Closhen D, Berres M, Werner C, Engelhard K, Schramm P. Influence of beach chair position on cerebral oxygen saturation: a comparison of INVOS and FORE-SIGHT cerebral oximeter. *J Neurosurg Anesthesiol.* 2013 Oct;**25**(4):414–9.

37. Cox RM, Jamgochian GC, Nicholson K, et al. The effectiveness of cerebral oxygenation monitoring during arthroscopic shoulder surgery in the beach chair position: a randomized blinded study. *J Shoulder Elbow Surg.* 2018 Apr;**27**(4):692–700.

38. Kalmar AF, Dewaele F, Foubert L, et al. Cerebral haemodynamic physiology during steep Trendelenburg position and CO_2 pneumoperitoneum. *Br J Anaesth.* 2012 Mar;**108**(3):478–84.

39. Beck S, Ragab H, Hoop D, et al. Comparing the effect of positioning on cerebral autoregulation during radical prostatectomy: a prospective observational study. *J Clin Monit Comput.* 2021 Aug;**35**(4):891–901.

40. Casati A, Fanelli G, Pietropaoli P, et al. Monitoring cerebral oxygen saturation in elderly patients undergoing general abdominal surgery: a prospective cohort study. *Eur J Anaesthesiol.* 2007 Jan;**24**(1):59–65.

41. Casati A, Fanelli G, Pietropaoli P, et al. Continuous monitoring of cerebral oxygen saturation in elderly patients undergoing major abdominal surgery minimizes brain exposure to potential hypoxia. *Anesth Analg.* 2005 Sep;**101**(3):740–7.

42. Cowie DA, Nazareth J, Story DA. Cerebral oximetry to reduce perioperative morbidity. *Anaesth Intensive Care.* 2014 May;**42**(3):310–14.

43. Lin R, Zhang F, Xue Q, Yu B. Accuracy of regional cerebral oxygen saturation in predicting postoperative cognitive dysfunction after total hip arthroplasty: regional cerebral oxygen saturation predicts POCD. *J Arthroplasty.* 2013 Mar;**28**(3):494–7.

44. Ni C, Xu T, Li N, et al. Cerebral oxygen saturation after multiple perioperative influential factors predicts the occurrence of postoperative cognitive dysfunction. *BMC Anesthesiol.* 2015 Oct 26(15):156.

45. Murniece S, Soehle M, Vanags I, Mamaja B. Near infrared spectroscopy based clinical algorithm applicability during spinal neurosurgery and postoperative cognitive disturbances. *Medicina (Kaunas).* 2019 May 21;**55**(5):E179.

46. Kim J, Shim J-K, Song JW, Kim E-K, Kwak YL. Postoperative cognitive dysfunction and the change of regional cerebral oxygen saturation in elderly patients undergoing spinal surgery. *Anesth Analg.* 2016 Aug;**123**(2):436–44.

47. Trafidło T, Gaszyński T, Gaszyński W, Nowakowska-Domagała K. Intraoperative monitoring of cerebral NIRS oximetry leads to better postoperative cognitive performance: a pilot study. *Int J Surg.* 2015 Apr;**16**(Pt A):23–30.

48. Meng L, Xiao J, Gudelunas K, et al. Association of intraoperative cerebral and muscular tissue oxygen saturation with postoperative complications and length of hospital stay after major spine surgery: an observational study. *Br J Anaesth.* 2017;**118**(4):551–62.

Body Volumes and Fluid Kinetics

Robert G. Hahn

Anatomy

The human body consists of billions of cells bathing in a water solution with a salt concentration similar to that of prehistoric seawater. The fluid volume residing inside the cells is called the *intracellular fluid (ICF) volume* and represents approximately 35–40% of the body weight. The fluid volume outside the cells in called the *extracellular fluid (ECF) volume* and corresponds to 20% of the body weight.

The fluid volumes outside and inside the cells are separated by the semipermeable *cell membrane*, which mainly operates by active pumping functions. However, water moves passively across the cell membrane in response to changes in *osmolality*, which can be manipulated by the clinician. Osmolality is the number of particles dissolved in the water solution and is a powerful driving force for water distribution. Hence, administration of a fluid with a higher osmolality than 295 milliosmoles (mosmol) per kg (*hypertonic* fluid) withdraws water from the ICF to the ECF, while infusion of a fluid having a lower osmolality than 295 mosmol/kg (*hypotonic* fluid) creates a movement of water volume in the opposite direction. However, most infusion fluids are *isotonic*, which means that they do not redistribute water across the cell membrane.

The ECF consists of the two body fluid volumes, the *plasma* and the *interstitial fluid*, which correspond to approximately 4% and 16% of the body weight, respectively. They are separated by the *capillary membrane*, which is highly permeable to water, electrolytes, and small molecules, such as glucose and amino acids. Erythrocytes do not pass at all. Proteins leave the plasma slowly and, together with intravascular fluid, circulate through the interstitial fluid space and return to the plasma via the *lymphatic system*. Fluid distribution across the capillary membrane can be manipulated by modifying the small addition to the osmolality given by large-sized molecules, mainly plasma proteins. This part of the osmolality is quantified by the *colloid osmotic (oncotic) pressure* (Fig. 6.1).

Crystalloid fluids lack oncotic properties as they contain only small molecules that easily pass the capillary membrane. By contrast, *colloid fluids* contain large-sized molecules that have a slow transcapillary passage and, therefore, a prolonged intravascular persistence.

Hormones

The body fluids circulate constantly. The blood volume is pumped around the entire cardiovascular system within one minute. Many hormonal and neurological mechanisms maintain the body fluid volumes within narrow limits. *Vasopressin* (AVP) is secreted from the neurohypophysis in response to hyperosmolality and hypotensive hemorrhage. Elevated fluid pressure in the cardiac atrium and ventricle stimulates secretion of *atrial natriuretic*

67

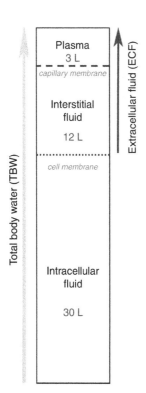

Figure 6.1 Schematic drawing of the body fluid compartments. A black and white version of this figure will appear in some formats. For the color version, please refer to the plate section.

peptide (ANP) and *brain natriuretic peptide* (BNP), which accelerate the urine flow and the capillary filtration of albumin. *Cortisol* and *aldosterone* are steroid hormones that are secreted in greater amounts in response to trauma. They cause retention of water and sodium by acting on the kidney. *Renin*, which is secreted in response to arterial hypotension, raises the plasma concentration of aldosterone.

The sympathetic nervous impulses are of interest for fluid balance as they constrict arterioles, which raises peripheral resistance. Sympathetic impulses also increase venous return by constricting large veins and stimulate release of *noradrenaline* and *adrenaline* to the blood. These adrenal hormones cause vasoconstriction, although adrenaline also causes vasodilation in muscle tissue.

Water Turnover

The minimal recommended intake of water in humans is 25–30 mL/kg per 24 hours. Children have a higher metabolic activity and therefore require more fluid. The water intake is needed to compensate for evaporation from the skin and lungs (*insensible water losses*), as well as for maintaining a baseline urine flow sufficient for the excretion of metabolic waste products.

The need for fluid is increased during general anesthesia due to associated vasodilation, which increases the "unstressed" blood volume. An increase of the plasma volume by fluid administration restores venous return, and but might need to be complemented by a vasoconstrictor. Moreover, local disturbances of tissue perfusion easily develop due to the depression of the autonomous system, which can be counteracted by plasma volume expansion.

Physiological mechanisms aimed to combat derangements of the body fluid volumes may also be partially blunted during general anesthesia. Most delicate is a loss of blood volume (*hypovolemia*), which is compensated by vasoconstriction up to a hemorrhage of 1 L of blood. Loss of ECF volume is called *volume depletion* and occurs in diarrhea, ileus, and diabetic ketoacidosis. Here, 3–4 L, or even more, can be lost before shock ensues. The tolerance for ICF losses is poorly known but is likely to be greater than for volume depletion.

Anthropometry

Empirical relationships may be used to estimate the size of the body fluid compartments at baseline. The simplest rules state that the plasma volume corresponds to 4% of the body weight, BV is 7% of the body weight, and ECF volume makes up 20% of the body weight. Total body water represents 45–50% of the body weight in the adult female. The percentage is 60% in young adult men but 50% in older men. Children have a higher percentage. Such rules are simple but useful for the clinician to remember.

More precise information can be obtained by *regression equations*. These are typically based on tracer measurements of body fluid volumes performed by external tracer substances in large numbers of humans. Below is an example of such equations for estimation of the blood volume (BV) in women and men:[1]

$$BV\ (L,\ female) = 0.03308\ weight\ (kg) + 0.3561\ height^3(m) + 0.1833$$

$$BV\ (L,\ male) = 0.03219\ weight\ (kg) + 0.3669\ height^3(m) + 0.6041$$

Central Blood Volume

Measurement of the *intrathoracic* or *central blood volume* is possible with certain modern hemodynamic monitoring systems, such as the PiCCO™. These apparatuses are used mainly to measure central flow rates and blood pressures, but the central blood volume is provided as an adjunct output. A central venous pressure line or arterial catheterization is needed to obtain the data on body fluid volumes. Measurement of the central blood volume is of interest because it is more clearly related to hypovolemia-related physiological responses than the total circulating blood volume.

Bioimpedance

Bioimpedance (BIA) means that a series of weak electrical currents of different frequency are run through the body, typically between the arm to the foot.[2] The method is based on that current has more difficulty passing through large amounts of water than small amounts. Provided that the body weight is known, an estimate of both the ICF and ECF volumes can be obtained as various frequencies pass through and outside cells with varying ease.

BIA might be applied while the patient is in bed before and after surgery, but rarely perioperatively due to the risk of mechanical and electrical interference. In the author's experience, BIA can provide useful data only for groups and has a place mainly as an adjunct to more precise methods.

Exogenous Tracers

Estimates of body fluid volumes by using externally introduced *tracers* are of interest in basic research, but are rarely used clinically. A tracer substance known to distribute solely within one body fluid compartment is injected into the blood and the size of the compartment calculated under steady-state conditions by means of *dilution* of the substance. The basic equation for such calculations is:

$$\text{Size of compartment} = \frac{\text{Injected dose of tracer}}{\text{Plasma concentration of tracer}}$$

Examples of such tracers include bromide and iohexol for measurements of the ECF volume. Radio-iodated albumin and indocyanine green (ICG) are used for measurement of the plasma volume.

Bromide has a very slow turnover, which means that the measurement might be problematic to repeat several times. *Iohexol* has a shorter half-life, only 100 minutes, but this also implies that an estimation of the ECF volume must be based on several plasma samples to account for the elimination. Sampling cannot start within 30–40 minutes of the tracer because the kinetics shows a clear distribution phase.[3]

The *total body water* (sum of ECF and ICF) can be measured with water isotopes, which include *tritium* (radioactive) and *deuterium* (not radioactive). Even distribution of these molecules in the body water requires about 3 hours to be completed.

An alternative approach is to use *ethanol*, but the relatively short half-life requires frequent sampling in blood or, alternatively, in the expired air.[4]

The *plasma volume* has frequently been measured by radioactive *iodated albumin*. After 10 minutes of distribution of the injected substance, 3–4 samples are usually taken over 30–40 minutes to account for the exponential elimination.

Evans Blue is a dye that binds to plasma albumin, just like radioactive iodine. The concentration is measured by light absorption.

Indocyanine green (ICG) is another dye that binds to plasma albumin. The half-life is only 3 minutes due to rapid uptake by the liver.[5] Therefore, ICG can be used both to measure liver blood flow and plasma volume. The short half-life makes the transit time of the tracer from the site of injection to the liver to be of importance to the calculations.[6] The short half-life also makes ICG the plasma volume tracer of choice in patients where the body fluid volumes are not in perfect steady state.[6]

The red blood cell volume can be quantified by marking erythrocytes in the bloodstream with *chromium*, *technetium*, or *carbon monoxide*. The total blood volume is then extrapolated by comparing the red cell mass with the hematocrit.

The size of the interstitial fluid space and the ICF volume cannot be measured by tracers. They are inferred from differences between body fluid spaces that can be measured, that is, the plasma volume, the ECF volume, and the total body water.

The tracers mentioned so far are of limited use in perioperative medicine because their half-life is quite long. They also require steady-state conditions, rarely present in the surgical setting. A probable exception is indocyanine green tracer because steady state is then needed for only a few minutes.

If applied during steady-state conditions. the tracer methods have an accuracy of between 1% (total body water) and 10% (radio-iodinated albumin).

A challenge when measuring both the plasma and erythrocyte volumes at the same time is that their proportions indicate a hematocrit that differs from the measured hematocrit in peripheral blood. A correction factor ("hematocrit factor") of 0.91 has been introduced to correct for the discrepancy. Hence, the plasma volume measured by labeling of albumin with a tracer is believed to be 9% smaller than the measured value. The hematocrit factor appears to be quite stable under various physiological circumstances [7] but has been given many different interpretations over the years.

Endogenous Tracers

The distribution of *infused fluid* between the ICF and ECF and between the plasma and the interstitial fluid can be estimated by using the serum sodium concentration (SNa) and the blood hemoglobin concentration (Hb) as biomarker.

Sodium. If all infused fluid and sodium (Na), as well as all voided amounts are known, the change in ICF volume can be estimated based on the assumption that Na is evenly distributed in the ECF volume, which makes up 20% of the body weight. From time 0 to time t, we get:

$$\Delta ICF = ECF + (infused - voided)volume - \frac{\left(SNa^*ECF - (added - voided)Na\right)}{SNa(t)}$$

This *mass balance equation* has mostly been used to calculate the intracellular distribution of electrolyte-free irrigating fluid, but it estimates the intracellular distribution of any infusion fluid as well.[8]

This equation can also be used to calculate the absolute size of the ECF provided that hypertonic saline is infused.[9]

Hemoglobin. Erythrocytes have a slow turnover (120 days) and remain in the bloodstream during fluid therapy. Therefore, changes in Hb mirror short-term relative changes in the blood volume (BV). The common approach is to estimate the BV at baseline (BV_o) by anthropometry and then multiply with the relative change in Hb to obtain an estimate the BV at a later time t (BV_t).

The change in blood volume is given by:

$$\Delta BV = BV_o(Hb_o / Hb_t) - BV_o$$

The amount of infused fluid that is retained in the blood is then given by:

$$Fluid\ retained\ (\%) - 100^*\Delta BV / infused\ volume$$

The fraction of fluid retained over time is the *efficiency.*

If the urinary output is known, the difference between the infused volume and the sum of the urine and blood volumes represents the change in interstitial fluid volume.

The Hb dilution concept can be developed to account for blood loss, if known. This is (usually) necessary when calculating fluid shifts based on Hb during surgery. We then calculate the total Hb mass and subsequently subtracts all losses (or adds transfused erythrocytes). The Hb mass in an adult is close to 1 kg.

$$Hb_o mass = BV_o Hb_o$$

$$BV_t = (Hb_o mass - loss\ of\ Hb\ mass)/Hb_t$$

These simple equations can be entered into a pocket calculator and may be helpful for the clinician when assessing whether a patient is hypervolemic or hypovolemic. The calculations can be applied repeatedly during surgery without loss of accuracy.[10]

The basic relationships shown above can, in turn, be developed to quantify the efficiency of one or several infusion fluids during ongoing surgery. The following modification of the approach uses a multiple regression equation to separate the effects of various factors that influence the blood volume.

$$\Delta BV = A\ (infused\ fluid\ volume) - B\ (blood\ loss)$$

Data may be entered for an entire operation or for shorter periods of time. For example, this approach was used to quantify the separate efficiencies of 20% albumin and lactated Ringer's on the plasma volume during cystectomy.[11]

The Hb method may be more difficult to apply in animals than in humans because several species (such as sheep and dogs) have reservoirs of erythrocytes in the spleen that are mobilized in stressful situations, including hemorrhage. In humans, such recruitment is negligible.[12]

Fluid Volume Kinetics

Drug regimens are commonly based on pharmacokinetic analysis. For this purpose, the Hb mathematics presented above have been elaborated upon to create a pharmacokinetic system for the analysis and simulation of the distribution and elimination of infusion fluids. Serial analyses of the Hb concentration in whole blood (20–40 samples) are then re-calculated to represent the plasma dilution over time that results from an infusion, the reason being that the plasma rather than whole blood equilibrates with other body fluids. The plasma dilution data are then fitted to the solutions of differential equations in a kinetic model aimed to describe (reasonably well) what happens in the body (Fig. 6.2).

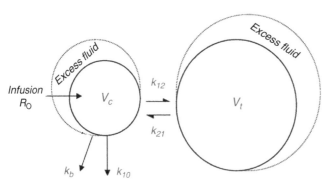

Figure 6.2 Schematic drawing of the model used for volume kinetic analysis.

A pharmacokinetic model is not usually interpreted in physiological terms, but much evidence supports the idea that volume kinetics reflects the distribution of infused fluid between body fluid compartments. Benefits with the volume kinetic approach is that dynamic events can be studied and that the kinetic parameters may be used to simulate experiments not performed. While volume kinetics can be used for scientific studies of fluid programs, the frequent Hb sampling makes it unsuitable for patient monitoring in the clinic. Non-invasive Hb is not currently accurate enough to serve this purpose.[13]

The Kinetic Model. The distribution of fluid between a *central* and a *peripheral* compartment (V_c and V_t, respectively) is governed three *rate constants*, k_{12}, k_{21}, and k_{10}. These are aimed to quantify the transcapillary leakage of fluid, the redistribution of fluid (mainly by the lymph), and the urinary excretion, respectively. A fluid volume kinetic analyses based on carefully measured data becomes more precise on inclusion of a fourth rate constant, k_b, which represents accumulation of infused fluid in a body space of unknown origin that is redistributed to the plasma at a very slow rate. This internal loss of fluid from the kinetic system to a "non-functional" space becomes more important when the urinary excretion is low, such as during general anesthesia. [14] The structural background to this space is probably that the interstitium consists of a free-fluid phase and a colloid-rich phase, of which the latter is difficult to expand but binds water more tightly.[15,16]

Crystalloid Fluid. Key findings with volume kinetics include that crystalloid fluid has a distribution phase of 30 minutes, which makes the plasma volume expansion much better than the usually assumed efficiency of 15–20% during an infusion and up to 30 minutes thereafter. As expected, the distribution phase is most apparent for short and brisk infusions (Fig. 6.3). However, infusion of small volumes of crystalloid fluid, such as 2–5 mL/kg over 15–30 minutes, undergoes little distribution, suggesting that a clear increase of the capillary hydrostatic pressure and the plasma dilution is needed to expand the interstitial matrix. High-rate infusions (>50 mL/min) slows the redistribution and, thus, has an intrinsic capacity to cause tissue edema.

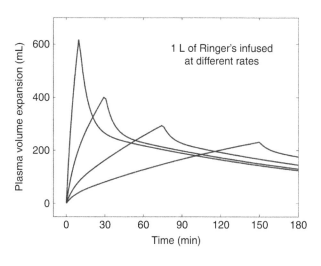

Figure 6.3 The volume expansion of the central body fluid space (the plasma) when 1 L of crystalloid fluid is infused at different rates. Simulations based on kinetic parameters derived from 30 infusion experiments of crystalloid electrolyte fluid in 10 conscious male volunteers published in *Medicina* 2017;**53**:233–41.

The rate of distribution slows down temporarily during the induction phase of epidural, spinal, and general anesthesia, which has been attributed to the accompanying reduction of the arterial pressure. The distribution of fluid even becomes arrested when the mean arterial pressure becomes established at 20 mmHg below baseline, which does not resolve until a new Starling equilibrium is established. How quickly that point is reached depends on the rate of infusion and/or the capillary refill. By contrast, measurements performed during induction of spinal anesthesia without hypotension shows a normal distribution profile.

The half-life of a crystalloid fluid is between 20 and 50 minutes in conscious volunteers and is usually longer in males. However, the plasma volume expansion will last longer as fluid is redistributed to the plasma from the interstitial fluid space. Based on the urine flow rate, the elimination is approximately 10 times longer during general anesthesia than in the conscious state. The main cause appears to be the lowered mean arterial pressure. Stimulating the alpha-1-receptors with norepinephrine and phenylephrine and blocking the beta-1-receptors with esmolol increases the urinary excretion during surgery, but it is still far from being as effective as the elimination in the conscious state.[17] The patient's capacity to handle infused fluid in the postoperative setting appears to be much better and is almost the same as in volunteers.

Plain 5% glucose and 2.5% glucose with electrolytes expand the plasma volume to the same degree as Ringer's lactate, but the expansion disappears faster post-infusion due to uptake of glucose and water into the body cells.

Arrested return of distributed crystalloid fluid (low k_{21}) creates a situation with hypovolemia and tissue edema. This unfortunate combination is an occasional finding but has been described in pre-eclampsia (humans), sepsis (sheep), and the transurethral resection syndrome (pigs).[14]

Colloid Fluid. Iso-oncotic colloid fluids do not have a distribution phase and expand the plasma volume by almost the same volume as the infused. Their plasma half-life is several hours as determined by the capillary leakage of the infused macromolecule (albumin, starch, or dextran).

Infusion of 20% albumin recruits three times the infused volume to the plasma. However, the plasma volume expansion is only doubled because some of the recruited fluid is subject to urinary excretion.[18] Although debated, the traditional view is that the interstitium is the source of the recruited fluid. The maximum plasma volume expansion occurs 10–20 minutes after an infusion ends. The half-life is very long (8–15 h) both in volunteers and in patients who have undergone surgery. A half-life of this magnitude implies that the induced plasma volume expansion lasts until the following day.[19]

Flow Rates. The output from a volume kinetic analysis is best illustrated by a plot, but the flow rates between the body fluid volumes can also be calculated directly. The flow of infused fluid from the plasma to the interstitium is given by the product of k_{12} and the volume expansion of V_c at any time and the return flow by the product of k_{21} and the volume expansion of V_t.

An example can be based on the kinetic parameters shown in Table 6.1, which were also used to create Figure 6.3. When plasma volume expansion is 500 mL, capillary leakage occurs at a rate of $500 \times 102.4 \times 10^{-3} = 51$ mL/min, urinary excretion

Table 6.1 Population kinetic parameters based on infusion experiments with crystalloid fluid in male volunteers. Covariate effects are omitted.

Kinetic parameter	Covariate	Best estimate	CV%
tvV_c (mL)	-	3 835	4.5
tvk_{12} ($10\text{–}3\ min^{-1}$)	-	102.4	9.3
tvk_{21} ($10\text{–}3\ min^{-1}$)	-	48.7	13.1
tvk_{10} ($10\text{–}3\ min^{-1}$)	-	15.4	9.3
tvk_b ($10\text{–}3\ min^{-1}$)		2.5	21.7

From *Medicina* 2017;53:233–41.
tv, typical value; CV, between-subject coefficient of variation.

at a rate of $500 \times 15.4 \times 10^{-3} = 7.7$ mL/min. The model must provide an estimate of the volume expansion of V_t before the rate of that redistribution of fluid (mainly via the lymph) can be calculated.

References

1. Nadler SB, Hidalgo JU, Bloch T. Prediction of blood volume in normal human adults. *Surgery.* 1962;**51**:224–32.

2. Chung YJ, Kim EY. Usefulness of bioelectrical impedance analysis and ECW ratio as guidance for fluid management in critically ill patients after operation. *Sci Rep.* 2021;**11**:12168.

3. Zdolsek J, Lisander B, Hahn RG. Measuring the size of the extracellular space using bromide, iohexol and sodium dilution. *Anesth Analg.* 2005;**101**:1770–7.

4. Norberg Å, Sandhagen B, Bratteby L-E, et al. Do ethanol and deuterium oxide distribute into the same water space in healthy volunteers? *Alcohol Clin Exp Res.* 2001;**25**:1423–30.

5. Menschen S, Busse MW, Zisowsky S, Panning B. Determination of plasma volume and total blood volume using indocyanine green: a short review. *J Med.* 1993;**24**:10–27.

6. Polidori D, Rowley C. Optimal back-extrapolation method for estimating plasma volume in humans using the indocyanine green dilution method. *Theor Biol Med Model.* 2013;**10**:48.

7. Chaplin H Jr, Mollison PL, Vetter H. The body/venous hematocrit ratio: its constancy over a wide hematocrit range. *J Clin Invest.* 1953;**32**:1309–16

8. Hahn RG, Drobin D. Rapid water and slow sodium excretion of Ringer's solution dehydrates cells. *Anesth Analg.* 2003;**97**:1590–4.

9. Hahn RG, Giménez-Milà M. Comparison between two solute equations and bioimpedance for estimation of body fluid volumes. *Intensive Care Med Exp.* 2022;**10**:7.

10. Hahn RG. Blood volume at the onset of hypotension in TURP performed during epidural anaesthesia. *Eur J Anaesth.* 1993;**10**:219–25.

11. Löffel L, Hahn RG, Engel D, Wuethrich PY. Intraoperative intravascular effect of lactated Ringer's solution and hyperoncotic albumin during hemorrhage in cystectomy patients. *Anesth Analg.* 2021;**133**:413–22.

12. Ebert RV, Stead EA. Demonstration that in normal man no reserves of blood are mobilized by exercise, epinephrine, and hemorrhage. *Am J Med Sci.* 1941;**201**:655–64.

13. Hahn RG, Wuethrich PY, Zdolsek JH. Can perioperative hemodilution be monitored with non-invasive measurement of blood hemoglobin? *BMC Anaesthesiol.* 2021;**21**:138.

14. Hahn RG. Understanding volume kinetics. *Acta Anaesthesiol Scand.* 2020;**64**:570–8.

15. Haljamäe H. Anatomy of the interstitial tissue. *Lymphology.*1978; **11**:128–32.

16. Aukland K, Reed RK. Interstitial-lymphatic mechanisms in the control of extracellular fluid volume. *Physiol Rev.* 1993;**73**:1–78.

17. Li Y, Zhu HB, Zheng X, et al. Low doses of esmolol and phenylephrine act as diuretics during intravenous anesthesia. *Crit Care.* 2012;**16**:R18.

18. Zdolsek M, Hahn RG, Zdolsek JH. Recruitment of extravascular fluid by hyperoncotic albumin. *Acta Anaesthesiol Scand.* 2018;**62**:1255–60.

19. Zdolsek M, Wuethrich PY, Gunnström M, et al. Plasma disappearance rate of albumin when infused as a 20% solution. *Crit Care.* 2022;**26**:104.

Crystalloid Fluids

Robert G. Hahn

The term *crystalloid fluid* refers to sterile water solutions that contain small molecules, such as salt and glucose, which crystallize when dried. These solutes easily pass through the capillary membrane, which is the thin fenestrated endothelium that divides the plasma volume from the interstitial fluid volume. This process of solute distribution brings along water. Hence, the volume of a crystalloid fluid is spread throughout the extracellular fluid (ECF) space.

Crystalloid fluid is relevant for several strategies. The majority of the crystalloid fluid used in the perioperative period aims to hydrate only the ECF space and is then used as *resuscitation fluid*. The fluid contains only electrolytes and compensates for anesthesia-induced vasodilation, small to moderate blood losses, and urinary excretion. Although evaporation consists of electrolyte-free water, such fluid losses are relatively small and can also be compensated by crystalloid electrolyte solutions.

Solutions containing glucose are typically used as *maintenance fluid*, which means that they support the normal requirement for water (25–30 mL/kg per 24 h in an adult). These fluids hydrate both the ECF and the intracellular fluid (ICF) spaces, as the uptake of glucose to the cells bring along water by virtue of osmosis. Glucose solutions may be used during the pre- and postoperative periods but rarely during ongoing surgery.

0.9% Saline

A 0.9% solution of saline is often called physiological or "normal." The osmolality is 308 milliosmoles (mosmol) per kg but, due to dilution by the plasma proteins, the fluid becomes isotonic (295 mosmol/kg) when infused into the bloodstream. However, 0.9% saline is still "unbalanced" because no attempt has been made to mimic the electrolyte composition of the ECF. The fluid contains a marked surplus of chloride ions and no buffer (Table 7.1). The "strong ion difference" of the fluid is zero, while being +38 in the plasma. This dilution of the plasma by 0.9% saline decreases the strong ion difference, which creates metabolic acidosis.[1,2] The pH is depressed to below the normal range if more than 2 L of 0.9% saline are infused.

Isotonic saline is the most widely used infusion fluid in Europe and probably worldwide, although the indications are limited. In adults, 0.9% saline should be reserved for patients with hyponatremia and hypochloremic metabolic alkalosis, as in disease states associated with vomiting. The fluid has a more accepted role for perioperative fluid therapy in children where the risk of subacute postoperative hyponatremia is a more serious concern than in adults.

A 0.9% saline solution is excreted more slowly than both lactated and acetated Ringer's solutions. Therefore, the volume effect ("efficiency") of the fluid to be about 10% greater compared with the Ringer's solutions (Fig. 7.1). The reason for the slow elimination is probably that the surplus of chloride ions has a vasoconstrictive effect on the renal blood vessels.

Table 7.1 Composition of plasma and the most common crystalloid solutions

	Osmolality (mosmol/kg)	pH	Na⁺ (mmol/L)	K⁺ (mmol/L)	HCO₃⁻ (mmol/L) equivalent	Cl⁻ (mmol/L)	Glucose (mmol/L)
Plasma	295	7.40	140	3.6–5.1	30	100	5
0.9% saline	308	5.0	154	0	0	154	0
7.5% saline	2400	3.5–7.0	1 250	0	0	1 250	0
Lactated Ringer's	274	6.5	130	4	30	110	0
Acetated Ringer's	270	6.0	130	4	30	110	0
Plasma-Lyte[a]	295	7.4	140	5	27	98	0
Glucose (5%)	278	5.0	0	0	0	0	278
Glucose (2.5%) + electrolytes	280	6.0	70	0	25	45	139

[a] Plasma-Lyte A also contains 23 mmol/L of gluconate.
The infusion fluids may contain small amounts of electrolytes like magnesium and calcium.

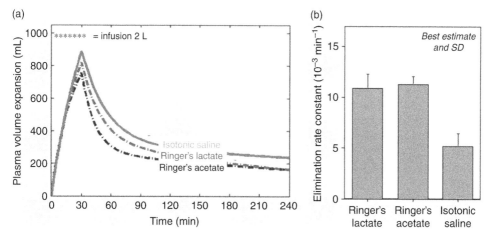

Figure 7.1 (a) Plasma volume expansion from infusion of 2 liters of isotonic saline, Ringer's lactate and Ringer's acetate in 10 healthy volunteers. Each curve is based on the modeled average plasma dilution from experiments performed in 10 male volunteers multiplied by the plasma volume at baseline as estimated by anthropometry. ******* symbolizes the time period when fluid is being infused.

(b) The rate of elimination of the three fluids. The half-life is the inverse of the shown elimination rate constant times 0.693. Hence, the half-life is about 60 min for the Ringer's solutions and 130 min for isotonic saline. Recalculations of data from Ref. [5] using a mixed models analytical program (Phoenix NLME). A black and white version of this figure will appear in some formats. For the color version, please refer to the plate section.

A 0.9% saline solution might cause abdominal pain when infused in healthy volunteers, which is not the case for lactated Ringer's.[1] Small prospective [2] and large retrospective [3] studies have shown that surgical complications are more common after open abdominal operations where 0.9% saline has been infused compared to balanced electrolyte fluid. However, the difference is disputed [4] and the use of 0.9% saline instead of a balanced Ringer's solution does not seem to increase the perioperative mortality.

Saline solution is devoid of calcium, which means that the fluid can be infused together with packed erythrocytes where citrate is used as a preservative. Large volumes of saline dilute the plasma calcium level, which can be an untoward effect because hypocalcemia decreases myocardial contractility. Therefore, calcium needs to be substituted if large volumes of isotonic saline are provided. No precise limit is known but should be in the range of 4 L in an adult.

Saline may also be marketed as hypertonic solutions at strengths of 3% and 7.5% solution. The first is mainly intended as a means of raising the serum sodium concentration in in-hospital patients and to reduce the intracranial pressure in neurotrauma patients. The latter is used for plasma volume expansion in emergency care, although the benefits have been questioned. In volunteers, 7.5% saline is four times more effective as a plasma volume expander than 0.9% saline.[5]

Ringer's Solution

Ringer's solution is a composition created by Sydney Ringer in the 1880s to be as similar as possible to the ECF. Alexis Hartmann later added a lactate buffer to the fluid and made it Hartmann's solution, or "lactated" Ringer's solution.

Today Ringer's solution is used with the addition of buffer in the form of *lactate* or *acetate*, of which the former is most common. Both ions are metabolized to bicarbonate in the body, albeit with certain differences. Lactate is metabolized in the liver and the kidneys with the aid of oxygen and under production of bicarbonate and carbon dioxide. Acetate is metabolized faster, and in most tissues, but it consumes only half as much oxygen per mole of produced bicarbonate compared with lactate. Hence, lactate slightly increases the oxygen consumption [6] and might also raise plasma glucose, particularly in diabetic patients.[7] Large amounts of lactated Ringer's confuse assays used to monitor lactic acidosis.

Both lactate and acetate are vasodilators. Rapid administration aggravates the reduction of the systemic vascular resistance that normally occurs in response to volume loading. However, adverse effect is hardly noticeable with the small amounts (28–30 mmol/L) present in the Ringer's solutions marketed for intravenous use. Both lactate and acetate are also fuels, although the calorific content in 1 L of any Ringer's solution is quite low (approximately 5 kcal).

Acetate is a more efficient buffer in the presence of a compromised circulation and in shock,[8] but differences between lactate and acetate in other settings are negligible.

Pharmacokinetics

During intravenous infusion the Ringer's solutions distribute from the plasma to the interstitial fluid space in a process that requires 25–30 minutes for completion. The distribution half-life is approximately 8 minutes [9] (see Fig. 7.1). The pharmacodynamics of the Ringer's solutions is strongly related to their capacity to expand the ECF volume.

Distribution: Infusing 300–400 mL at a rate of 10–20 mL/min will distribute fluid almost exclusively over the plasma volume.[10] This is rather due to the high compliance for volume expansion of the interstitial matrix than to a limiting effect of the capillary membrane. A higher rate of infusion overcomes the low compliance of the interstitial gel. When the rate of infusion is raised (50 mL/min and higher) the return of fluid from the interstitium to the plasma becomes progressively retarded,[11] which is probably due to loss of stiffness of the matrix.

Kinetic studies have separated one peripheral compartment that equilibrates quickly with the plasma from a second peripheral compartment of approximately the same size that equilibrates much more slowly with the plasma. Accumulation of fluid in this slow-equilibrating compartment is most apparent when the urinary excretion is low, such as during surgery.[12] Free fluid can even accumulate in lacunes in the interstitium if an infusion is provided fast enough to overcome the normally negative interstitial fluid pressure. This creates *pitting edema*, which might destruct the cytoarchitecture of vital organs if widespread (Fig. 7.2).

Elimination: The elimination (by voiding) in volunteers is so rapid that the fluid may exhibit one-compartment kinetics, which has been interpreted to imply that the fluid is distributed only to the plasma and to areas of the interstitial fluid space with the highest compliance for volume expansion. By contrast, elimination is greatly retarded during surgery where Ringer's always exhibits two-compartment kinetics.[9] Infusion of 2 L of Ringer's in volunteers is followed by elimination of 50–80% of the fluid within 2 hours, whereas the corresponding figure in anesthetized patients is only 10–20%.

(a)   (b)

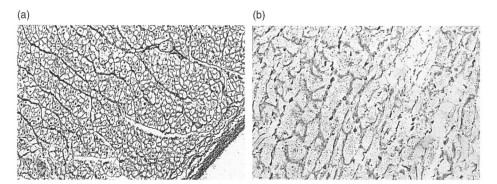

Figure 7.2 (a) Normal cytoarchitecture of a pig´s heart after receiving 150 mL/kg of mannitol 3% over 90 min. Lumina of the vessels are preserved (x 200).
(b) Destroyed cytoarchitecture in the subendocardium in a mouse that died after receiving 300 mL/kg of 0.9% saline over 60 min. The reticular fibers are fragmented and degenerated (x 600). Light microscopy with Gordon and Sweet's silver impregnation for reticulum fibers. Photographs were taken during the studies reported in *APMIS* 200;108:487–95, and *J Surg Res* 2001;95:114–25. A black and white version of this figure will appear in some formats. For the color version, please refer to the plate section.

Clinical Use

The Ringer's solutions may be used to replace preoperative losses of fluid due to diarrhea or bowel preparation. In contrast, vomiting should be replaced by 0.9% saline. They are commonly used (in a volume of approximately 500 mL) to compensate the blood volume for the expansion of the vascular tree that occurs from induction of both regional and general anesthesia.

Ringer's may also be used to compensate for hemorrhage up to 20% of the blood volume provided that the blood hemoglobin concentration remains above the transfusion trigger. The Ringer's solutions reverse the compensatory changes in blood pressure and sympathetic tone resulting from hypovolemia. There are numerous reports confirming that rapid infusion of Ringer's is a life-saving treatment in excessive hemorrhage due to the resulting expansion of the plasma volume. The commonly recommended dosage is to infuse three times as much Ringer's as the amount of blood lost (3:1 principle). If the patient's legs are placed in stirrups, a 2:1 replacement scheme can be used, with the last third given as a bolus infusion when the legs are lowered from the stirrups.[13]

By contrast, crystalloid fluid cannot reverse drug-induced hypotension. If a crystalloid bolus has no effect in reversing hypotension during surgery, the anesthetist should change strategy and lighten the anesthesia, or else institute treatment with an adrenergic drug, rather than providing several liters of crystalloid fluid.

There are concerns about the use of Ringer's in *brain injury*, because the fluid is slightly hypotonic (270 mosmol/kg) and increases brain cell mass when the central nervous system is traumatized.

The Ringer's solutions should be infused cautiously in patients with *renal insufficiency* since these patients may not be able to excrete an excess amount of crystalloid fluid.

The buffered Ringer's solutions contain 2 mmol/L of calcium and, therefore, cause coagulation in the infusion line if given together with erythrocytes preserved with citrate. This agent operates as an anticoagulant by binding calcium, which is a co-factor in the coagulation process.

The rate and volume of infused Ringer's solutions vary considerably during surgery. Overall, the volumes used in clinical practice today are lower than they were in the 1980s and 1990s. The most widely used basic rate of infusion to provide is 3–4 mL//kg/h, that is, approximately 250 mL/h in an adult male. In major surgery, a widely advocated concept is to provide a basic rate of 2 mL//kg/h of one of the buffered Ringer's solutions and then to increase the fluid administration whenever stroke volume decreases by >10% (*goal-directed fluid therapy*). The risk of postoperative nausea is increased if Ringer's solution is provided at a rate of only 2 mL//kg/h with no additional fluid.[14]

Adverse Effects

The rate of infusion of crystalloid fluid should be adjusted according to the patient's *cardiovascular status*. In healthy adult females very rapid infusions of Ringer's (2 L over 15 min) caused swelling sensations, dyspnea and headache.[15] This rate (133 mL/min) should not be exceeded in the absence of blunt hypovolemia. No symptoms were observed after infusing the same volume more slowly.

Too rapid volume loading might be complicated by instant *pulmonary edema*. There is also a risk of pulmonary edema developing in the postoperative period if the total volume infused during the day of surgery amounts to 7 L or more.[16]

Volume loading with 3 L of lactated Ringer's in volunteers (mean age 63 years) reduced the forced expiratory capacity and the peak flow rate.[17]

Outcome studies using prospective registration of postoperative adverse events have demonstrated that crystalloid fluid administration during colonic surgery should be closer to 4 mL/kg/h than 12 mL/kg/h.[18] The larger volumes of crystalloid electrolyte fluid promote postoperative complications such as impaired wound healing and pneumonia. However, the optimal rate of infusion for various surgeries is still controversial, which is mostly due to a study by Myles et al. which showed that liberal fluid therapy carries a lower risk of increasing plasma creatinine postoperatively than smaller volumes.[19] The conclusions of this study have been debated.[20]

During major surgery, the fluid therapy should not follow a predetermined protocol but be guided by individual and frequent hemodynamic measurements during and after the procedure.

Plasma-Lyte

Plasma-Lyte is constructed to further refine the "balanced" composition of acetated Ringer's solution. Here, the sodium and chloride concentrations are virtually identical to those of human plasma, and the osmolality is the same as of the plasma (see Table 7.1).

In addition to acetate, Plasma-Lyte contains the negatively charged ion gluconate to maintain the ionic balance. While acetate is a widely used buffer in medical practice, gluconate is best known as being a chelate in oral calcium tablets. However, gluconate has been in widespread use as a taste improver in the food industry for more than 100 years. Gluconate is also a part of our intermediary metabolism, and an amount corresponding to the content of 4 L of Plasma-Lyte is produced each day in the human body. Gluconate has a poor buffering effect and is non-toxic. Both acetate and gluconate are metabolized as energy, but gluconate is to a greater extent excreted in the urine.

Plasma-Lyte is used in the same indications as the buffered Ringer's solution. The fluid should be considered also in trauma patients and in children due to the iso-osmotic composition. Plasma-Lyte causes very few aberrations of the plasma electrolytes since the ionic composition is more similar to the ECF fluid than any of the other crystalloid electrolyte solutions.[21,22]

Plasma-Lyte is, just as 0.9% saline, devoid of calcium, which makes the fluid possible to infuse in the same intravenous line as erythrocytes preserved with citrate. Calcium may need to be substituted when more than 4 L of the fluid have been administered due to dilution of the plasma calcium concentration.

Glucose Solutions

There is a twofold purpose of infusing *glucose* (dextrose) solutions. The first is to prevent blunt starvation, which aids wound healing, well-being and recovery. The second purpose is to provide free water to hydrate the ICF space. Glucose solutions are the mainstay of such treatments in debilitated patients who cannot be fed orally.

Providing intravenous glucose always carries the risk of inducing hyperglycemia. Plasma glucose > 10 mmol/L increases the risk of postoperative infection [23,24] and osmotic diuresis develops when plasma glucose is 12–15 mmol/L, which implies that the kidneys lose control of the fluid and electrolyte excretion. Moreover, more pronounced cerebral damage occurs in the event of cardiac arrest.[25] Therefore, the management of glucose infusions requires knowledge, attention and responsibility.

The body's handling of glucose is impaired during trauma and surgery due to the development of *insulin resistance*. Figure 7.3 shows which plasma glucose concentrations can be expected from various rates of infusion of glucose 5% before, during and after surgery in relatively healthy non-diabetic subjects, standardized to a body weight of 70 kg. Anesthetists who use glucose 2.5% simply double the rates, which can be considered as first choice when starting an infusion.[26]

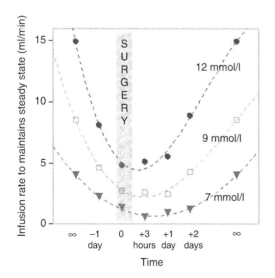

Figure 7.3 Plasma steady-state glucose concentrations (isobars) resulting from various rates of infusion of glucose 5% (y-axis) for various points in time during the perioperative period. The rates are standardized for a patient having a body weight of 70 kg, Computer simulation based on kinetic data from: *BJA* 2004;67:72–81, *BJA* 2003;90:600–7, *Br J Anaesth* 2005;94:30–8, *Trials* 2012;13:97 and *Theor Biol Med Model* 2013;10:48.

Glucose 5% is indicated after surgery when the patient cannot eat and drink. Glucose is sometimes infused before surgery when the operation is started late in the day, and in some hospitals also as a 2.5% solution during the surgical procedure. However, there is little reason to routinely administer glucose perioperatively as hormonal changes associated with surgery sufficiently maintain the blood glucose level. Moreover, shorter preoperative fasting and fast-track surgery with early postoperative mobilization have limited the use of intravenous glucose treatment in routine surgery.

Electrolytes are often added to the glucose solutions used for maintenance fluid therapy, that is, during the postoperative phase. Many preparations already contain half the electrolyte content of a balanced Ringer's solution. In other cases, sodium and potassium are added based on measurements of the plasma concentrations of these ions.

Hypertonic glucose solutions (10% and 20%) must be monitored by measurements of the plasma glucose concentration and frequently need to be supplemented with exogenous insulin. These fluids are used for more ambitious supplementation of calories in postoperative and intensive care settings.

Glucose metabolism yields CO_2, and the accompanying increased breathing might be a problem in debilitated patients with impaired lung function.

When used for *maintenance therapy*, a glucose solution should provide the basic need of electrolytes. As a rule, 1 mmol of sodium and 1 mmol of potassium per kilo body weight per 24 hours should be given. A safe rate of administration of potassium is 10 mmol per hour, which can be increased to 20 mmol per hour if the electrocardiogram is monitored.

It is not advisable to abruptly stop a glucose infusion that has been given at high rate due to the risk of *rebound hypoglycemia*. This is an issue when, for example, parenteral nutrition is turned off, during labor and Cesarean section.

Repeated infusion of electrolyte-free glucose solution (usually plain 5%) might induce *subacute hyponatremia*. This complication usually develops 2–3 days after surgery and is characterized by neurological disturbances, nausea and vomiting.[27] When symptoms appear, serum sodium is usually between 120 and 130 mmol/L (normal level 138–140 mmol/L).

Mannitol

Mannitol is an isomer of glucose that is eliminated only by renal excretion. The molecule remains essentially in the ECF fluid. The half-life is approximately 130 minutes but can be much longer in the presence of impaired kidney function.

The clinical use of mannitol for intravenous administration is restricted to a plain 10% or 20% solution (in some countries only 15%), which induces diuresis in failing, oliguric kidneys. The mechanism is that the renal excretion of mannitol occurs by virtue of osmotic diuresis, by which the body loses water.

The hypertonic nature of the mannitol solutions has made it a means of acutely reducing the intracranial pressure in patients with *head trauma*. The volume used is then 500–750 mL, of which half is given as a bolus infusion.

The marked increase in ECF volume makes infusion of hypertonic mannitol contraindicated in congestive heart failure. Like all hypertonic fluids, mannitol 15% should not be administered together with erythrocyte transfusions.

Mannitol in an iso-osmotic 5% solution is used as an irrigating fluid in transurethral surgery when monopolar electric current is used for cutting.

References

1. Williams EL, Hildebrand KL, McCormick SA, Bedel MJ. The effect of intravenous lactated Ringer's solution vs. 0.9% sodium chloride solution on serum osmolality in human volunteers. *Anesth Analg*. 1999;**88**:999–1003.

2. Wilkes NJ, Woolf R, Mutch M, et al. The effects of balanced versus saline-based hetastarch and crystalloid solutions on acid-base and electrolyte status and gastric mucosal perfusion in elderly surgical patients. *Anesth Analg*. 2001;**93**:811–16.

3. Shaw AD, Bagshaw SM, Goldstein SL, et al. Major complications, mortality, and resource utilization after open abdominal surgery. 0.9% saline compared to Plasma-Lyte. *Ann Surg*. 2012;**255**:821–9.

4. Maheshwari K, Turan A, Makarova N, et al. Saline versus lactated Ringer's solution: the Saline or Lactated Ringer's (SOLAR) Trial. *Anesthesiology*. 2020;**132**:614–24.

5. Drobin D, Hahn RG. Kinetics of isotonic and hypertonic plasma volume expanders. *Anesthesiology*. 2002;**96**:1371–80.

6. Ahlborg G, Hagenfeldt L, Wahren J. Influence of lactate infusion on glucose and FFA metabolism in man. *Scand J Clin Lab Invest*. 1976;**36**:193–201.

7. Thomas DJB, Albertini KGMM. Hyperglycaemic effects of Hartmann's solution during surgery in patients with maturity onset diabetes. *Br J Anaesth*. 1978;**50**:185–8.

8. Kveim M, Nesbakken R. Utilization of exogenous acetate during canine hemorrhagic shock. *Scand J Clin & Lab Invest*. 1979;**39**:653–8.

9. Hahn RG. Understanding volume kinetics. *Acta Anaesthesiol Scand*. 2020;**64**:570–8.

10. Hahn RG, Bahlmann H, Nilsson L. Dehydration and fluid volume kinetics before major open abdominal surgery. *Acta Anaesthesiol Scand* .2014;**58**:1258–66.

11. Hahn RG, Drobin D, Zdolsek J. Distribution of crystalloid fluid changes with the rate of infusion: a population-based study. *Acta Anaesthesiol Scand*. 2016;**60**:569–78.

12. Hahn RG. Fluid escape to the "third space" during anesthesia, a commentary. *Acta Anaesthesiol Scand*. 2020;**65**:451–6.

13. Hahn RG. Blood volume at the onset of hypotension in TURP performed during epidural anaesthesia. *Eur J Anaesth*. 1993;**10**:219–25.

14. Apfel CC, Meyer A, Orphan-Sungur M, et al. Supplemental intravenous crystalloids for the prevention of postoperative nausea and vomiting. *Br J Anaesth*. 2012;**108**:893–902.

15. Hahn RG, Drobin D, Ståhle L. Volume kinetics of Ringer's solution in female volunteers. *Br J Anaesth*. 1997;**78**:144–8.

16. Arieff AI. Fatal postoperative pulmonary edema. Pathogenesis and literature review. *Chest*. 1999;**115**:1371–7.

17. Holte K, Jensen P, Kehlet H. Physiologic effects of intravenous fluid administration in healthy volunteers. *Anesth Analg*. 2003;**96**:1504–9.

18. Nisanevich V, Felsenstein I, Almogy G, et al. Effect of intraoperative fluid management on outcome after intraabdominal surgery. *Anesthesiology*. 2005;**103**:25–32.

19. Myles PS, Bellomo R, Corcoran T, et al.; Australian and New Zealand College of Anaesthetists Clinical Trials Network and the Australian and New Zealand Intensive Care Society Clinical Trials Group. Restrictive versus liberal fluid therapy for major abdominal surgery. *N Engl J Med*. 2018;**378**:2263–74.

20. Bahlmann H, Hahn RG. IV fluids for major surgery: comment. *Anesthesiology*. 2019;**131**:1367–8.

21. Chua H-R, Venkatesh B, Stachowski E, et al. Plasma-Lyte 148 vs 0.9% saline for fluid resuscitation in diabetic ketoacidosis. *J Crit Care*. 2012;**27**:138–45.

22. Hadimioglu N, Saadawy I, Saglam T, Ertug Z, Dinckan A. The effect of different crystalloid solutions on acid-base balance and early

kidney function after kidney transplantation. *Anesth Analg.* 2008;**107**:264–9.

23. Hanazaki K, Maeda H, Okabayashi T. Relationship between perioperative glycemic control and postoperative infections. *World J Gastroenterol.* 2009;**15**:4122–5.

24. Kwon S, Thompson R, Dellinger P, et al. Importance of perioperative glycemic control in general surgery: a report from the Surgical Care and Outcomes Assessment program. *Ann Surg.* 2013;**257**:8–14.

25. Siemkowicz E. The effect of glucose upon restitution after transient cerebral ischemia: a summary. *Acta Neurol Scand.* 1985;71 417–27.

26. Sjöstrand F, Edsberg L, Hahn RG. Volume kinetics of glucose solutions given by intravenous infusion. *Br J Anaesth.* 2001;**87**:834–43.

27. Ayus JC, Wheeler JM, Arieff AI. Postoperative hyponatremic encephalopathy in menstruant women. *Ann Intern Med.* 1992;**117**:891–7.

Chapter

8

Colloid Fluids

Robert G. Hahn

The term *colloid fluid* refers to a sterile water solution with added macromolecules that pass through the capillary wall only with great difficulty. The osmotic strength of macromolecules is not great, so a colloid fluid must also contain electrolytes to be non-hemolytic. As long as macromolecules reside within the capillary walls, their contribution to the total osmolality (the *colloid osmotic pressure*) is still sufficient to maintain a large proportion (or all) of the infused fluid volume inside the bloodstream.

Colloid fluids are used as plasma volume expanders and have more long-lasting effect than crystalloid fluids. They carry a risk of allergic reactions not shared by crystalloid fluids. Therefore, smaller blood losses should be replaced by crystalloid fluid, and colloids are withheld until 10% of the blood volume has been lost. If fluid overload is not at hand, the clinician may continue to use Ringer's solution as volume replacement until the transfusion trigger is reached. However, switching to a colloid fluid may help to reduce postoperative morbidity.[1]

The colloids should be mixed in balanced electrolyte solutions and not in saline. The reason for this is the metabolic acidosis induced by saline, but the changeover is important only if 2–3 L of the colloid is administered. However, even minor acidosis from the saline in a colloid fluid adds on to acidosis caused for other reasons.

Overall, the use of colloid solutions has declined in recent years. The change is due to the disclosure of adverse renal effects on the kidneys from the use of artificial colloids in the intensive care setting. Moreover, the better plasma volume expanding effect compared with crystalloids has been questioned when fluid therapy is extended over several days in intensive care patients.

Albumin is currently the most widely accepted colloid fluid in the clinic.

Albumin

Albumin is the most abundant protein in plasma and, therefore, has an important role in maintaining the intravascular colloid osmotic pressure. Albumin has a molecular weight of 70 kDa. Albumin solutions are prepared from the blood of donors and have a strength of 3.5%, 4%, or 5%, and are even available as a hyperoncotic 20% preparation.

Pharmacokinetics

Albumin 5% expands the plasma volume by 70–80% of the infused volume. In healthy volunteers, the plasma volume expansion fades away slowly according to a mono-exponential function.

An infusion of 10 mL/kg of albumin 5% increases the serum albumin concentration by 10%, which remains unchanged for more than 8 hours.[2] Restoration of the normal blood volume is governed by translocation of albumin molecules from the plasma to the interstitial fluid space. Moreover, the plasma volume expansion per se has a diuretic effect. The albumin is gradually transported back to the plasma via lymphatic pathways. By contrast, 20% albumin increases the blood volume by twice the infused volume.

Exogenous albumin has an intravascular half-life of approximately 10 hours, while the plasma volume expansion is somewhat shorter.[3] However, a recent analysis points out that the capillary leakage rate easily becomes erroneously high in complex clinical settings due to protein exudation, blood loss, and variations in blood volume; the correct half-life of exogenously administered albumin is probably closer to 16 hours.[4] Support for this leakage rate is received from some, but not from all, previous studies.[5,6]

Clinical Use

Albumin is a "natural" colloid and remains an effective means of restoring the plasma volume and normal hemodynamics in hypovolemic shock.

Despite high cost and limited supply in most countries, the use of albumin in adults has undergone a revival in recent years. The main reason in that the adverse effects of the artificial colloids on kidney function do not seem to be shared by albumin.[7] The plasma volume expansion lasts until the following day.

Albumin also has a scavenger effect that is appreciated in intensive care. Acute reduction of plasma albumin is a sign of *capillary leak* in inflammatory disorders, such as sepsis. The leakage rate of endogenous albumin is normally 5% per hour but can be considerably higher in septic patients.[8] The reason seems to be breakdown (shedding) of the glycocalyx layer of the endothelium, which otherwise binds plasma proteins and other colloid particles more firmly to the vascular system.[9] However, no increase in capillary leakage rate of albumin occurred when 20% albumin was infused in patients with a moderately severe inflammatory response (Fig. 8.1). This may suggest that exogenous albumin may have a normalizing effect of an accelerated capillary leakage rate.[4]

In intensive care, albumin infusions have been used to treat *hypoalbuminemia*.[10] This therapy has gradually been taken out of practice as low plasma albumin is a sign of severe disease rather than a medical problem in itself. The added albumin will soon be subject to catabolism and used in the same way as amino acids in the body.

Albumin may be used to replace excessive albumin losses in special medical conditions, such as nephritis.

Hyperoncotic (20%) albumin does not improve survival in septic patients (ALBIOS study),[7] but both ALBIOS and the earlier SAFE study suggested a survival benefit for albumin treatment in patients with septic shock.[7,11]

Hyperoncotic (20%) albumin operates as a diuretic even without concomitant administration of furosemide. The effectiveness appears to be only marginally affected by low arterial pressure,[12] whereas impairment of the diuretic response by hypotension is quite strong for crystalloid fluid.

Starch

Hydroxyethyl starch (HES) consists of polysaccharides and is prepared from plants such as grain or maize. The use of HES has declined during the past decade due to reports of renal

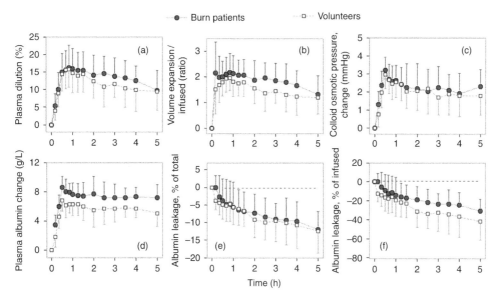

Figure 8.1 Blood variables during and after a 30-min infusion of 3 mL/kg of 20% albumin (approximately 200 mL) in 15 healthy volunteers and in 15 post-burn patients. The plasma C-reactive protein concentration averaged 2 mg/L in the volunteers and 86 mg/L in the post-burn patients. All data are the mean (SD). From *Crit Care* 2020;**24**:191.

injury in septic patients, but the preparations still have a prominent role in perioperative care in many countries.

Chemistry

HES is the only type of colloid preparation that has undergone company-driven development to achieve refinement during the past 30 years. Several different formulations may be marketed, both old and new. They vary in concentration, usually being 6% or 10%. They also vary in chemical composition with respect to molecular weight, the number of hydroxyethyl groups per unit of glucose (substitution), and the placement of these hydroxyethyl groups on the carbon atoms of the glucose molecules (C2/C6 ratio).

The variability in chemical composition determines the differences in clinical effect between the solutions. Over the past decades, the trend has been to use molecules of smaller size to reduce the half-life and the risk of hemorrhagic complications. *Hetastarch* contains the largest molecules (450 kDa) and *pentastarch* contains intermediate-sized molecules (260 kDa). The most recently developed HES preparations have an even lower molecular size, on average 130 kDa. The degree of substitution may be low (0.45–0.60) or high (0.62–0.70) and the C2/C6 ratio is low if less than eight.

The preparations are usually described with the key characteristics of molecular size and substitution, with or without being followed by the C2/C6 ratio. Hence, currently the most widely promoted HES preparations are denoted HES 130/0.4/9:1 (Voluven from Fresenius-Kabi) and HES 130/0.62/6:1 (Venofundin from B. Braun). A modern adaptation is to mix the HES in balanced crystalloid solutions instead of in 0.9% saline, which is to be preferred when several fluid bags are prescribed.

The degree of substitution is the key determinant for half-life. Higher molecular size increases the risk of adverse effects in the form of anaphylactoid reactions, coagulopathy, and postoperative itching.

HES (6%) mixed in hypertonic (7.5%) saline has been marketed for emergency and trauma situations. Such a solution expands the plasma by much more than the infused volume, by virtue of osmotic volume transfer from the ICF space.

Pharmacokinetics

A 6% HES solution in iso-osmotic saline or balanced electrolytes expands the plasma volume by as much as the infused volume (Fig. 8.2). Considerable variability in this respect may be encountered when administered to intensive care patients.[13]

The *elimination* of the HES molecules is a complex issue. They have a spectrum of sizes of which the smallest (<60–70 kDa) are quickly eliminated by renal excretion. Larger molecules first need to be cleaved by endogenous alpha-amylase into smaller fragments before being excreted, a process that increases the osmotic strength per gram of polysaccharide. The HES molecules are also subjected to phagocytosis by the reticuloendothelial system, and remnants may be found in the liver and spleen even after several years. Hence, the half-life of the HES molecules does not correspond closely with the plasma volume expansion over time.

The half-life of the HES molecules in Venofundin was 3.8 h when administered to volunteers.[14] The product monograph from the manufacturer (Fresensius Kabi, 2007) claims that plasma half-life of the HES molecules in Voluven is 1.4 hours and that approximately 60% of them can later be recovered in the urine. The decay of the plasma volume expansion for HES 130/0.4 (Voluven) occurred with a half-life of 2 hours in the study of volunteers illustrated in Figure 8.1.[15] The intravascular persistence of the fluid volume is much shorter than the half-life of the HES molecules, which suggests that the molecules reside outside the circulation for many hours before being eliminated.

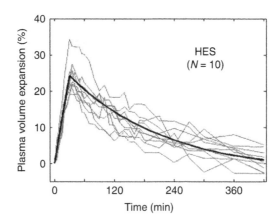

Figure 8.2 Plasma volume expansion from infusion of 10 mL/kg of hydroxyethyl starch 130/0.4 (Voluven) over 30 min in 10 male volunteers. The thick curve is the modeled average and the thin lines each of the underlying experiments. The volume of distribution can be calculated based on this plot by extrapolating the modeled curve to zero time and use as the denominator in a ratio where the dose is the numerator; this appears to be 3 L, which is close to the estimated plasma volume. Based on data from *Crit Care* 2013;**17**:R104.

As for crystalloid fluids, the effect duration is markedly longer when given to replace hemorrhage.[16]

The elimination of crystalloid fluid is known to be greatly retarded by anesthesia and surgery, but there is no data on the rate of elimination of colloid fluid volumes in the perioperative setting.

Clinical Use

Hydroxyethyl starch is recommended for plasma volume expansion in bleeding patients. The colloid is not indicated for use in intensive care in Europe.

The first 10–20 mL should be infused slowly and the patient closely observed with respect to allergic reactions, which are rare and less severe than for dextran.

The highest recommended dose of Voluven is 3.5 L per day in an adult of 70 kg. Only half as much should be allowed for dextran and HES preparations that contain larger molecules.

Although small-sized HES (130 kDa) preparations have a shorter persistence in the blood, they have the same clinical efficacy as median-sized HES preparations while being safer.[17]

The "Starch Debate"

Europe has suffered a debate on the clinical use of HES in clinical medicine. Four studies published between 2001 and 2012 showed a greater increase in plasma creatinine concentration, greater need for renal replacement therapy, and/or a poorer outcome in septic patients treated with HES as compared with gelatin or crystalloid fluid.[18–21] The only study with mixed diagnoses was the CHEST study, which is, however, the least convincing of these trials.[21]

Critics argue that HES exerts a dose-dependent toxic effect on the kidneys. Defenders point out that these trials never compared the fluids when used as first-line treatment, and that the administration often deviated from clinical practice. Moreover, sepsis is a very special clinical situation and outcome data associated with the use of drugs should not be uncritically extrapolated to other patient groups.

In late 2013 the European Medicines Agency put limitations on the use of HES in Europe. From then on, these colloids can only be used within the EU to combat hypovolemia in bleeding patients and not at all in the intensive care setting. Sepsis, burn injuries, and renal failure are contraindications. Treatment should be initiated only if crystalloids are insufficient. The lowest effective dose should be used, and treatment be continued for the shortest period of time and no longer than 24 hours. Serum creatinine must be monitored in the aftermath of the HES treatment.[22]

Several later meta-analyses and studies of surgical patients have not convincingly confirmed that HES promotes postoperative kidney injury. However, outcome results are mixed [23] and, in 2022, the US Food and Drug Administration issued the far-reaching warnings on the use of HES, as Europe did in 2013.[24]

Gelatin

Gelatin solutions consist of polypeptides from bovine raw material. This colloid was already in use during World War I and since then has mostly been used in Great Britain and its former colonies. Gelatin is considered to have a fairly good plasma volume-expanding effect, similar to that of HES.[25] The duration is shorter (approximately 2 h) due to the relatively small size of the molecules (average 30 kDa), which makes them excretable by the kidneys. Mild anaphylactoid reactions occur at a frequency of 0.3%, which is relatively high, but severe reactions are rare.[26] The effect of gelatin on blood coagulation is small.

Gelatin had a bad reputation for some years due to the risk of spreading slow virus diseases such as "mad cow disease." To prevent this problem, the gelatin preparations are now heated to high temperature before sale.

There are two marketed solutions: Haemaccel, which contains 3.5% gelatin, and Gelofusine, which is a plasmion-succinylated gelatin mixed in isotonic saline. The latter is the most widely used gelatin today. The solution is slightly hypo-osmotic (274 milliosmoles [mosmol] per kg) and contains 154 mmol/L of sodium but only 120 mmol/L of chloride, whereby hyperchloremic acidosis will be less of a problem compared with Voluven and 0.9% saline.

Dextran

Long chains of glucose molecules (polysaccharides) are synthesized by bacteria to serve as macromolecules in the group of infusion fluids called the *dextrans* (sometimes abbreviated as DEX). As with albumin, the osmolality of a water solution containing only the macromolecules is quite low and necessitates that electrolytes are added as well.

The used dextran solutions have an average molecular weight of 70 kDa (dextran 70) or 40 kDa (dextran 40), and concentrations used are 3%, 6%, or 10%. The most widely used, 6% dextran 70, expands the plasma volume with the same volume as the infused amount, while initially being somewhat stronger. The plasma volume expansion subsides with a half-life of almost 3 hours. A solution of 10% dextran 40 expands the plasma volume by twice the infused volume. The half-life is shorter than for dextran 70.

The dextran molecules are either excreted by the kidneys or metabolized by an endogenous hydrolase (dextranase) to carbon dioxide and water.

The dextrans decrease blood viscosity and improve microcirculatory blood flow. This can sometimes be noted by visual inspection of the cut surface in a surgical wound as oozing – small vessels seem to open and bleed more. This might be disturbing to the surgeon. The total blood loss does not seem to be increased in surgery with an expected small blood loss, while dextran more clearly increases the blood loss during major surgery where the hemorrhage is expected to be on the high side.[27]

Dextran in hypertonic (7.5%) saline has been available in some countries as an effective plasma volume expander in emergencies and pre-hospital trauma care. The dose is 4 mL/kg and should be provided as a fluid bolus. One unit of 250 mL is usually given.

The literature about dextran is extensive but mostly authored during the 1960s and 1970s. By contrast, the literature about gelatin is very limited despite gelatin being the oldest of the colloids, introduced during World War I.

Clinical Use

Dextran 70 is used to expand the plasma volume and/or to prevent thromboembolism. Dextran 40 is used to improve the microcirculation after vascular surgery. The maximum dose is 1.5 g/(kg day), which corresponds to 1.5–2.0 L of 6% dextran 70 in an adult. Hemorrhagic complications may ensue if larger amounts are given.

There is a risk of *anaphylaxis* developing in patients having irregular antibodies to dextran. This complication occurs in a frequency of 0.27%,[26] but severe reactions can be prevented by dextran molecules of very small size (1 kDa). This pre-treatment is performed by giving an intravenous injection of dextran 1, which blocks the irregular antibodies ("hapten binding"), just before dextran 40 or 70 is infused.

The use of dextran for plasma volume support has dwindled in recent years. The reasons are lack of company promotion, the increased hemorrhage in major surgery, and scattered availability of dextran 1 to prevent anaphylactic reactions.

Plasma

Human plasma should be used to administer coagulation factors and only as a last resort as a plasma volume expander. However, plasma volume expansion is much more variable with plasma than with albumin 5%.[2] The difference is probably due to increased capillary leak caused by occasional cross-reactions with the recipient's immunological system. Other drawbacks with the use of human plasma include the high occurrence of fever reactions (3–4%), the risk of anaphylaxis in patients with hereditary IgA deficiency, and the rare but dangerous complication called "transfusion-related acute lung injury" (TRALI).

Therapeutic Window for Colloids

When to use a colloid fluid has always been a matter of opinion, but adhering exclusively to one or the other does not seem to be rational.

The use of colloids is always hampered by a risk of anaphylaxis, which occurs even from very small doses, and a risk of coagulopathy, which requires infusion of at least 1 L of colloid. The cost of colloid therapy is also higher. Therefore, crystalloid fluid should be the first-line fluid for plasma volume support during surgery. However, the risk of anaphylaxis can be accepted when the administered amount of crystalloid is so large that their adverse effects appear in a statistically increased frequency.

Crystalloids prolong the gastrointestinal recovery time when >2 L has been infused [28] and there is a statistically increased risk of complications when the volume exceeds 3 L.[29] Several other studies support that the risk of adverse effects increases when gradually more crystalloid fluid is infused, and 3 L seems to be a well-founded limit suggesting that the clinician should seriously consider switching to a colloid fluid. On doing so, the aggregate risk of postoperative complications may be reduced.[1]

Calculations based on this view suggests that colloid fluid is only indicated when the preoperative blood hemoglobin concentration is greater than 120 g/L.[30] Patients with a lower blood hemoglobin reach the transfusion trigger before 3 L of crystalloid is administered.

Volume Equivalents between Colloids and Crystalloids

The potency of colloid and crystalloid fluids can be compared by simulations based on volume kinetic parameters (for details, see the Chapter 6, "Body Volumes and Fluid Kinetics"). The respective plasma volume–expanding potencies during surgery have been studied in different settings since the mid-1990s. Simulations based on such data show a time-dependency. At the end of a 30-minute infusion, an iso-oncotic colloid fluid (in this case, Voluven) expands the plasma 1.5 times more than a crystalloid. Thirty minutes after the infusion ends, the distribution of the crystalloid has increased the ratio to 2.5 times, but the ratio becomes reduced over time due to the pronounced anesthesia-induced inhibition of excretion of crystalloid fluid that is due to the anesthesia.

These differences are greater in the conscious state than during general anesthesia, owing to the depression of the turnover of crystalloid fluid that occurs due to the low arterial pressure during anesthesia. An exception is the occurrence of a sharp decrease in arterial pressure, which is usually the case during induction of anesthesia. In that setting, all infused crystalloid fluid is temporarily retained in the plasma.

Albumin (20%) is twice as potent as iso-oncotic colloids and the ratios between the colloid/crystalloid potencies mentioned above should then be doubled.[3]

Using a non-kinetic regression model, 20% albumin had a five times higher potency than Ringer's lactate as plasma volume expander during major surgery.[31]

References

1. Joosten A, Delaporte A, Ickx B, et al. Crystalloid versus colloid for intraoperative goal-directed fluid therapy using a closed-loop system: a randomized, double-blinded, controlled trial in major abdominal surgery. *Anesthesiology*. 2018;**128**:55–66.

2. Hedin A, Hahn RG. Volume expansion and plasma protein clearance during intravenous infusion of 5% albumin and autologous plasma. *Clin Sci*. 2005;**106**:217–24.

3. Zdolsek M, Hahn RG. Kinetics of 5% and 20% albumin: a controlled crossover trial in volunteers. *Acta Anaesthesiol Scand*. 2022;**66**:847–58.

4. Zdolsek M, Wuethrich PY, Gunnström M, et al. Plasma disappearance rate of albumin when infused as a 20% solution. *Crit Care*. 2022;**26**:104.

5. Karanko MS, Laaksonen VO, Meretoja OA. Effects of concentrated albumin treatment after aortocoronary bypass surgery. *Crit Care Med*. 1987; **15**:737–42.

6. Norberg Å, Rooyackers O, Segersvärd R, Wernerman J. Leakage of albumin in major abdominal surgery. *Crit Care*. 2016;**20**:113.

7. Caironi P, Tognoni G, Masson S, et al. Albumin replacement in patients with severe sepsis or septic shock. *New Engl Med*. 2014;**370**:1412–21.

8. Fleck A, Raines G, Hawker F, et al. Increased vascular permeability: a major cause of hypoalbuminaemia in disease and injury. *Lancet*. 1985;**325**:781–4.

9. Woodcock TE, Woodcock TM. Revised Starling equation and the glycocalyx model of transvascular fluid exchange: an improved paradigm for prescribing intravenous fluid therapy. *Br J Anaesth*. 2012;**108**:384–94.

10. Marik PE. The treatment of hypoalbuminemia in the critically ill patient. *Heart Lung*. 1993;**22**:166–70.

11. The SAFE Study Investigators. A comparison of albumin and saline for fluid resuscitation in the intensive care unit. *New Engl J Med*. 2004;**350**:2247–56.

12. Gunnström M, Zdolsek J, Hahn RG. Plasma volume expansion and fluid kinetics of 20% albumin during general anesthesia and surgery lasting for more than 5 hours. *Anesth Analg*. 2022;**134**:1270–9.

13. Christensen P, Andersson J, Rasmussen SE, Andersen PK, Henneberg SW. Changes in circulating blood volume after infusion of hydroxyethyl starch 6% in critically ill patients. *Acta Anaesthesiol Scand*. 2001;**45**:414–20.

14. Lehmann GB, Asskali F, Boll M, et al. HES 130/0.42 shows less alteration of pharmacokinetics than HES 200/0.5 when

dosed repeatedly. *Br J Anaesth.* 2007;**98**:635–44.

15. Hahn RG, Bergek C, Gebäck T, Zdolsek J. Interactions between the volume effects of hydroxyethyl starch 130/0.4 and Ringer's acetate. *Crit Care.* 2013;**17**:R104.

16. James MF, Latoo MY, Mythen MG, et al. Plasma volume changes associated with two hydroxy ethyl starch colloids following acute hypovolaemia in volunteers. *Anaesthesia.* 2004;**59**:738–42.

17. Ickx BE, Bepperling F, Melot C, Schulman C, van der Linden PJ. Plasma substitution effects of a new hydroxyethyl starch HES 130/0.4 compared with HES 200/0.5 during and after extended acute normovolaemic haemodilution. *Br J Anaesth.* 2003;**91**:196–202.

18. Schortgen F, Lacherade LC, Bruneel F, et al. Effects of hydroxyethyl starch and gelatine on renal function in severe sepsis: a multicentre randomised study. *Lancet.* 2001;**357**:911–16.

19. Brunkhorst FM, Engel C, Bloos F, et al. Intensive insulin therapy and pentastarch resuscitation in severe sepsis. *N Engl J Med.* 2008;**358**:125–38.

20. Perner A, Haase N, Guttormsen AB, et al. Hydroxyethyl starch 130/0.42 versus Ringer's acetate in severe sepsis. *N Engl J Med.* 2012;**367**:124–34.

21. Myburgh JA, Finfer S, Bellomo R, et al. Hydroxyethyl starch or saline for fluid on intraoperative oliguria resuscitation in intensive care. *N Engl J Med.* 2012;**367**:1901–11.

22. European Medicines Agency. Hydroxyethyl starch solutions for infusion. 2014.

23. Futier E, Garot M, Godet T, Biais M, et al. Effect of hydroxyethyl starch vs saline for volume replacement therapy on death or postoperative complications among high-risk patients undergoing major abdominal surgery: The FLASH randomized clinical trial. *JAMA.* 2020;**323**:225–36.

24. Landow, L, Wei S, Song L, Goud R, Cooper, K. Recent U.S. Food and Drug Administration labeling changes for hydroxyethyl starch products due to concerns about mortality, kidney injury, and excess bleeding. *Anesthesiology.* 2022;**136**:868–70.

25. Awad S, Dharmavaram S, Wearn CS, Dube MG, Lobo DN. Effects of an intraoperative infusion of 4% succinylated gelatinee (Gelofusine®) and 6% hydroxyethyl starch (Voluven®) on blood volume. *Br J Anaesth.* 2012;**109**168–76.

26. Laxenaire MC, Charpentier C, Feldman L. Anaphylactoid reactions to colloid plasma substitutes: incidence risk factor mechanisms. A French multicenter prospective study. *Ann Fr Anesth Reanimat.* 1994;**13**:301–10.

27. Rasmussen KC, Hoejskov M, Johansson PI, et al. Coagulation competence for predicting perioperative hemorrhage in patients treated with lactated Ringer's vs. Dextran–a randomized controlled trial. *BMC Anesthesiol.* 2015;**15**:178.

28. Li Y, He R, Ying X, Hahn RG. Ringer's lactate, but not hydroxyethyl starch, prolongs the food intolerance time after major abdominal surgery; an open-labelled clinical trial. *BMC Anesthesiology.* 2015;**15**:2.

29. Varadhan KK, Lobo DN. Symposium 3: A meta-analysis of randomised controlled trials of intravenous fluid therapy in major elective open abdominal surgery: getting the balance right. *Proc Nutr Soc* .2010;**69**:488–98.

30. Hahn RG. Why crystalloids will do the job in the operating room. *Anaesthesiol Intensive Ther.* 2014;**46**:342–9.

31. Löffel L, Hahn RG, Engel D, Wuethrich PY. Intraoperative intravascular effect of lactated Ringer's solution and hyperoncotic albumin during hemorrhage in cystectomy patients. *Anesth Analg.* 2021;**133**:413–22.

Chapter 9

The Role of Plasmatic Viscosity

Pedro Cabrales, Amy G. Tsai, Judith Martini
and Marcos Intaglietta

Introduction

Blood transfusion is unique in medicine since it was never subjected to rigorous clinical trials associated with today's medical interventions. It is assumed to be safe and efficacious, which is mostly the case for immediate results. However, it increases patient mortality by 8–10% per decade per unit transfused.[6,15] This is due to the difference in time scales between how transfusion decisions are made and monitored, occurring in the span of days, often involving practitioners not primarily responsible for the patient's long-term health, which evolves over periods of decades.[27]

Blood transfusions are usually carried out when central blood hematocrit (Hct) or blood hemoglobin (Hb) concentration and blood surface oxygen partial pressure (spO_2) reach a lower limit labeled "transfusion trigger," and proceeds once blood group data ensure donor/recipient compatibility. Parameters and limiting values defining the "transfusion trigger" are still debated leading to a variability regarding the quantity ranging labeled from "restrictive" to "liberal."

The transfusion trigger strives to be "physiological" and reflects the patient's systemic oxygen delivery (DO_2) relative to its value in normal conditions. However, DO_2 measurements are complex and challenging in intensive care scenarios. Mahecic et al. [19] summarized currently proposed transfusion trigger parameters, including electrocardiogram data, central/mixed venous O_2 saturation, and near infrared spectroscopy to measure oxygen-specific tissue hypoxia; however, Hct, Hb and spO_2 remain the primarily used parameters.

Blood transfusion is a well-honed procedure, usually giving patients a rapid sensation of well-being; however, it is not risk-free.[29,28] It is expensive and requires an important societal commitment to making blood available. The quantity of blood used could be reduced significantly since normal DO_2 is four times the mammalian demand, while transfusions are made at a Hct that provides twice the DO_2 demand. This might be due to physiological evidence indicating the reduction in blood unloading O_2 into the tissue after delivering 60% of normal DO_2. However, this limitation is not reported in experimental studies of hemodilution when Hb decreased below 7–8 g/dL Hb, suggesting that blood transfusion practice may be missing critical information.

Blood Transfusion as a Microcirculatory Mechanics Phenomenon

We hypothesize that analysis of hemodilution/anemia and its correction by blood transfusion does not yet include current findings on how O_2 is transported and regulated in the microcirculation, particularly the capillaries.

The development of instrumentation and methods for studying the microvasculature in conditions that reproduce its physiological state [25] significantly modified earlier micro-vascular structure and function perceptions. These methods measure flowing blood hydraulic pressure, flow velocity, microvascular diameter dynamics, blood and tissue pO_2 with micrometer spatial resolution, microvessel Hct, functional capillary density [FCD, number of capillaries with red blood cell (RBC) passage over a period] and microvascular wall nitric oxide (NO) concentration.

The studies show:

1) Capillaries are tunnels in the tissue, lined by endothelial cells whose thickness modulates inner capillary diameter as a function of local hydraulic capillary and osmotic phenomena mediated by the endothelial wall.[11]

2) Passage of RBCs through capillaries is determined by the capillary inner diameter, which varies due to endothelial swelling, which can proceed up to occluding the capillary, lowering FCD.

3) Tissue and organism survival primarily depends on FCD maintenance and is mostly unrelated to local tissue pO_2 [13] as shown in Figure 9.1a.

4) FCD is a function of capillary pressure and blood viscosity as shown in Figure 9.1b.

5) Tissue pO_2 is determined by O_2 gradients extending and decaying from the blood/tissue arteriolar interfaces.[31]

6) Systemic Hct persists until arterioles reach 100 microns and then is reduced by 80% in the capillaries, returning to its systemic level in the venules [17] as shown in Figure 9.2.

7) Blood viscosity is a linear function of plasma viscosity and a quadratic function of Hct according to equation (1).

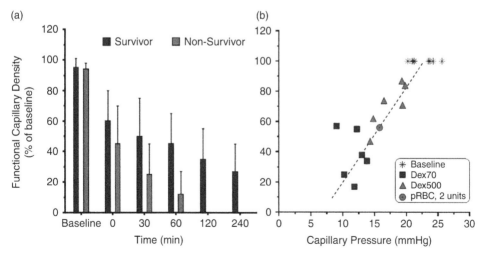

Figure 9.1 (a) Survival vs. functional capillary density (FCD) (% of control) during 4 hr hemorrhagic shock and FCD association with capillary pressure in extreme hemodilution.[13] (b) FCD as a function of capillary pressure in extreme hemodilution with high and low viscosity plasma expanders and blood transfusion in shock resuscitation. It is apparent blood transfusion provides a marginal increase in microvascular pressure in the treatment of profound anemia by comparison to hyperviscous resuscitation.[2]

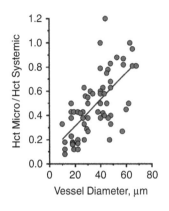

Figure 9.2 Distribution of hematocrit (Hct) in microvessels of cat mesentery as a function of vessel diameter in in vivo conditions. This distribution is due to hydrodynamic effects at bifurcations lowering systemic Hct as vessels branch.[17,18]

These findings show that the Krogh model for O_2 transport does not apply to capillaries since their blood/tissue O_2 gradients needed to supply the tissue are too small to sustain tissue O_2 consumption, a function provided by arterioles. Furthermore, tissue survival is critically dependent on maintaining an FCD threshold, as shown in Figure 9.1a, needed to clear the tissue from products of metabolism, comprising large molecules with low diffusion constants, whose accumulation poisons the tissue.

A critical finding on the regulation of arteriolar blood flow and the tissue O_2 supply evolved from the observation of A. Schretzenmayr, 1932, that the dog femoral artery dilated when flow increased, reported by J.A. Bevan.[1] Subsequently, Fazio et al. [7] found that increasing Hct due to using diuretics increased carotid artery diameter of hypertensive patients, proposing the blood viscosity role as a factor in regulating vessel wall vasodilator release. Melkumyants et al. [24] demonstrated that blood flow velocity modulates arteriolar diameter.

Increased flow velocity and increased viscosity increase shear stress σ on the vascular wall and was proposed to cause the release of the dilation agent by the vascular wall, identified by Furchgott and Zawadzki [9] to be nitric oxide (NO). Chávez-Negrete et al. [4] analyzed blood NO levels in hypertensive patients treated with diuretics, finding that mean arterial pressure (MAP) decreased significantly in proportion to the simultaneous increase of Hct and blood NO levels closing the loop in these considerations.

This background is relevant to transfusion medicine because introducing packed red blood cells (pRBCs) into the circulation increases blood viscosity, increasing the heart workload and DO_2, while simultaneously increasing σ and NO production, causing vaso-dilation via the NO pathway, thus lowering the aforementioned increased flow resistance and workload. The outcome of these competing effects was modeled by Li et al.,[16] showing that DO_2 in progressive normovolemic hemodilution is maximal at Hct 55% of normal, is maintained above normal up to Hct ~14%, and reduces by 50% at Hct ~11%, while Habler and Messmer [10] reported DO_2 being maximal at Hct 82% of normal, remained above normal down to Hct 28%, and was 50% of normal at Hct 11% in experimental dog studies.

Notably, limited bleeding, which lowers Hct, has been used since antiquity to improve patient's conditions, a justifiable practice if increasing DO_2 by 10–15% is expected to have a significant effect in the circulation where DO_2 is usually 400% of the basal requirement.

Missing Factors in Blood Transfusion Decisions

The practice of blood transfusion mostly focuses on monitoring/maintaining blood O_2 *carrying* capacity, rather than blood O_2 *delivery* capacity, due to the complexity and costs of obtaining additional data, particularly cardiac output. Ambiguities also arise in evaluating patient pO_2, using devices that average values from the skin's surface as overlaying micro-vessels whose blood pO_2 varies from near systemic to the lowest values in the organism (Intaglietta et al. [12]). Therefore, Hct and pO_2 values used to evaluate a patient's DO_2 status may not provide definitive information on realistic O_2 deficits nor address the O_2 delivery status.

The question therefore arises about what additional information could be used to more precisely define a patient's DO_2, how to apply this in handling anemia by blood transfusion, and whether alternative approaches could provide adequate or better O_2 supply.

The Ubiquitous, Paradoxical Role of Blood Plasma Viscosity

We propose that the missing factor in practicing blood transfusion is the evaluation and manipulation of a patient's blood plasma viscosity, [14] specifically differentiating between effects due to changes of blood viscosity due to increasing Hct versus effects due to specifically changing plasma viscosity.

The Hct distribution in the microvascular network changes from systemic after 100–80 μm diameter arterioles, lowering to ~1/5 of systemic in the capillaries as shown in Figure 9.2.[18] Zimmerman et al. [32] report blood viscosity μ_{blood} being a function of Hct and plasma viscosity μ_{plasma} according to equation (1):

$$\mu_{blood} = \mu_{plasma}\left(1 + 0.0049\,\mathrm{Hct} + 0.0017\,\mathrm{Hct}^2\right), \tag{1}$$

where Hct is uniform in blood vessels > 100 μm diameter, while plasma viscosity equally affects the whole circulation, including capillaries. Changes in Hct minimally affect capillary blood viscosity, where Hct is 5× lower than systemic, becoming even smaller when anemia reduces Hct according to equation (1).

The Biomechanical Factor from the Capillary Circulation

The velocity gradient at the blood/vessel interface generates shear stress σ proportional to the local blood viscosity and the shear rate at the wall, the overall effect being proportional to the vascular area, which increases as blood passes through progressive bifurcation levels.

A precise evaluation of how σ is distributed in the tissue is a virtually impossible task, requiring meticulous microscopic measurements of vascular geometry, and related flow velocities and Hct measurements in large number of microvessels in the tissue mostly inaccessible to microscopic measurements. However information on the required data may be obtained from the meticulous work of Franklin Mall, [20] who reported numerical estimate of the anatomical data in arterioles and capillaries, which in combination with the data of Figure 9.2 and equation (1) allows calculating $\sigma_{arterioles}$ and $\sigma_{capillaries}$ for changes of plasma viscosity due to introducing a high viscosity plasma expander versus increasing blood viscosity by transfusion of pRBCs to increase Hct.

We note that σ_i is due to the total flow $\mathbf{Q}$ which is constant for each bifurcation level $\mathbf{i}$, blood viscosity μ_i, and blood vessel radius $\mathbf{R_i}$ according to:

$$\sigma_i = \frac{4Q\mu_i}{R_i^3}, \tag{2}$$

where the total shear stress Σ generated by an arteriole and its ensuing capillaries is given by the sum of products of shear stress given by equation (2) times the respective arteriolar a_{art} and capillary a_{cap} surface areas on contact with the flowing blood yielding:

$$\Sigma = [a_{art}\sigma_{art} + a_{cap}\sigma_{cap}] = 4Q\frac{a_{art}\mu_{art}}{R_{art}^3}\left[1 + \frac{R_{art}^3}{R_{cap}^3}\frac{a_{cap}}{a_{art}}\frac{\mu_{cap}}{\mu_{art}}\right] \tag{3}$$

We carry out calculations to compare Σ generated in the microcirculation when treating anemia by: 1) Transfusing 2 pRBCs units, and, 2) increasing plasma viscosity to 2 cP by transfusing a viscogenic plasma expander. Q is assumed to remain constant, σ_{art} and σ_{cap} calculated using equation (2) and viscosities are calculated using equation (1) with Hct obtained from Figure 9.2.

Regarding Figure 9.2, we make the approximation that central Hct is constant down to ~95 μm diameter arterioles, and reduces linearly as shown in the smaller branches. We further propose that in the anemic subject Hct follows the same pattern, and reduces linearly in the smaller branches, reducing to zero Hct at a common intersection for all Hcts, as shown.

We use the data of Mall for the dog mesentery for comparing the effects of the plasma viscosity change versus Hct change for varying the total shear stress and therefore the increase in NO availability in the tissue. Accordingly, the microcirculation the dog mesentery is reported to be composed of 0.2 cm long × 0.002 cm diameter arterioles, each branching ultimately supplying blood to 300 capillaries, 0.1 cm long × 0.0008 cm diameter, whereby capillary surface area is 2.4× that of the arteriolar supply. Equation (3) allows estimating the total shear stress Σ to which the microvascular endothelium is subjected per arteriole for each of the two forms of microvascular viscosity enhancement, showing that the total shear stress generated by increasing plasma viscosity is 60% greater than that generated by 2 units pRBC transfusion.

We propose that this effect significantly increases NO production causing dilation, increasing blood flow velocity and DO_2, an effect not available in transfusing pRBCs.

Experimental Evidence on the Relation between Endothelial Microvascular NO Concentration, Endothelial Shear Stress, and Microvessel Flow Velocity

Our calculation is based on simplifications of physiological data that fundamentally require experimental verification. In this context, we studied the two transfusion modalities in the in vivo microcirculation of the awake hamster window chamber model [26] rendered 50% anemic by exchange transfusion with hamster plasma or dextran 70 kDa. Treatments with hyperviscous plasma infusion or RBC transfusion were used for restoring DO_2 24 hours after induction of anemia. Window chamber flow parameters were assumed to correspond to systemic parameters and studied 4 hours after the induction of anemia. Flow changes measured in the large arterioles (diameter > 100 μm) were assumed to reflect systemic changes. Viscosities were measured at the experiment's end using a Brookfield viscometer.

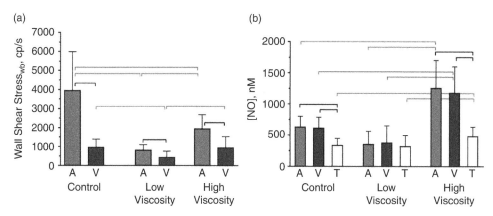

Figure 9.3 Measurement of vessel wall shear stress (a) and vascular NO concentration (b) in the arterioles, venules, and tissue in the microcirculation of awake hamsters hemodiluted to ~25% normal hematocrit (Hct) using low viscosity dextran 70 kDa and high viscosity dextran 500 kDa. Brackets denote statistical significance.

We used human equivalent hamster blood pRBC units of 65% Hct, and 500 kDa dextran dissolved in Ringer's lactate was used as a plasma expander to increase plasma viscosity to 2.0 cP. Mean arterial blood pressure was measured via a carotid artery indwelling catheter, also used for pRBC and dextran 500 infusions.

Our results (Fig. 9.3) confirm our hypothesis and preliminary calculations showing the significant increase in shear stress and NO bioavailability due to using high viscosity plasma expansion. They were reported in the literature as a means to treat extreme hemodilution (i.e., central Hct 25% of normal), a significantly more severe condition than hemodilution-induced 50% anemia. We consider these findings critical since extreme hemodilution is an extreme condition, which, not properly addressed, causes the lethal FCD fall shown in Figure 9.1.

Summary and Conclusions

We show that blood transfusion has limited effectiveness in treating 50% anemia compared with plasma viscosity enhancement since it primarily addresses the increase in Hct rather than DO_2. The effectiveness of pRBC transfusion should also be viewed considering that 25% of transfused RBCs are destroyed 24 hours post-transfusion, increasing Hb blood concentration 2× over normal, reducing the 2 RBC units to 1.5. Notably, it has been stated that transfusing 1.0 unit of blood has no greater effect on the recipient than the same loss of blood on the donor.

Our studies (Fig. 9.4) were completed using various dosages of 60% pRBCs, the commercial plasma expander Hextend (6% hetastarch in lactated Ringer's), and an experimental super-viscous hyaluronan-based macromolecular solution to treat 50% anemic hamsters. We show that using high viscosity plasma is equivalent to or better than pRBCs to restore DO_2. Notably, Hextend is a readily available, low-cost product, of apparently universal use and long shelf life. The practicality of use can ultimately be extended in considering that clinically resuscitation is always with fluid first to restore blood volume, and secondly to restore DO_2, while this approach could easily combine both procedures.

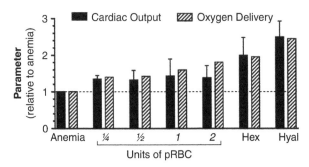

Figure 9.4 Summary of studies showing cardiac output and DO_2 in 50% anemic awake hamsters, transfused with packed red blood cells (pRBCs) and Hextend (Hex), increasing plasma viscosity to 2.0 cP, and an experimental hyaluronan high viscosity plasma expander (Hyal), increasing plasma viscosity to 2.5 cP. Note that cardiac output is independent of the pRBC volume transfused, and that since 1/4 unit has the same cardiac output effect as 2 units, the change in flow due to transfusion appears to be independent of the change of O_2 transport.

Our findings show the difference in results between increasing DO_2 by increasing Hct, which does not majorly change microvascular DO_2, versus increasing plasma viscosity, which directly and significantly stimulates NO generation, promoting vasodilatation, increasing FCD, microvascular flow, and DO_2, while lowering O_2 demand.[30]

Paradoxically, plasma and blood viscosity increase is usually associated with pathological conditions. However, we show that elevation of **both** parameters results in increased perfusion and lower peripheral vascular resistance. Increasing plasma viscosity has a generalized beneficial effect on microvascular function, as shown by de Witt et al. [5] in brain perfusion studies. Elevation of plasma viscosity induces sustained NO-mediated dilation in the hamster cremaster microcirculation, in vivo, due to increased capillary flow velocity induced by vasodilation, as shown by Cabrales et al.[3]

In extreme hemodilution, blood viscosity is insufficient to pressurize the capillary to a level that ensures adequate FCD, which we show is corrected by increasing plasma viscosity up to 2.2 cP. Conversely, blood transfusion changes central blood viscosity with minuscule effects on capillary viscosity, and while blood transfusion increases blood viscosity, the increased Hct also increases NO scavenging. decreasing the effectiveness of the induced vasodilatation.

In anemia, low capillary pressure induces endothelial swelling and lowers FCD, which can be reversed by increasing capillary pressure. Application of these findings to hemorrhagic shock treatment leads to hyperosmotic-hyperviscous resuscitation as a modality for recovery of microvascular function.[2,22]

One must keep in mind, though, that hyperviscous resuscitation fluids, such as starches, have a substantial impact on blood coagulation.[8] Starches interfere with fibrinogen polymerization, thereby decreasing clot firmness, an event that is undesirable in a severely bleeding patient.[23,21] Further studies are therefore needed to address this issue and eventually come up with a fluid design that incorporates hyperviscous properties without side effects on the coagulation system.

In conclusion, since normal $DO_2 = 4 \times DO_{2rest}$, where DO_{2rest} is the DO_2 required by the organism at rest, we propose that hyperviscous plasma expanders provide a new, economic and effective treatment of anemia that could ultimately extend anemia survival while lowering the transfusion trigger from the present $2 \times DO_{2rest}$ to the natural limit of $1 \times DO_{2rest}$. This gain is due to their ability to restore FCD, a critically ignored function for tissue survival not provided by blood transfusion, thus proposing that their deployment could ultimately double the usefulness and availability of the world blood supply.

References

1. Bevan JA. Shear stress, the endothelium and the balance between flow-induced contraction and dilation in animals and man. *Int J Microcirc Clin Exp.* 1997;**17**:248–56.

2. Cabrales P, Tsai AG, Intaglietta M. Is resuscitation from hemorrhagic shock limited by blood oxygen-carrying capacity or blood viscosity? *Shock.* 2007;**27**:380–9.

3. Cabrales P, Tsai AG, Intaglietta M. Microvascular pressure and functional capillary density in extreme hemodilution with low and high plasma viscosity expanders. *Am J Physiol.* 2004;**287**:H363–H373.

4. Chávez-Negrete AJ, Rojas-Uribe M, Gallardo-Montoya JM, Intaglietta M. Hemorrheologic effect of diuretics in the control of blood pressure in the hypertensive patient. *Rev Med Inst Mex Seguro Soc.* 2017;**55**:S343–S349.

5. De Witt C, Schafer C, von Bismarck P, Bolz SS, Pohl U. Elevation of plasma viscosity induces sustained NO-mediated dilation in the hamster cremaster microcirculation in vivo. *Pflügers Arch.* 1997;**434**:354–61.

6. Engoren MC, Habib RH, Zacharias A, et al. Effect of blood transfusion on long-term survival after cardiac operation. *Ann Thorac Surg* 2002;**74**:1180–6.

7. Fazio M, Bardelli M, Macaluso L, et al. Mechanics of the carotid artery wall and baroreflex sensitivity after acute ethanol administration in young healthy volunteers. *Clin Sci (Lond).* 2001;**101**:253–60.

8. Fries D, Haas T, Klingler A, et al. Efficacy of fibrinogen and prothrombin complex concentrate used to reverse dilutional coagulopathy–a porcine model. *Br J Anaesth.* 2006;**97**:460–7.

9. Furchgott RF, Zawadzki JV. The obligatory role of endothelial cells in the relaxation of arterial smooth muscle by acetylcholine. *Nature.* 1980;**288**:373–6.

10. Habler OP, Messmer KF. The physiology of oxygen transport. *Transfus Sci.* 1997;**18**:425–35.

11. Intaglietta M, de Plomb EP. Fluid exchange in tunnel and tube capillaries. *Microvasc Res.* 1973;**6**:153–68.

12. Intaglietta M, Johnson PC, Winslow RM. Microvascular and tissue oxygen distribution. *Cardiovasc Res.* 1996;**32**:632–43,.

13. Kerger H, Saltzman DJ, Menger MD, Messmer K, Intaglietta M. Systemic and subcutaneous microvascular PO2 dissociation during 4-h hemorrhagic shock in conscious hamsters. *Am J Physiol.* 1996;**270**:H827–H836.

14. Késmárky G, Kenyeres P, Rábai M, Tóth K. Plasma viscosity: a forgotten variable. *Clin Hemorheol Microcirc.* 2008;**39**:243–6.

15. Koch CG, Li L, Duncan AI, et al. Transfusion in coronary artery bypass grafting is associated with reduced long-term survival. *Ann Thorac Surg.* 2006;**81**:1650–7.

16. Li W, Tsai AG, Intaglietta M, Tartakovsky DM. A model of anemic tissue perfusion after blood transfusion shows critical role of endothelial response to shear stress stimuli. *J Appl Physiol (1985).* 2021;**131**:1815–23.

17. Lipowsky HH, Firrell JC. Microvascular hemodynamics during systemic hemodilution and hemoconcentration. *Am J Physiol.* 1986;**250**:H908–H922.

18. Lipowsky HH, Usami S, Chien S. In vivo measurements of "apparent viscosity" and

microvessel hematocrit in the mesentery of the cat. *Microvasc Res.* 1980;**19**:297–319.

19. Mahecic TT, Dünser M, Meier J. RBC transfusion triggers: is there anything new? *Transfus Med Hemother.* 2020;**47**(5) 361–8.

20. Mall F. Die Blut- und Lymphwege im Dünndarm des Hundes. *Ber Sachs Ges Akad Wiss.* 1887;**14**:153.

21. Martini J, Cabrales P, Fries D, Intaglietta M, Tsai AG. Effects of fibrinogen concentrate after shock/resuscitation: a comparison between in vivo microvascular clot formation and thromboelastometry. *Crit Care Med.* 2013;**41**:e301–8.

22. Martini J, Cabrales P, Tsai AG, Intaglietta M. Mechanotransduction and the homeostatic significance of maintaining blood viscosity in hypotension, hypertension and haemorrhage. *J Intern Med.* 2006;**259**:364–72.

23. Martini J, Maisch S, Pilshofer L, et al. Fibrinogen concentrate in dilutional coagulopathy: a dose study in pigs. *Transfusion.* 2014;**54**:149–57.

24. Melkumyants AM, Balashov SA, Khayutin VM. Endothelium dependent control of arterial diameter by blood viscosity. *Cardiovasc Res.* 1989;**23**:741–7.

25. Papenfuss HD, Gore RW, Gross JF. Effect of variable hydraulic conductivity on

transcapillary fluid exchange: application to the microcirculation of rat intestinal muscle. *Microvasc Res.* 1980;**19**:263–76.

26. Papenfuss HD, Gross JF, Intaglietta M, Treese FA. A transparent access chamber for the rat dorsal skin fold. *Microvasc Res.* 1979;**18**:311–18.

27. Shander A, Bracey AW Jr., Goodnough LT, et al. Patient blood management as standard of care. *Anesth Analg.* 2016;**123**(4):1051–3.

28. Shander A, Friedman T. The yin and yang of blood transfusion. *Turk J Anaesthesiol Reanim.* 2017;**45**:122–3.

29. Shander A, Javidroozi M, Ozawa S, Hare GM. What is really dangerous: anaemia or transfusion? *Br J Anaesth.* 2011;**107**(1):i41–59.

30. Shen W, Xu X, Ochoa M, et al. Role of nitric oxide in the regulation of oxygen consumption in conscious dogs. *Circ Res.* 1994;**75**:1086–95.

31. Tsai AG, Friesenecker B, Mazzoni MC, et al. Microvascular and tissue oxygen gradients in the rat mesentery. *Proc Nat Acad Sci.* 1998 **95**:6590–5.

32. Zimmerman R, Tsai AG, Salazar Vazquez BY, et al. Posttransfusion increase of hematocrit per se does not improve circulatory oxygen delivery due to increased blood viscosity. *Anesth Analg.* 2017;**124**(5):1547–54.

Chapter 10

Acid–Base Issues in Fluid Therapy

Niels Van Regenmortel, Wouter Rosseels,
and Paul W.G. Elbers

It is widely appreciated that the administration of intravenous fluids can exert an effect on the human acid–base status. In this chapter, we will try to elucidate the mechanisms behind this phenomenon and elaborate how it can be avoided by so-called balanced solutions. Finally, we will discuss whether there is a clinical impact of adopting an acid–base neutral fluid strategy.

An Introduction to the Stewart Approach

While the following introduction should be sufficient to provide the reader with the necessary basics to understand the effect of fluid infusion on a patient's acid–base state, a more elaborate explanation can be found in dedicated scientific literature.[1]

There are three popular methods to assess derangements in acid–base physiology. These are the bicarbonate-centered approach, the bases excess method and the Stewart approach. Essentially, these are all mathematically compatible. However, for patients with many co-existing acid–base disorders, the Stewart approach arguably provides the best insight. A potential drawback lies in its perceived complexity. Yet, as discussed below, it completely demystifies the interaction between acid–base balance and electrolyte physiology and hence the acid–base effects of fluids. The Stewart approach argues that bicarbonate does not play a causal role in acid–base disturbances. Instead, acid–base and electrolyte balances are governed by a number of physicochemical equations, derived from basic principles of physics and chemistry (Table 10.1). These must be satisfied simultaneously.

Two important concepts thus emerge. First, water is abundantly present in the body and is a virtually inexhaustible source of $[H^+]$ formation or reuptake. This is described by the water equilibrium equation. Second, as all equations must be simultaneously satisfied, it follows that only three independent parameters will ultimately determine the final equilibrium of water dissociation, and therefore also $[H^+]$ or pH. This can be mathematically expressed as:

$$[H^+]^4 + [H^+]^3 \times ([K_A] + [SID]) + [H^+]^2 \times (([K^A] \times ([SID] - [A_{TOT}]) \\ - (K_C \times PCO_2 + K'_W))) + [H^+] \times (K_A \times (K_C \times PCO_2 + K'_W) \\ + K_3 \times K_C \times PCO_2) - K_A \times K_3 \times K_C \times PCO_2 = 0$$

For bedside purposes, it is sufficient to remember that this daunting equation may be functionally represented as $[H^+] = f(PCO_2, [SID], A_{TOT})$. This implies that $[H^+]$ (and also $[HCO_3^-]$) are dependent parameters, which can only be modified by changes in the three independent parameters above.

Table 10.1 The Stewart equations

Water dissociation equilibrium	$[H^+] \times [OH^-] = K'_W$
Weak acid dissociation equilibrium	$K_A \times [HA] = [H^+] \times [A^-]$
Conservation of mass for "A"	$A_{TOT} = [A^-] + [HA]$
Bicarbonate ion formation equilibrium	$[PCO_2] \times K_C = [H^+] \times [HCO_3^-]$
Carbonate ion formation equilibrium	$[K_3] \times [HCO_3^-] = [H^+] \times [CO_3^{2-}]$
Electrical neutrality equation	$SID + [H^+] - [HCO_3^-] - [A^-] - [CO_3^{2-}] - [OH^-] = 0$

All equations reflect chemical equilibriums that need to be satisfied simultaneously. K items represent constants. Units are mEq/L for ions, mM for HA and A_{TOT} and kPa or mmHg for PCO_2. SID, strong ion difference.

PCO_2, **the partial pressure of CO_2.** It follows from the Stewart equations that if PCO_2 increases, $[H^+]$ must increase as well. This is not different from other approaches to acid–base physiology.

[SID], the strong ion difference. Strong ions are essentially completely dissociated and thus exist in charged form only. Important examples include Na^+, K^+, Ca^{2+}, Mg^{2+}, Cl^-, lactate and ketoacids. In contrast, weak ions can exist in charged and uncharged forms at the same time. Examples include HCO_3^-, albumin and inorganic phosphate. The strong ion difference is the difference between the sum of the strong cations and the sum of the strong anions. In plasma, [SID] is mainly determined by $[Na^+]$ and $[Cl^-]$ and its normal value lies around 40 mEq/L. It follows from the Stewart equations that if SID decreases, $[H^+]$ must increase and vice versa. Any pathological process that disturbs the balance between strong cations and strong anions will thus directly affect pH. This includes lactic acidosis, ketoacidosis, renal acidosis, vomiting-induced alkalosis, contraction alkalosis and most importantly iatrogenic fluid administration.

[A_{TOT}], the total amount of weak acids. Weak acids are molecules that exist in incompletely ionized forms. They are grouped as A_{TOT}, the total amount of weak acids, and consist mainly of plasma proteins. From an acid–base perspective, albumin and to a lesser extent phosphate are the most important contributors. It follows from the Stewart equations that if A_{TOT} increases, $[H^+]$ must also increase. This implies that hypoalbuminemia of any cause contributes to alkalosis. Similarly, hyperphosphatemia, as seen in renal failure, causes acidosis.

The effect of the different parameters on acidity is summarized in Figure 10.1. It is easily appreciated that a decrease in [SID] exerts the strongest effect.

Impact of Fluids on Acid–Base Status

The Pivotal Role of Crystalloid [SID]

If a patient is being resuscitated with large amounts of fluids, plasma strong ion difference will be forced in the direction of the [SID] of the fluid. For example, NaCl 0.9% has a [SID] of 0 mEq/L. Thus, giving large amounts of NaCl 0.9% will lower the normal plasma [SID]. This directly causes $[H^+]$ to rise and thus acidosis. Therefore, it is important to consider [SID] when choosing fluids for resuscitation.

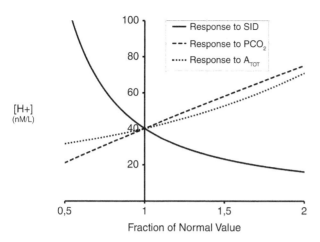

Figure 10.1 Spider plot showing the dependence of plasma pH on changes in the three independent variables: strong ion difference (SID) (normal value = 40 mEq/L), pCO_2 (normal value = 40 mmHg) and total concentration of non-volatile weak acids (A_{TOT}) (normal value = 17.2 mM/L).

Importantly, it is the [SID] rather than the chloride content per se that causes this effect. Hyperchloremic acidosis is a poor descriptor since it considers only chloride. Theoretically, it would be perfectly possible to produce a solution that is more hyperchloremic than plasma and yet would (seemingly paradoxically) lead to metabolic alkalosis, provided it contained enough cations to increase the [SID]. A fluid containing 120 mEq/L of chloride and 160 mEq/L of sodium in the absence of other strong ions is an example of such a solution. On the other hand, the use of a chloride-free solution will not per se avoid acidosis. For example, glucose and dextrose 5% do not contain any chloride and also lack strong cations, leading to a [SID] of 0 mEq/L. The acid–base effect of such a solution will be the same as NaCl 0.9% (maybe slightly less important due to an increased distribution of the fluid towards the intracellular compartment).

The only way to avoid fluid-based manipulations of the acid–base equilibrium is by using fluids that respect the human [SID] after being administered. We call these solutions "balanced," and their common characteristic lies in the fact that they contain more strong cations (mostly sodium) than strong anions (mostly chloride) and the electrical "gap" hereby created is filled by alkalinizing anions, like lactate, acetate and gluconate among others. These agents, sometimes called "buffers" (which is not the completely correct term from a chemical point of view), are metabolized after administration, exposing the solution's in vivo [SID] (versus the [SID] "in the bag," which is often 0 since lactate acts as strong anion). Classic examples of balanced solutions are Ringer's acetate and Hartmann's solution. More recent formulations are Plasma-Lyte® (Baxter, Deerfield, IL, USA) or Sterofundin ISO® (B. Braunn, Melsungen, Germany). An overview of the most common fluids with their respective [SID] is given in Table 10.2.

A relevant question is at which in vivo [SID] a solution would be completely acid–base neutral. An intuitive answer would be a [SID] comparable to that of human plasma, around 40 mEq/L. This is not correct though, as fluid administration does not only manipulate the patient's [SID], but also another independent variable, A_{TOT}, while pCO_2 is kept constant due to respiration. Morgan et al. experimentally deduced that a solution that does not alter acid–base profile needs to have a [SID] of 24 mEq/L.[2,3] Gattinoni and Carlesso et al. confirmed this finding mathematically and argued that to avoid a change in pH by diluting plasma with fluids, the [SID] of the solution has to equal the patient's bicarbonate

Table 10.2 Composition and [SID] of fluids that are frequently used across Europe. Not all solutions are available in every country

		Nutrients	Cations (mEq/L)				Anions (mEq/L)									
		Glucose (g)	Na^+	K^+	Ca^{2+}	Mg^{2+}	Cl^-	HPO_4^{2-}	HCO_3^-	Lactate	Acetate	Gluconate	Malate	SID (mEq/L)	pH	Osmolarity (mOsm/L)
Unbalanced — Hypotonic	Glucose 5%	50	0	0	0	0	0	0	0	0	0	0	0	0	4.20	278
	NaCl 0.45% in glucose 5%	50	77	0	0	0	77	0	0	0	0	0	0	0	4.30	432
	GNaK[1]	50	51	40	0	0	91	0	0	0	0	0	0	0	4.50	460
	Glucidion[2]/Bionolyte[3] 5%	50	68.4	26.8	0	0	95.2	0	0	0	0	0	0	0	4.80	467
Isotonic	NaCl 0.9%	0	154	0	0	0	154	0	0	0	0	0	0	0	5.50	308
Hypertonic	NaCl 0.9% in glucose 5%	50	154	0	0	0	154	0	0	0	0	0	0	0	3.5–6.5	585
	Tutofusin[1]	0	140	5	5	3	153	0	0	0	0	0	0	0	4.3–6.5	300
	NaCl 3%	0	513	0	0	0	513	0	0	0	0	0	0	0	5.50	1 026
	Mannitol 15%	0	0	0	0	0	0	0	0	0	0	0	0	0	4.5–7	823
Colloid	Voluven[3]	0	154	0	0	0	154	0	0	0	0	0	0	0	4–5.5	308
Balanced — Hypotonic	Glucion 5%[1]	50	54	26	0	5.2	55	12.4	0	25	0	0	0	30	4.90	447
	Rehydrex[3] 5%	50	70	0	0	0	45	0	0	0	25	0	0	25	6	440
	Hartmann's/Ringer's Lactate#	0	131	5	4	0	111	0	0	29	0	0	0	29	5–7	278
	Ringer's Acetate	0	130	5.4	1.8	2	112	0	0	0	27	0	0	27	6–8	276

Category	Solution													
Isotonic	Sterofundin ISO/Ringerfundin[2]	0	145	4	5	2	127	0	0	24	0	5	29	5.1–5.9	309
	Plasma-Lyte[1]	0	140	5	0	3	98	0	0	27	23	0	50	7.40	295
	Ionolyte[3]	0	137	4	0	3	110	0	0	34	0	0	34	6.9–7.9	286
	Sodium bicarbonate 1.3%	0	154	0	0	0	0	154	0	0	0	0	154	7–8.5	308
Hyper-tonic	Sodium bicarbonate 8.4%	0	1 000	0	0	0	0	1 000	0	0	0	0	1 000	7.0 – 8.5	2 000
Colloid	Gelofusine[2]	0	154	0	0	0	120	0	0	0	0	0	34*	7.1–7.7	274
	Geloplasma[3]	0	152	5	0	3	100	0	30	0	0	0	64*	7.1–7.7	287
	Gelaspan/Isogelo[2]	0	151	4	2	2	103	0	0	24	0	0	56*	7.1–7.7	284
	Volulyte[3]	0	137	4	0	3	110	0	0	34	0	0	34	5.7–6.5	287
	Tetraspan[2]	0	140	4	5	2	118	0	0	24	0	5	33§	5.6–6.4	296

[1] • Baxter, Deerfield, IL, USA
[2] • B. Braun, Melsungen, Germany
[3] • Fresenius Kabi, Bad Homburg, Germany
* Also contains weak acids and thus has an impact on A_{TOT}
# Slightly different formulations exist
§ Information according to product information leaflet. Electrolyte charge does not match acetate charge.

concentration.[4,5] Plasma-Lyte® has a higher in vivo SID of 50 mEq/L and could thus theoretically lead to metabolic alkalosis (also see below). On the other hand, its high [SID] can be useful in situations where hyperchloremic or other forms of metabolic acidosis are already present or in case of concomitant use of unbalanced solutions like NaCl 0.9%, for example, as diluents for medication.

Alkalinizing Agents in Balanced Solutions

A variety of alkalinizing agents for use in balanced solutions is currently available. Acetate, lactate and gluconate are the most important compounds; malate is also sometimes used.

The most frequently used metabolizable anion in crystalloid solutions remains lactate, an application that was discovered by Alexis Hartmann. In a recent animal trial, it was shown to be inferior to other agents in severe hemorrhagic shock, possibly due to an increased lactate concentration that may inhibit glycolysis and hereby energy production. In moderate hemorrhagic shock, however, it was directly metabolized hereby possibly ameliorating cardiac function and improving survival.[6]

Acetate initially got a bad reputation as an alkalinizing agent after being used in fluids for hemodialysis, where it notoriously caused vasodilation and impaired cardiac contractility, leading to cardiovascular instability. The doses that were used, however, importantly surpassed acetate's metabolization rates. In intravenous fluid management, it is nowadays generally regarded as safe.[7] It was shown to be rapidly metabolized without adverse events in an animal model of severe hemorrhagic shock.[8]

Little is known about the clinical effects of gluconate, although it is commonly used in the food industry. In a recent study, Plasma-Lyte, an acetate/gluconate-based balanced solution, was compared with Ringer's lactate in the resuscitation of critically ill burn patients. Unexpectedly in view of its higher in vivo [SID], not more metabolic alkalosis was observed with the use of Plasma-Lyte compared with Ringer's lactate.[9] A possible explanation is the slow metabolism of gluconate, which is largely excreted unchanged in urine. More hypocalcemia was observed under Plasma-Lyte, possibly explained by the chelation of calcium due to gluconate and by the absence of calcium in Plasma-Lyte (compared with Ringer's). Close monitoring of calcium levels during resuscitation with large amounts of Plasma-Lyte should therefore be considered.

Acid–Base Effects of Colloid Solutions

An important fact to acknowledge is that the acid–base effect of some colloid solutions is not only determined by their [SID], but that the colloid itself can be a source of A_{TOT}. For example gelatins are proteins that exert weak acid activity. In the bag, their net negative charge leads to a positive [SID] of the carrier crystalloid solution. Gelofusine® (B. Braun, Melsungen, Germany), a succinylated gelatin, contains 154 mEq/L sodium and 120 mEq/L chloride, while the gelatin itself accounts for remainder of the negative charge to ensure electroneutrality. Technically this makes the gelatins "spontaneously" balanced solutions, although sometimes their core crystalloid solutions can be balanced at well. Their effect on acid–base status is difficult to predict: at least until the gelatin molecules are metabolized they exert an acidifying effect through an increase in A_{TOT}. Human albumin, whether in a concentration of 4%, 5% or 20%, follows the same principle. Hydroxy-ethyl starches have no weak acid activity which makes their [SID] solely dependent on that of their carrier fluids. In an attempt to optimize these products, last generation starches were improved by balancing their vehicle solution. E.g., Volulyte® is Voluven® (both from Fresenius Kabi, Bad Homburg, Germany) in a balanced core solution. An overview of the most frequently used colloids can be found in Table 10.2.

The Treatment of Metabolic Alkalosis

A high plasma [SID], as for example seen after the loss of chloride-rich gastric juice due to vomiting or nasogastric drainage, leads to metabolic alkalosis. NaCl 0.9% would be a fair treatment choice in an attempt to reduce [SID]. The use of fluids with a negative [SID] could be an even more effective strategy. To create such fluids, strong anions should present in higher concentrations that strong cations. Solutions containing ammonium chloride are good examples. In some parts of the world dedicated preparations such as Multion Gastrique® (Baxter, Deerfield, IL, USA) are available.

The Importance of Fluid pH and Bicarbonate Content

Two common misconceptions can easily be dispelled in the light of the Stewart approach. The first is presumed effect of the pH of a solution – thus its [H^+] concentration – on acid–base status. The law of mass – on which the Stewart approach is based upon – dictates that protons cannot be added to or removed from aqueous media, but that they appear from the dissociation of water when forced to by the concentration of (the independent variables) [SID], A_{TOT} and pCO_2. The pH of a solution is a characteristic that is relevant for the tolerability of intravenous administration, but has no predictable effect on acid–base equilibrium. Another inaccurate concept is that of the dilution of bicarbonate as the cause of metabolic acidosis due to fluid loading. Bicarbonate is a weak anion and its concentration is again a dependent variable according to Stewart's theory. It will be generated from its main source, CO_2 (as the endpoint of aerobic metabolism) in an amount based upon the "gap" created by [SID]. Simplifying this process by calling it bicarbonate dilution is more than a terminological flaw, it goes against basic physical chemistry. Moreover, when administering sodium bicarbonate as an alkalinizing agent, it is the strong cation sodium, administered without any strong anion, that increases plasma [SID] and leads to the correction of metabolic acidosis. Bicarbonate should merely be seen as a fellow companion, its only role lying in ensuring electrical neutrality of the solution. Proof of this concept can be experienced in the often encountered phenomenon that sodium bicarbonate is less effective in correcting metabolic acidosis in a patient with hypernatremia.

The Clinical Relevance of Balanced Solutions

Numerous reports, most of them dating back to the 1990s, show a clear relationship between fluid therapy and the occurrence of metabolic acidosis.[10–12] Also the role of balanced solutions in avoiding this fall in base excess and resulting in a more stable acid–base profile was established in different patient populations many years ago.[13] The clinical relevance of these findings on the other hand was debated and openly doubted, especially in the light of a lack of high quality evidence.[14,15] It was the presumed negative effect of hyperchloremia on kidney function, induced by vasoconstriction of the afferent arteriole of the renal glomerulus, that lead to persistent research.[16] At first, the only available data that showed an impact on clinically relevant endpoints came from animal studies and experiments in normal volunteers. [17–20] Nephrological literature provided further, although circumstantial, evidence for the deterioration of kidney function when long-term hyperchloremic metabolic acidosis was left untreated.[21] In an experimental setting, the effects of fluid type on renal parameters could be reproduced in humans.[22]

Until recently, there was a lack of randomized-controlled trials using clinical rather than biochemical endpoints. This changed in 2013, with the multi-center, cluster-randomized, double-crossover trial, SPLIT (0.9% Saline versus Plasma-Lyte 148 for intensive care unit (ICU) fluid therapy) failed to demonstrate a difference in the incidence of acute kidney injury (RIFLE stage I or F) in ICU patients receiving Plasma-Lyte compared with NaCl 0.9%.[23] The interpretability was complicated by the low median volume that was administered (a median of 2 litres), especially since 2 litres of non-study fluid resuscitation fluid (mostly Plasma-Lyte with a SID of 50 mEq/L) had already been administered before randomization. In the SOLAR trial (Saline versus Lactated Ringer's solution), Maheshwari and colleagues compared the relative safety of saline and lactated Ringer's solution in patients undergoing elective orthopaedic and colorectal surgery. After 1.9 L of study fluid, no significant difference was observed in the primary composite outcome of hospital mortality and major postoperative complications (including acute kidney injury), [24] The BaSICS trial failed to demonstrate a difference in 90-day mortality after exposing 10 520 ICU patients to a cumulative median volume of 2.9 L of either NaCl 0.9% versus Plasma-Lyte (of which 1.5 L were administered on the first day after enrollment). The PLUS trial (Plasma-Lyte 148 versus saline) was performed in over 5000 patients who received either Plasma-Lyte 148 or NaCl 0.9% for a longer duration than in previous trials (median volume 3.9 (IQR 2–6.7) litres over 6 (IQR 3–10) days. No difference in the primary outcome of 90-day mortality was observed. [25]

Other studies yielded positive results when comparing Plasma-Lyte with NaCl 0.9%. In the SMART trial (Isotonic Solutions and Major Adverse Renal Events Trial), conducted in 5 units of a large academic ICU, the use of balanced crystalloids did reduce the incidence of the primary outcome of MAKE30 in comparison with NaCl 0.9%. MAKE30 is a composite endpoint of death, the initiation of renal replacement therapy and persistent renal dysfunction defined as a doubling of creatinine. This effect was larger in patients with sepsis and in those who had been exposed to larger volumes of crystalloids.[26] A similar result was observed in a parallel study conducted by the same researchers in non-critically ill adults presenting in the emergency department.[27]

An overview of the most important clinical studies on the use of balanced solutions in the ICU is shown in Table 10.3. A possible explanation for the discrepancy in clinical outcomes might be the overrepresentation of elective surgical patients in different trials. Surgical patients tend to be relatively healthy, and the fluid volumes needed for resuscitation are often lower. Patients in the SMART trial were predominantly admitted for sepsis or respiratory failure requiring invasive ventilation, exposing them to a higher a priori risk of acute injury and mortality. Also, it is possible that statistical power to detect a mortality difference is not sufficient, even in studies including thousands of patients. A meta-analysis conducted in 2021 concluded that the estimated effect of using balanced solutions compared with NaCl 0.9% in critically ill adult patients ranges from a relative reduction of 9% to a relative increase of 1% in the risk of death, with a high probability that the average effect of using balanced crystalloids is to reduce mortality.[28]

Table 10.3 Overview of the large studies comparing balanced solutions with NaCl 0.9% in the ICU

Study	Type	Intervention	Number of pts	Exposure	Primary outcome
Yunos et al., *JAMA* 2012 [29]	Before & After	Chloride poor vs. chloride rich	1 533 APACHE II mean score 16	Chloride 700 → 500 mmol per patient	RIFLE incidence/ class; RRT[*]
SPLIT, *JAMA* 2015 [30]	Double-blind RCT	Plasma-Lyte vs NaCl 0.9%	2 278 APACHE II mean score 14	Median 2 L study fluid after 2 L pre-study	RIFLE I or F
SMART, *NEJM* 2018 [31]	Cluster-randomized RCT	Plasma-Lyte vs NaCl 0.9%	15 802 Predicted mortality 9.5%	1 (IQR 0–3.2) L study fluid after 0L pre-study	MAKE30 (mortality, RRT, doubling of creatinine)[*]
BaSICS, *JAMA* 2021 [32]	Double-blind RCT	Plasma-Lyte vs NaCl 0.9%	11 052 APACHE II mean score 12	1.5 L in 24 h, 2.1 L *in toto*	90 d mortality
PLUS, *NEJM* 2022 [33]	Double-blind RCT	Plasma-Lyte vs NaCl 0.9%	5 037 APACHE II mean score 19	3.9 L over 6 d	90 d mortality

IQR, interquartile range; 0L, zero liters; RRT, renal replacement therapy.
* Indicates statistical significance.

Future studies might benefit from restricting enrollment to patients predicted to receive large volumes of crystalloids in the ICU to determine the critical dose beyond which the acid-effect would become clinically relevant. Awaiting more uniform results, individual patient characteristics together with cost and availability of the fluids may determine the choice for balanced solutions.

References

1. Kellum J, Elbers P, eds. *Stewart's Textbook of Acid-Base*, 2nd ed. Lulu.com.

2. Morgan TJ, Power G, Venkatesh B, et al. Acid-base effects of a bicarbonate-balanced priming fluid during cardiopulmonary bypass: comparison with Plasma-Lyte 148. A randomised single-blinded study. *Anaesth Intensive Care.* 2008;**36**(6):822–9.

3. Morgan TJ, Venkatesh B, Hall J. Crystalloid strong ion difference determines metabolic acid-base change during acute normovolaemic haemodilution. *Intensive Care Med.* 2004;**30**(7):1432–7.

4. Carlesso E, Maiocchi G, Tallarini F, et al. The rule regulating pH changes during crystalloid infusion. *Intensive Care Med.* 2011;**37**(3):461–8.

5. Gattinoni L, Carlesso E, Maiocchi G, et al. Dilutional acidosis: where do the protons come from? *Intensive Care Med.* 2009;**35**(12):2033–43.

6. Hofmann-Kiefer KF, Chappell D, Kammerer T, et al. Influence of an acetate- and a lactate-based balanced infusion solution on acid base physiology and hemodynamics: an observational pilot study. *Eur J Med Res.* 2012;**17**:21.

7. Phortmueller CA, Fleischmann E. Acetate-buffered crystalloid fluids: current knowledge, a systematic review. *J Crit Care.* 2016;**35**:96–105.

8. Rohrig R, Wegewitz C, Lendemans S, Petrat F, de Groot H. Superiority of acetate compared with lactate in a rodent model of severe hemorrhagic shock. *J Surg Res.* 2014;**186**(1):338–45.

9. Chaussard M, Depret F, Saint-Aubin O, et al. Physiological response to fluid resuscitation with Ringer lactate versus Plasmalyte in critically ill burn patients. *J Appl Physiol.* 2020;**128**:709–14.

10. Liskaser FJ, Bellomo R, Hayhoe M, et al. Role of pump prime in the etiology and pathogenesis of cardiopulmonary bypass-associated acidosis. *Anesthesiology.* 2000;**93**(5):1170–3.

11. O'Dell E, Tibby SM, Durward A, et al. Hyperchloremia is the dominant cause of metabolic acidosis in the postresuscitation phase of pediatric meningococcal sepsis. *Crit Care Med.* 2007;**35**(10):2390–4.

12. Scheingraber S, Rehm M, Sehmisch C, et al. Rapid saline infusion produces hyperchloremic acidosis in patients undergoing gynecologic surgery. *Anesthesiology.* 1999;**90**(5):1265–70.

13. Waters JH, Gottlieb A, Schoenwald P, et al. Normal saline versus lactated Ringer's solution for intraoperative fluid management in patients undergoing abdominal aortic aneurysm repair: an outcome study. *Anesth Analg.* 2001;**93**(4):817–22.

14. Handy JM, Soni N. Physiological effects of hyperchloraemia and acidosis. *Br J Anaesth.* 2008;**101**(2):141–50.

15. Roth JV. What is the clinical relevance of dilutional acidosis? *Anesthesiology.* 2001;**95**(3):810–2.

16. Hansen PB, Jensen BL, Skott O. Chloride regulates afferent arteriolar contraction in response to depolarization. *Hypertension.* 1998;**32**(6):1066–70.

17. Aksu U, Bezemer R, Yavuz B, et al. Balanced vs unbalanced crystalloid resuscitation in a near-fatal model of hemorrhagic shock and the effects on renal

oxygenation, oxidative stress, and inflammation. *Resuscitation*. 2012;**83**(6):767–73.

18. Kellum JA, Song M, Almasri E. Hyperchloremic acidosis increases circulating inflammatory molecules in experimental sepsis. *Chest*. 2006;**130**(4):962–7.

19. Wilcox CS. Regulation of renal blood flow by plasma chloride. *J Clin Invest*. 1983;**71**(3):726–35.

20. Williams EL, Hildebrand KL, McCormick SA, et al. The effect of intravenous lactated Ringer's solution versus 0.9% sodium chloride solution on serum osmolality in human volunteers. *Anesth Analg*. 1999;**88**(5):999–1003.

21. de Brito-Ashurst I, Varagunam M, Raftery MJ, et al. Bicarbonate supplementation slows progression of CKD and improves nutritional status. *J Am Soc Nephrol*. 2009;**20**(9):2075–84.

22. Chowdhury AH, Cox EF, Francis ST, et al. A randomized, controlled, double-blind crossover study on the effects of 2-L infusions of 0.9% saline and Plasma-Lyte(R) 148 on renal blood flow velocity and renal cortical tissue perfusion in healthy volunteers. *Ann Surg*. 2012;**256**(1):18–24.

23. Young P, Bailey M, Beasley R. Effect of a buffered crystalloid solution vs saline on acute kidney injury among patients in the intensive care unit. *JAMA*. 2015;**314**(16):1701–10.

24. Maheshwari K, Turan A, Makarova N, et al. Saline versus lactated Ringer's solution – The Saline or Lactated Ringer's (SOLAR) trial. *Anesthesiology*. 2020;**132**;614–24.

25. Finfer S, Micallef S, Hammond N, et al. Balanced multielectrolyte solution versus saline in critically ill adults. *N Eng J Med*. 2022;**386**(9):815–26.

26. Semler MW, Self WH, Wanderer JP, et al. Balanced crystalloids versus saline in critically ill adults. *N Eng J Med*. 2018;**378**(9):829–39.

27. Self WH, Semler MW, Wanderer JP, et al. Balanced cystalloids versus saline in noncritically ill adults. *N Eng J Med*. 2018;**378**(9):819–28.

28. Hammond NE, Zampieri FG, Di Tanna GL, et al. Balanced crystalloids versus saline in critically ill adults – a systematic review with meta-analysis. *NEJM Evid*. 2022;**1**(2).

29. Yunos NM Bellomo R, Hegarty C, et al. Association between a chloride-liberal vs chloride-restrictive intravenous fluid administration strategy and kidney injury in critically ill adults. *JAMA*. 2012;**308**(15):1566–72.

30. Young P, Bailey M, Beasley R, et al.; SPLIT Investigators. Effect of a buffered crystalloid solution vs saline on acute kidney injury among patients in the intensive care unit: the SPLIT randomized clinical trial. *JAMA*. 2015;**314**:1701–10.

31. Semier MW, Self WH, Wanderer JF, et al.; SMART Investigators and the Pragmatic Critical Care Research Group. Balanced crystalloids versus saline in critically ill adults. *N Engl J Med*. 2018;**378**(9):829–39.

32. Zampieri FG, Machado FR, Biondi RS, et al.; BaSICS Investigators and the BRICNet members. Effect of intravenous fluid treatment with a balanced solution vs 0.9% saline solution on mortality in critically ill patients: the BaSICS randomized clinical trial. *JAMA*. 2021;**326**:1–12.

33. Finfer S, Micallef S, Hammond N, et al.; PLUS Study Investigators; Australian New Zealand Intensive Care Society Clinical Trials Group. Balanced multielectrolyte solution versus saline in critically ill adults. *N Engl J. Med*. 2022;**386**:815–26.

11 Outcome and Organ Dysfunction after Major Surgery

Eryn R. Thiele, Chelsea A. Patry, Susan M. Walters
and Amanda M. Kleiman

Perioperative physicians, including surgeons and anesthesiologists, with the help of other specialists have made major strides in improving safety through improvements in knowledge, surgical techniques, equipment, medications, and other tools utilized in the perioperative period. Despite this work, the risk of mortality for adult patients undergoing noncardiac surgery remains greater than 1% with morbidity still quite common. Morbidity and mortality in the perioperative period are often related to perioperative organ dysfunction thought to be associated with the effects of surgery and anesthesia on the body. Nearly all organ systems may be affected perioperatively, with the derangements ranging from mild and temporary to permanent and potentially catastrophic. This chapter will review the impact of cardiac and non-cardiac surgery on individual organ systems and explore some of the effects of these perturbations on perioperative morbidity and mortality.

Neurological

The most devastating neurological complication in the perioperative period is stroke. The incidence of perioperative stroke in non-cardiac surgery ranges from 0.1% to 1.9% while the incidence in cardiac and major vascular surgery is 1.9% to 9.7%.[1,2] Further defining the timeline, most strokes occur during the 24 hours after surgery, with 5% to 15% of these perioperative strokes occurring immediately within the postanesthesia care unit (PACU).[3] Perioperative stroke results in both a higher mortality and an increase in morbidity.

Stroke mortality in the nonsurgical setting is 12.6%; however, the impact of a stroke is much higher when it occurs in the perioperative setting.[4] Perioperative stroke was associated with an 8-fold increase in perioperative mortality within 30 days of surgery.[5] Moreover, patients with nonfatal perioperative strokes required help with activities of daily living, and more than 50% were transferred to a long-term care facility.[6] As with non-perioperative strokes, the speed at which a perioperative stroke is treated is essential. Each hour from initial symptom to artery puncture carried with it a 5.3% absolute decrease in likelihood of functional independence as well as an absolute decrease in functional outcome.[7]

Two additional neurological sequelae that are often intertwined but separate entities are postoperative delirium (POD) and postoperative cognitive dysfunction (POCD). POD typically develops acutely after surgery, lasts hours to days, and manifests as disturbances in attention and changes in cognition.[8] Patients, surgical and nonsurgical, who experience delirium have a higher overall mortality rate with the estimated 1- and 6-month mortality rate in elderly nonsurgical patients as 14% and 22%, respectively.[9] Further studies indicated duration of delirium was the strongest independent factor in both ventilator time and intensive care unit (ICU) length of stay.[10]

Similarly, POCD is a decrease in cognitive function as compared with preoperatively that is associated with surgery affecting thought processes including executive function, attention, and concentration.[11] The decline in cognitive dysfunction is long term and can be measured via neuropsychological testing.[11] Data suggest that the development of POCD is associated with poor outcomes, which are strongly associated with preoperative cognitive function, particularly in elderly patients. The development of POCD after cardiac surgery results in a 10-fold increase in mortality and an over 7-fold risk of permanent cognitive decline including dementia.[12]

Cardiac

Major adverse cardiac events (MACE) play a significant role in adverse clinical outcomes following all surgical procedures. While there is no standard definition, MACE typically includes myocardial ischemia, heart failure, recurrent angina, need for cardiovascular intervention, and arrhythmias.[13] Studies have demonstrated that the incidence of MACE is 3% after major non-cardiac surgery and that the presence of MACE increases the risk of both in-hospital death and ischemic stroke.[14] Furthermore, myocardial ischemia is the most common cause of 30-day mortality after non-cardiac surgery.[15]

Traditionally, clinicians used clinical signs and symptoms alone to identify MACE. Advancements in laboratory tests, however, as well as more specific biomarkers have improved the ability to detect cardiovascular abnormalities. The use of high-sensitivity cardiac troponin (hs-cTn) assays, for example, have made it possible to better identify myocardial injury.[16] The higher the peak troponin value after non-cardiac surgery, the higher the risk of death.[17] Importantly, even sub-clinical, asymptomatic increases in troponin are associated with increased risk of mortality.[15] Additionally, the use of plasma brain natriuretic peptide (BNP) and plasma N-terminal pro-BNP (NT-proBNP) can be used to differentiate cardiac and non-cardiac causes of dyspnea, better diagnose heart failure, and potentially to predict outcomes after non-cardiac surgery, and length of stay.[18–19]

Postoperative atrial fibrillation (POAF) is one of the most common perioperative arrhythmias. The incidence of new onset POAF in patients undergoing cardiac surgery ranges from 18% to 32% while the incidence is closer to 1% to 2% in non-cardiac surgeries. Regardless of type of surgery, new onset POAF results in an increased risk of stroke, hospital length of stay, and both in-hospital and post-discharge mortality up to 1 year. Specifically, in non-cardiac surgical patients, POAF nearly triples the risk of stroke at 5 years.[20]

Gastrointestinal

Postsurgical gastrointestinal dysfunction, most commonly presenting as ileus, is one of the most common recognized adverse outcomes. In patients presenting for gastrointestinal surgery, a postoperative ileus can increase a patient's length of stay by 4.9–8.4 days, burdening both the patient and increasing hospital costs.[21] Though not as frequent, patients undergoing non-gastrointestinal surgeries also suffer from gastrointestinal complications and worsening postoperative outcomes, potentially placing the patient at increased risk of other complications including deep venous thrombosis, myocardial infarction, aspiration pneumonia, sepsis, and death, although causality is difficult to determine with largely retrospective studies.[22]

The postoperative gastrointestinal dysmotility that evolves into an ileus is mediated by inflammation, neural reflexes, and neurohumoral peptides. Specifically in abdominal surgery, the inflammatory response is due to manipulation and direct trauma.[23] For non-abdominal procedures, the mechanism is believed to originate from ischemia and the translocation of cytokines from the site of surgical trauma. Additionally, inhibitory neural reflexes act via noxious spinal afferent signals, increasing sympathetic activity in the gastrointestinal tract.[24] Nitric oxide, other vasoactive intestinal polypeptides, and possibly substance P are also thought to act as inhibitory neurotransmitters, slowing gut motility.[25]

While less common, other gastrointestinal complications including gastrointestinal bleeding, mesenteric ischemia, and bowel obstruction can be devastating. For example, in patients undergoing cardiac surgery, mesenteric ischemia occurs in up to 0.31% of cases, but is associated with mortality rates as high as 77%. In this same population, hemorrhage occurs in 0.52% of patients with an associated 18% mortality.[26] Bowel obstruction has a similar incidence and mortality to hemorrhage.

Hepatic

Unlike extensively studied organ systems such as the cardiovascular or gastrointestinal system, much is unknown as to the effect of perioperative hepatic dysfunction on surgical outcomes. Likewise, there are no useful treatments for hepatic injury. The elimination of halothane has greatly decreased the rate of perioperative major hepatic dysfunction; however, researchers have found that after cardiac surgery requiring cardiopulmonary bypass, 10% of patients will develop hyperbilirubinemia, which is associated with a significant increase in mortality risk. Perioperative hyperbilirubinemia has been associated with increased duration of inotropic support, mechanical ventilation requirement, and both ICU and overall length of hospital stay.[27] Periprocedural hepatic dysfunction and its effect on postoperative outcomes remains a pertinent research opportunity.

Endocrine

Perturbations in glucose metabolism, namely hyperglycemia, in the perioperative period are an extensively studied phenomena, with known detrimental effects on patient outcomes. Surgery and general anesthesia lead to a neuroendocrine stress response, with a release of hormones such as epinephrine, glucagon, cortisol, and growth hormone, as well as inflammatory cytokines. The release of these factors cause metabolic derangements including insulin resistance, decreased glucose utilization, impaired insulin secretion, and protein catabolism – all leading to hyperglycemia.[28] Within the realm of cardiac surgery, perioperative hyperglycemia is associated with worsened neurocognitive dysfunction, an increased rate of infection, an increased rate of respiratory complications, and lower 5-year survival rate.[29] In patients undergoing general, vascular, and urological surgery, intraoperative hyperglycemia is associated with surgical site infection, pneumonia, urinary tract infections, and sepsis.[30] In the orthopedic patient population, hyperglycemia confers an increased risk of both surgical site and periprosthetic infection.[31] Unfortunately, strict glucose control also does not appear to be the answer with significant evidence in the non-surgical population without an improvement in outcomes and a single study in operative patients with an association between strict glucose control and an increased risk of death and stroke.[32] Further studies are needed to determine the optimal blood glucose goal in different patient populations.

Conversely, hypoglycemia portends poor outcomes as well. In cardiac surgery, postoperative hypoglycemia is associated with both morbidity (increased number of wound infections and longer length of stay) and mortality, although it is unknown if this is causal or the result of adverse events.[32]

Pulmonary

Postoperative pulmonary complications (PPC) represent one of the most common perioperative complications, with an incidence of 1–33% depending on patient-related and surgical factors.[33] Postoperative pulmonary complications within the first week after surgery range from atelectasis and need for supplemental oxygen to pleural effusions, pneumonia, respiratory failure, reintubation, and acute respiratory distress syndrome (ARDS).[33–34] Any primary pulmonary complication significantly increases the risk of mortality in both cardiac and non-cardiac surgery.[33] A study examining postoperative pulmonary dysfunction in cardiac surgery patients found those patients to have higher serum creatinine and lactate, longer mechanical ventilation, higher infection rates, and higher incidence of low cardiac output states, in addition to higher mortality.[34] Risk factors for development of a PPC include age, proximity of surgery to the thorax, where pain can disrupt postoperative pulmonary mechanics, frailty, long-standing poor cardiopulmonary health, smoking, and obesity.[33–36]

Twenty years ago, the Acute Respiratory Distress Syndrome Network (ARDSNet) found that lung injury in critically ill patients was a modifiable risk factor for adverse outcomes by demonstrating that low tidal volume ventilation in the setting of ARDS improved mortality.[36] These "lung protective" strategies have been widely adopted with the definition of ARDS evolving over time to focus on timing, chest imaging, oxygenation, and the severity (measured by the ratio of blood oxygenation:fractional inspired oxygen concentration). The incidence of ARDS in surgical patients is fortunately low, approximately 0.2%, but the concept of poor gas exchange also explains the etiology of more common PPCs.[33]

Multiple opportunities exist to prevent the development of PPCs. Enhanced recovery pathways are increasingly used to provide preoperative access to smoking cessation and preoperative evaluation clinics, intraoperative lung protective ventilation, epidural and multimodal analgesia, and goal directed fluid therapy, and postoperative enhancement of respiratory mechanics with incentive spirometry and non-invasive ventilatory support.[37] These interventions are diverse and multidisciplinary but can have a profound impact on individual patient outcomes and overall healthcare burden.

Renal

Acute kidney injury (AKI) correlates with elevated morbidity and mortality, longer hospital stay and cost in the short term and increased risk of chronic renal insufficiency in the long term. A systematic definition for acute kidney injury was established in 2004 with the Risk, Injury, Failure, Loss, End-stage renal disease (RIFLE) criteria with modifications made in response to the significance of small changes in creatinine on mortality with the addition of the Acute Kidney Injury Network (AKIN) criteria. Patient factors related to a heightened risk of perioperative AKI include pre-existing preoperative creatinine elevation and chronic kidney disease, African American race, advanced age, congestive heart failure, insulin-dependent diabetes, pulmonary disease, obesity, and peripheral vascular disease.[38]

In non-cardiac surgery, around 6% of patients have an AKI perioperatively. Even minor changes in creatinine (25–49% above baseline) postoperatively have been found to increase the risk of death of at least 2-fold and increase length of stay by around 2 days.[39] In one large retrospective cohort, at 1 year postoperatively over a quarter of patients with AKI died compared with only 6% of patients without AKI, a hazard ratio for death of 2.96.[40]

AKI in cardiac surgery is a well-known phenomenon given prolonged ischemic times, creation of microemboli, risk of hypotension, cardiopulmonary bypass, and associated use of inotropes and vasopressors. A recent meta-analysis found the risk of AKI in this population to be 25–30%, increasing morbidity and mortality, length of stay, and cost. [41] Long-term morbidity is also increased, with patients suffering AKI after elective cardiac surgery having more than double the cumulative risk of death at 5 years than patients without AKI.[42]

Adequate resuscitation with balanced crystalloids, maintaining oxygen carrying capacity with transfusion, and avoidance of nephrotoxic agents have been related to reduction of acute kidney injury risk. Other modifiable risk factors include glycemic control and nutritional support.[38] Early identification and prevention are opportunities for reduction in AKI burden.

Ophthalmologic

Perioperative visual loss (POVL) is a rare but crippling complication occurring primarily after spine or cardiac surgery.[44–45] The incidence of POVL following spine and cardiac surgery is between 0.03–0.2% and 0.06–0.113%, respectively.[44–45] Risk factors for POVL include anemia, microemboli, hypotension, globe compression, prone positioning, duration of surgery, duration of cardiopulmonary bypass, use of vasoactive infusions, and pre-existing vascular or ocular diseases including glaucoma. Increased volume administration has been linked to POVL following both spine and cardiac surgery, prompting a preference for colloid administration by some providers and American Society of Anesthesiologists Guidelines, despite that the benefits of colloid versus crystalloid are generally lacking.[44]

While POVL is not directly linked to increases in mortality, there is no doubt regarding the effect of POVL on morbidity, greatly impacting daily quality of life in these patients. This morbidity is particularly devastating in the patient populations primarily affected, adding to their significant preoperative morbidity. While some POVL resolves spontaneously, the majority is permanent, with treatment options including acetazolamide and corticosteroids being largely ineffective.[44] Similar to the previously discussed organ systems, prevention by avoiding major physiological and hemodynamic changes and other risk factors as much as feasible is recommended for patients undergoing prolonged spine and cardiac surgeries. In high-risk patient populations, it may also be prudent to counsel patients preoperatively regarding the risk of potential POVL.

Discussion/Conclusion

While recent advancements in surgery and anesthesia have improved outcomes, unfortunately the perioperative period is associated with organ system dysfunction ranging from mild, temporary derangements to debilitating, permanent injury associated with significant morbidity and mortality. Prior to elective surgery, clinicians should aim to identify risk factors for perioperative organ dysfunction and attempt to optimize patient comorbidities. However, optimizing intraoperative management including continued improvement in surgical techniques and anesthetic management may be more fruitful, especially for urgent and emergent procedures that are typically associated with a greater risk of organ dysfunction. Improvements in diagnostic tests may allow clinicians to better detect even clinically silent organ dysfunction, allowing for prediction of outcomes in at-risk populations and prompting earlier intervention to potentially mitigate more severe and permanent organ damage.

Unfortunately, randomized controlled trials are difficult to conduct in this population due to ethical issues, which limits the availability of strong prospective evidence for clinicians regarding perioperative organ dysfunction. Ultimately, however, more studies are needed to better characterize organ dysfunction in the perioperative period and to examine strategies to prevent or mitigate organ dysfunction and improve patient outcomes.

References

1. Bateman BT, Schumacher HC, Wang S, Shaefi S, Berman MF. Perioperative acute ischemic stroke in noncardiac and nonvascular surgery: incidence, risk factors, and outcomes. *Anesthesiology*. 2009;**110**:231–8.

2. Bucerius J, Gummert JF, Borger MA, et al. Stroke after cardiac surgery: a risk factor analysis of 16,184 consecutive adult patients. *Ann Thorac Surg*. 2003;**75**:472–8.

3. Sharifpour M, Moore LE, Shanks AM, et al. Incidence, predictors, and outcomes of perioperative stroke in noncarotid major vascular surgery. *Anesth Analg*. 2013;**116**:424–34.

4. El-Saed A, Kuller LH, Newman AB, et al. Geographic variations in stroke incidence and mortality among older populations in four US communities. *Stroke*. 2006;**37**:1975–9.

5. Mashour GA, Shanks AM, Kheterpal S. Perioperative stroke and associated mortality after noncardiac, nonneurologic surgery. *Anesthesiology*. 2011;**114**:1289–96.

6. Devereaux PJ, Yang H, Yusuf S, et al.; POISE Study Group. Effects of extended-release metoprolol succinate in patients undergoing non-cardiac surgery (POISE trial): a randomised controlled trial. *Lancet*. 2008;**371**:1839–47.

7. Fransen PS, Berkhemer OA, Lingsma HF, et al.; Multicenter Randomized Clinical Trial of Endovascular Treatment of Acute Ischemic Stroke in the Netherlands Investigators. Time to reperfusion and treatment effect for acute ischemic stroke: a randomized clinical trial. *JAMA Neurol*. 2016;**73**:190–6.

8. Deiner S, Silverstein JH. Postoperative delirium and cognitive dysfunction. *Br J Anaesth*. 2009;**103**(suppl 1):i41–6.

9. Cole MG, Primeau FJ. Prognosis of delirium in elderly hospital patients. *CMAJ*. 1993;**149**:41–6.

10. Riker RR, Shehabi Y, Bokesch PM, et al.; SEDCOM (Safety and Efficacy of Dexmedetomidine Compared With Midazolam) Study Group. Dexmedetomidine vs midazolam for sedation of critically ill patients: a randomized trial. *JAMA*. 2009;**301**:489–99.

11. Steinmetz J, Christensen KB, Lund T, Lohse N, Rasmussen LS; ISPOCD Group. Long-term consequences of postoperative cognitive dysfunction. *Anesthesiology*. 2009;**110**:548–55.

12. Inouye SK. Delirium in older persons. *N Engl J Med*. 2006;**354**(11):1157–65.

13. Poudel I, Tejpal C, Rashid H, Jahan N. Major adverse cardiovascular events: an inevitable outcome of ST-elevation myocardial infarction? A literature review. *Cureus*. 2019;**11**:e5280.

14. Smilowitz NR, Gupta N, Ramakrishna H, et al. Perioperative major adverse cardiovascular and cerebrovascular events associated with noncardiac surgery. *JAMA Cardiol.* 2017;**2**:181–7.

15. Devereaux PJ, Biccard BM, Sigamani A, et al.; Writing Committee for the VSI. Association of postoperative high-sensitivity troponin levels with myocardial injury and 30-day mortality among patients undergoing noncardiac surgery. *JAMA.* 2017;**317**:1642–1.

16. Thygesen K, Alpert JS, Jaffe AS, et al.; Executive Group on behalf of the Joint European Society of Cardiology/American College of Cardiology/American Heart Association/World Heart Federation Task Force for the Universal Definition of Myocardial Infarction. Fourth universal definition of myocardial infarction (2018). *Circulation.* 2018;**138**:e618–e51.

17. Devereaux PJ, Chan MT, Alonso-Coello P, et al.; Vascular Events In Noncardiac Surgery Patients Cohort Evaluation Study I. Association between postoperative troponin levels and 30-day mortality among patients undergoing noncardiac surgery. *JAMA.* 2012;**307**:2295–304.

18. Fox AA, Nascimben L, Body SC, et al. Increased perioperative B-type natriuretic peptide associates with heart failure hospitalization or heart failure death after coronary artery bypass graft surgery. *Anesthesiology.* 2013;**119**:284–94.

19. Park JH, Shin GJ, Ryu JI, Pyun WB. Postoperative B-type natriuretic peptide levels associated with prolonged hospitalization in hypertensive patients after non-cardiac surgery. *Korean Circ J.* 2012;**42**:521–7.

20. Gialdini G, Nearing K, Bhave PD, et al. Perioperative atrial fibrillation and the long-term risk of ischemic stroke. *JAMA.* 2014;**312**:616–22.

21. Iyer S, Saunders WB, Stemkowski S. Economic burden of postoperative ileus associated with colectomy in the United States. *J Manag Care Pharm.* 2009;**15**(6):485–94

22. Swong K, Johans S, Molefe A, et al. Unintended consequences after postoperative ileus in spinal fusion patients. *World Neurosurg.* 2019;**122**:e512-e515.

23. Peters EG, Pattamatta M, Smeets BJJ, et al. The clinical and economical impact of postoperative ileus in patients undergoing colorectal surgery. *Neurogastroenterol Motil.* 2020;**32**(8):e13862.

24. Barquist E, Bonaz B, Martinez V, et al. Neuronal pathways involved in abdominal surgery-induced gastric ileus in rats. *Am J Physiol.* 1996;**270**(4 Pt 2):R888–94.

25. Kalff JC, Schraut WH, Billiar TR, Simmons RL, Bauer AJ. Role of inducible nitric oxide synthase in postoperative intestinal smooth muscle dysfunction in rodents. *Gastroenterology.* 2000 **118** (2):316–27.

26. Chaudhry R, Zaki J, Wegner R, et al. gastrointestinal complications after cardiac surgery: a nationwide population-based analysis of morbidity and mortality predictors. *J Cardiothorac Vasc Anesth.* 2017;**31**(4):1268–74.

27. Sharma P, Ananthanarayanan C, Vaidhya N, et al. Hyperbilirubinemia after cardiac surgery: An observational study. *Asian Cardiovasc Thorac Ann.* 2015;**23** (9):1039–43.

28. Schricker T, Gougeon R, Eberhart L, et al. Type 2 diabetes mellitus and the catabolic response to surgery. *Anesthesiology.* 2005;**102**(2):320–6.

29. Greco G, Ferket BS, D'Alessandro DA, et al. Diabetes and the association of postoperative hyperglycemia with clinical and economic outcomes in cardiac surgery. *Diabetes Care.* 2016;**39**(3):408–17.

30. Shanks AM, Woodrum DT, Kumar SS, Campbell DA Jr, Kheterpal S. Intraoperative hyperglycemia is independently associated with infectious complications after non-cardiac surgery. *BMC Anesthesiol.* 2018;**18**(1):90.

31. Akiboye F, Rayman G. management of hyperglycemia and diabetes in orthopedic surgery. *Curr Diab Rep.* 2017;**17**(2):13.

32. Desai SP, Henry LL, Holmes SD, et al. Strict versus liberal target range for perioperative glucose in patients undergoing coronary artery bypass grafting: a prospective randomized controlled trial. *J Thorac Cardiovasc Surg.* 2012;**143**:318–25.

33. Johnston LE, Kirby JL, Downs EA, et al.; Virginia Interdisciplinary Cardiothoracic Outcomes Research (VICTOR) Center. Postoperative hypoglycemia is associated with worse outcomes after cardiac operations. *Ann Thorac Surg.* 2017;**103** (2):526–32.

34. Odor PM, Bampoe S, Gilhooly D, et al. Perioperative interventions for prevention of postoperative pulmonary complications: systematic review and meta-analysis. *BMJ.* 2020;**368**:m540.

35. Rady MY, Ryan T, Starr NJ. Early onset of acute pulmonary dysfunction after cardiovascular surgery: risk factors and clinical outcome. *Crit Care Med.* 1997;**25**:1831–9.

36. Warner DO. Preventing postoperative pulmonary complications: the role of the anesthesiologist. *Anesthesiology.* 2000;**92**:1467–72.

37. Acute Respiratory Distress Syndrome Network, Brower RG, Matthay MA, Morris A, et al. Ventilation with lower tidal volumes as compared with traditional tidal volumes for acute lung injury and the acute respiratory distress syndrome. *N Engl J Med.* 2000;**342**(18):1301–8.

38. Odor PM, Bampoe S, Gilhooly D, et al. Perioperative interventions for prevention of postoperative pulmonary complications: systematic review and meta-analysis. *BMJ.* 2020;**368**:m540.

39. Gumbert SD, Kork F, Jackson ML, et al. Perioperative acute kidney injury. *Anesthesiology.* 2020;**132**:180–204.

40. Kork F, Balzer F, Spies CD, et al. Minor postoperative increases of creatinine are associated with higher mortality and longer hospital length of stay in surgical patients. *Anesthesiology.* 2015;**123**:1301–11.

41. O'Connor ME, Hewson RW, Kirwan, CJ, et al. Acute kidney injury and mortality 1 year after major non-cardiac surgery. *Br J Surg.* 2017;**104**:868–76.

42. Hu J, Chen R, Liu S, et al. Global incidence and outcomes of adult patients with acute kidney injury after cardiac surgery: a systematic review and meta-analysis. *J Cardiothorac Vasc Anesth.* 2016;**30**:82–9.

43. Hansen MK, Gammelager H, Mikkelsen MK, et al. Post-operative acute kidney injury and five-year risk of death, myocardial infarction, and stroke among elective cardiac surgical patients: a cohort study. *Crit Care.* 2013;**17**:R292.

44. Kla KM, Lee LA. Perioperative visual loss. *Best Pract Res Clin Anaesthesiol.* 2016;**30** (1):69–77.

45. Raphael J, Moss HE, Roth S. Perioperative visual loss in cardiac surgery. *J Cardiothorac Vasc Anesth.* 2019;**33**(5):1420–9.

Chapter 12

Perioperative Goal-Directed Hemodynamic Therapy

Sean Coeckelenbergh, Brenton Alexander, Maxime Cannesson and Alexandre Joosten

Background

Modern anesthesia has revolutionized perioperative medicine and introduced countless technological advances that have greatly improved patient safety. Anesthesiologists are now specialists in both anesthesia administration and perioperative medicine. Although morbidity and mortality have decreased concomitantly, perioperative complications still occur. These negatively impact patient well-being and significantly increase healthcare costs.[1] In 2012, an observational study reported that perioperative mortality in Europe remained as high as 4%. The same study also underlined the limitations of current perioperative medicine and the need for improved patient care.[2] High-risk patients, defined either by their age, comorbidities, or the surgery itself, make up 15% of the global surgical population and 80% of perioperative deaths.[3] The overwhelming cause of death in these patients is fundamentally due to cellular hypoxia following an inadequate balance between oxygen delivery (Do_2) and tissue metabolic demand (Vo_2).[4] While this imbalance may occur due to a wide variety of etiologies, goal-directed hemodynamic therapy (GDHT) is a strategy that aims to correct this imbalance by determining hemodynamic targets and maintaining them with specific interventions. This strategy first appeared in the 1980s and remains a key topic in perioperative and intensive care medicine today. The improvement in patient outcome following GDHT implementation has pushed perioperative clinical management to evolve from optimizing inconsistent, practitioner dependent, hemodynamic targets to more standardized and evidence-based endpoints. Currently, some teams have highlighted the benefits of individualizing GDHT by setting arterial pressure and cardiac output (CO) targets to a patient's baseline preoperative values. Despite the many documented benefits of GDHT, there still remains controversy regarding its overall impact on patient outcome. In this chapter, we aim to explain and clarify these points by taking an in-depth historical perspective on the evolution of GDHT over the past four decades.

From Maximizing Oxygen Delivery to Optimizing Stroke Volume

In 1985, Schultz et al. published a randomized controlled trial (RCT) that demonstrated the benefits of hemodynamic *maximization* in patients undergoing hip fracture repair.[5] A total of 70 patients were randomized to receive either standard care or preoperative, intraoperative, and postoperative GDHT guided invasively using a Swan–Ganz catheter. Mortality decreased 10-fold from 29% in the standard care group to 2.9% in the GDHT group. The same year, another cohort study of 220 critically ill surgical patients compared those who survived with non-survivors and determined that, despite having similar initial vital signs, those who survived had improved cardiac function, better pulmonary reserve, lower pulmonary artery pressure, increased Do_2, and increased Vo_2. Non-survivors, on the other hand, developed lactic acidosis that was attributed to a defect in oxygen extraction due to microcirculatory alterations.[6] In 1988, Shoemaker et al. demonstrated the detrimental effect of perioperative tissue oxygen debt, defined as the measured Vo_2 minus the estimated Vo_2 requirements. In their study, all patients developed tissue oxygen debt during the intraoperative and immediate postoperative periods. While survivors quickly compensated for their tissue oxygen debt, it persisted and increased in non-survivors.[7] These studies led to the hypothesis that a hemodynamic approach that aimed to *maximize* Do_2 would decrease perioperative morbidity and mortality related to tissue hypoxia.

Shoemaker et al. tested this hypothesis in a population of high-risk surgical patients in an RCT that compared standard care with or without invasive hemodynamic monitoring to a Swan–Ganz guided supra-physiological group having the following hemodynamic goals: CI > 4.5 $L/min/m^2$, Do_2 > 600 ml/min and Vo_2 > 170 $ml/min/m^2$. Patients in the supra-physiological GDHT group had less postoperative complications, shorter intensive care unit (ICU) length of stay (LOS), and reduced mortality. In 1993, Boyd et al. confirmed this hypothesis in an RCT of 107 mostly surgical trauma patients.[8] They showed once again that maximizing patient Do_2 with a supra-physiological GDHT strategy in the preoperative, intraoperative, and postoperative periods led to decreased morbidity and mortality. In a follow-up study of these patients, the authors noted that long term survival was also greater in the supra-physiological GDHT group.[9] Shoemaker and his team then attempted to refine which patients would benefit most from this strategy and the ideal time to start hemodynamic maximization in various follow-up studies.[10–12]

Other teams, however, soon published conflicting results in studies using similar designs.[13–16] In their meta-analysis of 7 studies that included a total of 1016 patients, Heyland et al. reported that a GDHT strategy targeting supra-physiological CI, Do_2, and Vo_2 in critically ill patients was not associated with decreased mortality, with the possible exception of a preoperative approach.[17] Despite these contradictory results, the search for an ideal perioperative hemodynamic strategy led several authors to create simpler GDHT strategies, such as the maximization of DO_2 by focusing predominantly on CO. In 1995, one of the initial studies aimed at stroke volume (SV) maximization through the use of transesophageal Doppler. Investigators randomized 60 cardiac surgery patients with pre-served left ventricular ejection fraction (LVEF > 50%) to receive either standard care or 200 ml boluses of hydroxyethyl starch-based colloid every 15 minutes until SV was maximized.[18] Their results confirmed that maximizing CO led to decreased postoperative complications and hospital LOS. Studying gastric mucosal perfusion with tonometric assessment of gastric intramucosal pH, the authors also demonstrated improved splanchnic perfusion in the GDHT group. Two years later, Sinclair et al. demonstrated that in patients undergoing proximal femoral fracture repair, Doppler-guided stroke volume maximization decreased postoperative complications and shortened LOS.[19] In addition, half of the patients who developed splanchnic hypoxia did not have noticeable blood pressure decrease, which reaffirms the limitation of blood pressure as a predictor of tissue oxygenation. In the years that followed, many RCTs demonstrated that, when compared with fluid management guided by static parameters such as central venous pressure and heart rate, a GDHT strategy leads to decreased postoperative complications, less postoperative ileus, and shorter length of stay in various surgical populations.[20,21]

From 1985 to 2000, surgeons, intensivists and anesthesiologists pioneered strategies based on "supra-physiological" maximization of hemodynamics to improve outcome in high-risk patients.[22] Such strategies had their limitations, especially in patients unable to improve their hemodynamic status despite aggressive use of fluids, vasopressors, and inotropes.[23,24] Maximizing SV, for example, could lead to complications associated with fluid overload.[25] Using this line of logic and taking into consideration each individual patient's hemodynamic responses to various interventions, a better approach has since been described that aims to limit fluid infusion in order to *optimize*, and not *maximize*, SV. This approach adapts to each patient's fluid responsiveness and takes a more individualized and refined approach by moving beyond simply maximizing physiological variables.[26] In the following years, anesthesiologists would simplify these strategies with a strong focus mainly on CO optimization, while a concomitant paradigm shift would push fluid administration away from the arbitrary concept of "restrictive versus liberal fluid therapy" towards a more personalized "goal-directed" strategy.

Fluid Therapy: Breaking Away from the "Restrictive versus Liberal" Paradigm

Before Mythen et al.'s demonstration of the potential for SV optimization using colloids guided by transesophageal Doppler,[18] most anesthesiologists administered liberal amounts of fluid using static parameters such as blood pressure, heart rate, and central venous pressure. Arguments for a liberal approach included fluid losses from preoperative fasting, insensible losses, diuresis, hemorrhage, and third space redistribution. However, the clinical relevance of several of these phenomena, such as preoperative fasting deficits, insensible fluid losses, and "third spacing," have never been definitively demonstrated.[27] This realization and the increased evidence of the negative impact of excessive fluids led progressively towards a generalized shift from liberal to restrictive fluid management.[28,29]

At the start of the twenty-first century, numerous teams compared restrictive versus liberal fluid strategies.[30] In a multicenter RCT of 172 patients, Brandstrup et al. found that a restrictive approach (i.e., volume-to-volume compensation with a colloid), when compared with what at that time was standard care (i.e., 3–7 ml/kg/h crystalloid third space loss compensation with 1000–1500 ml of crystalloid for up to a 500 ml loss followed by colloid infusion for greater losses), was associated with decreased postoperative morbidity.[28] More recently, however, Myles et al. showed in a large trial of over 3000 patients that there was no difference in long-term outcome when comparing "restrictive versus liberal" approaches and that a restrictive approach could even be associated with a higher rate of acute kidney injury in high-risk patients during major abdominal surgery.[30]

This fluid management controversy, which has spanned over two decades, is in large part due to the lack of clear definitions of "restrictive" and "liberal." For example, the definitions of "restrictive" and "liberal" fluid regimens were quite different in all of the above studies. A better approach than using poorly defined gross categorizations would be to take a step back and look at the issue from another perspective: would it not be better to optimize the patient's cardiac preload using an individualized goal-directed fluid strategy?

Heart–Lung Interactions: Clear Goals for Fluid Administration

Despite its monitoring strengths, the pulmonary artery catheter is consistently limited by the significant invasiveness intrinsic to its placement. Other, less invasive tools, such as transesophageal Doppler, are available but have their own limitations (e.g., a considerable learning curve). Pulse contour technology derived from the heart–lung interactions, however, provides a means for both semi-invasive and completely non-invasive hemodynamic guidance of GDHT.[31] Moving forward, there is preliminary evidence that it is even possible to use smartphone technology to measure stroke volume or pulse pressure variation.[32–36] Cyclic increases in intrathoracic pressure during mechanical ventilation change both right and left ventricular afterload and preload. Increased intrathoracic pressure decreases venous return and pushes systemic arterial blood away from the heart and the chest. The decrease in intrathoracic pressure during expiration has the opposite effect. This leads to variations in stroke volume that can be indirectly seen as variations in arterial pulse pressure (i.e., the difference in systolic and diastolic blood pressure). These variations are greater in hypovolemic patients and decrease with fluid administration if the patient is fluid responsive.[37]

The most commonly used dynamic parameters derived from heart–lung interactions are pulse pressure variation (PPV), stroke volume variation (SVV), and the Pleth Variability Index (PVI). All have been proposed as useful tools to guide preload optimization strategies. [38–41] These dynamic parameters have been evaluated in multiple studies and are now an essential part of GDHT.[31] Although heart–lung interactions provide a means for evaluating fluid responsiveness, several conditions, in addition to mechanical ventilation, are needed for the monitor to provide valid information. For pulse contour analysis, patients must be in sinus rhythm, at least 8 ml/kg (ideal body weight) of tidal volume for the most validated thresholds to be accurate, and a heart rate to respiratory rate ratio greater than 3.6. Arrhythmias, aortic regurgitation, sternotomy, thoracotomy, and right ventricular failure all negatively impact the capacity of these parameters to predict fluid responsiveness.[42] Under recognized conditions, SVV and PPV can predict fluid responsiveness (i.e., preload dependence) if their values are above 12–13%.[31] If the values are under 9%, patients are almost certainly no longer fluid responsive and additional fluids may be inadequate. For 25% of patients, however, there is a "gray zone" where SVV and PVV values between 9% and 12% may or may not predict fluid responsiveness.[43]

Multiple studies have shown the benefits of SV and CO optimization during non-cardiac surgery, emphasizing the importance of applying this strategy in high-risk patients.[44] Despite the abundance of evidence for using such dynamic indicators of fluid responsiveness to guide perioperative preload optimization strategies, many practicing anesthesiologists still only use static parameters such as blood pressure, heart rate, diuresis, and central venous pressure.[45] Static parameters do not predict fluid responsiveness consistently and cannot guide a GDHT strategy reliably.[46] Clinician skepticism and poor compliance to GDHT protocols have thus been a major limitation in improving care in high-risk surgical patients.[47]

Current Perioperative GDHT Controversy

GDHT has thus been shown to improve both intraoperative hemodynamic parameters and patient outcome. Despite many publications demonstrating its benefits, GDHT remains a subject of heated debate, and large randomized trials continue to have mitigated results. [48–55] One example of this is a recent RCT demonstrating no improvement of GDHT during emergency laparotomy for abdominal surgery.[56] Several potential causes may be at the root of these discrepancies, the discussion of which is worth having.

Firstly, it is illusory to think that in the twenty-first century, when postoperative mortality ranges from 2 to 4% in high-risk surgery,[2] that one intervention can improve survival. Instead, it is of greater interest to investigate individual causes of morbidity, such as kidney injury, anastomotic leakage, infection, and other complications that strongly affect patient outcome and well-being. Secondly, it is important to underline that what is standard care today actually incorporates GDHT. Although there is still some resistance to implementing GDHT, indicators of fluid responsiveness, such as PPV, appear automatically on many contemporary monitors. Clinicians that have access to this information will consequently be influenced to administer fluids when they notice that PPV values are elevated even if they do not explicitly consider their hemodynamic management as goal-directed. As an example, in a recently published RCT by de Waal et al.,[49] the standard care group of anesthesiologists administered fluids to correct hypotension based on "local practice." Did they display PPV, a readily available indicator of fluid responsiveness, in certain centers? If so, this could in itself be considered goal-directed therapy in the standard care group. Similar to the sepsis GDHT trials, better standards of care, promoted by the initial publications that demonstrated improved outcome during GDHT, have led clinicians to change their practice and integrate advanced monitoring variables into their decision making and thus improve outcome in standard care groups. Finally, many studies, including de Waal's recent RCT, do not measure protocol compliance. If compliance is low in the GDHT group and clinicians have access to indicators of fluid responsiveness, finding a difference between groups is nearly impossible. Poor protocol compliance, unrealistic endpoints, and improved standard care (e.g., by implementing tools such as PPV) have thus significantly contributed to the current GDHT controversy.

Individualized Hemodynamic Therapy: The Next Step in Improving Patient Care?

Over the past four decades, the advances in hemodynamic monitoring and demonstrated benefits of GDHT have improved the standard of care (Fig. 12.1). Clinicians today consistently use blood pressure thresholds (e.g., 65 mmHg) for fluid and vasopressor administration and many also use indicators of fluid responsiveness such as PPV or SVV. This protocolized approach has decreased the high variability of patient care, such as a liberal or restrictive fluid administration, and may be part of the reason for non-significant results in recent publications. However, a novel approach to further improving patient care is now emerging: individualizing hemodynamics.[57–60]

Individualizing care entails that patient hemodynamics are optimized based on their baseline values. Instead of targeting the same threshold for every patient, blood pressure, stroke volume, and cardiac index are maintained within a small range of their preoperative values. Several studies have already pioneered this next step in GDHT. In a multicenter RCT, Futier et al. demonstrated that maintaining SBP within 10% of baseline values led to decreased postoperative morbidity.[61] Nicklas et al. individualized cardiac output by administering fluids and dobutamine to maintain the baseline pre-induction cardiac index.[62] They also demonstrated improved postoperative outcome in the individualized GDHT group. In a post-hoc secondary analysis, the authors also reported that intraoperative personalized GDHT reduced the incidence of acute myocardial injury compared with routine hemodynamic management in high-risk patients having major abdominal surgery. [55] Promising, individualized GDHT, however, is still dependent on protocol compliance.

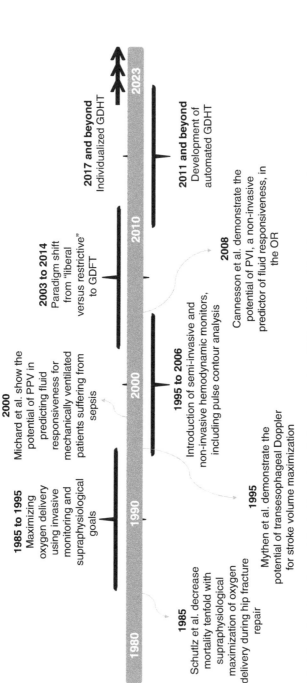

Figure 12.1 Evolution of perioperative goal-directed hemodynamic therapy over time. GDFT, goal-directed fluid therapy; PPV, pulse pressure variation; GDHT, goal-directed hemodynamic therapy; OR, operating room. A black and white version of this figure will appear in some formats. For the color version, please refer to the plate section.

Assisting clinicians with decision support or even closed-loop systems has also shown promise in maintaining individualized GDHT targets and may even further improve patient outcome.[63–73]

Conclusion

Perioperative GDHT has greatly evolved over the past four decades. Early hemodynamic management was marked by high variability in endpoints and, as a result, was very practitioner dependent. After the development of the concept of GDHT in the 1980s, paradigms such as restrictive and liberal fluid infusions began to lose credibility and perioperative care progressively became standardized (e.g., maintaining PPV under 13% and mean arterial pressure above 65 mmHg). Today, the current challenges of GDHT are the lack of compliance and the unique variability of each patient's physiology. By further individualizing hemodynamic targets and using systems to increase compliance (e.g., closed loops), we may be able to begin a new phase of GDHT that can further improve perioperative patient care and outcomes.

References

1. Pirson M, Dehanne F, Van den Bulcke J, et al. Evaluation of cost and length of stay, linked to complications associated with major surgical procedures. *Acta Clin Belg.* 2018;**73**(1):40–9.

2. Pearse RM, Moreno RP, Bauer P, et al. Mortality after surgery in Europe: a 7 day cohort study. *Lancet.* 2012;**380** (9847):1059–65.

3. Pearse RM, Harrison DA, James P, et al. Identification and characterisation of the high-risk surgical population in the United Kingdom. *Crit Care.* 2006;**10** (3):R81.

4. Bennett-Guerrero E, Welsby I, Dunn TJ, et al. The use of a postoperative morbidity survey to evaluate patients with prolonged hospitalization after routine, moderate-risk, elective surgery. *Anesth Analg.* 1999;**89**(2):514–19.

5. Schultz RJ, Whitfield GF, LaMura JJ, Raciti A, Krishnamurthy S. The role of physiologic monitoring in patients with fractures of the hip. *J Trauma.* 1985;**25** (4):309–16.

6. Bland RD, Shoemaker WC, Abraham E, Cobo JC, Hemodynamic and oxygen transport patterns in surviving and nonsurviving postoperative patients. *Crit Care Med.* 1985;**13**(2):85–90.

7. Shoemaker WC, Appel PL, Kram HB. Tissue oxygen debt as a determinant of lethal and nonlethal postoperative organ failure. *Crit Care Med.* 1988;**16** (11):1117–20.

8. Boyd O, Grounds RM, Bennett ED. A randomized clinical trial of the effect of deliberate perioperative increase of oxygen delivery on mortality in high-risk surgical patients. *JAMA.* 1993;**270** (22):2699–2707.

9. Rhodes A, Cecconi M, Hamilton M, et al. Goal-directed therapy in high-risk surgical patients: a 15-year follow-up study. *Intensive Care Med.* 2010;**36**(8):1327–32.

10. Fleming A, Bishop M, Shoemaker W, et al. Prospective trial of supranormal values as goals of resuscitation in severe trauma. *Arch Surg.* 1992;**127**(10):1175–1179; discussion 1179–81.

11. Shoemaker WC, Appel PL, Kram HB, Bishop MH, Abraham E. Sequence of physiologic patterns in surgical septic shock. *Crit Care Med.* 1993;**21** (12):1876–89.

12. Bishop MH, Shoemaker WC, Appel PL, et al. Relationship between supranormal circulatory values, time delays, and outcome in severely traumatized patients. *Crit Care Med.* 1993;**21**(1):56–63.

13. Tuchschmidt J, Fried J, Astiz M, Rackow E. Elevation of cardiac output and oxygen delivery improves outcome in septic shock. *Chest*. 1992;**102**(1):216–20.

14. Yu M, Levy MM, Smith P, et al. Effect of maximizing oxygen delivery on morbidity and mortality rates in critically ill patients: a prospective, randomized, controlled study. *Crit Care Med*. 1993;**21**(6):830–8.

15. Hayes MA, Timmins AC, Yau EH, et al. Elevation of systemic oxygen delivery in the treatment of critically ill patients. *N Engl J Med*. 1994;**330**(24):1717–22.

16. Gattinoni L, Brazzi L, Pelosi P, et al. A trial of goal-oriented hemodynamic therapy in critically ill patients. SvO2 Collaborative Group. *N Engl J Med*. 1995;**333** (16):1025–32.

17. Heyland DK, Cook DJ, King D, Kernerman P, Brun-Buisson C. Maximizing oxygen delivery in critically ill patients: a methodologic appraisal of the evidence. *Crit Care Med*. 1996;**24** (3):517–24.

18. Mythen MG, Webb AR. Perioperative plasma volume expansion reduces the incidence of gut mucosal hypoperfusion during cardiac surgery. *Arch Surg*. 1995;**130**(4):423–9.

19. Sinclair S, James S, Singer M. Intraoperative intravascular volume optimisation and length of hospital stay after repair of proximal femoral fracture: randomised controlled trial. *BMJ*. 1997;**315** (7113):909–12.

20. Phan TD, Ismail H, Heriot AG, Ho KM. Improving perioperative outcomes: fluid optimization with the esophageal Doppler monitor, a metaanalysis and review. *J Am Coll Surg*. 2008;**207**(6):935–41.

21. Bundgaard-Nielsen M, Secher NH, Kehlet H. "Liberal" vs. "restrictive" perioperative fluid therapy – a critical assessment of the evidence. *Acta Anaesthesiol Scand*. 2009;**53** (7):843–51.

22. Kern JW, Shoemaker WC. Meta-analysis of hemodynamic optimization in high-risk patients. *Crit Care Med*. 2002;**30** (8):1686–92.

23. Vallet B, Chopin C, Curtis SE, et al. Prognostic value of the dobutamine test in patients with sepsis syndrome and normal lactate values: a prospective, multicenter study. *Crit Care Med*. 1993;**21** (12):1868–75.

24. Rhodes A, Lamb FJ, Malagon I, et al. A prospective study of the use of a dobutamine stress test to identify outcome in patients with sepsis, severe sepsis, or septic shock. *Crit Care Med*. 1999;**27**(11):2361–6.

25. Challand C, Struthers R, Sneyd JR, et al. Randomized controlled trial of intraoperative goal-directed fluid therapy in aerobically fit and unfit patients having major colorectal surgery. *Br J Anaesth*. 2012;**108**(1):53–62.

26. Coeckelenbergh S, Van der Linden P, Rinehart J, Joosten A. Reply to: implementation of closed-loop-assisted intra-operative goal-directed fluid therapy during surgery. *Eur J Anaesthesiol*. 2019;**36** (4):304–5.

27. Chappell D, Jacob M, Hofmann-Kiefer K, Conzen P, Rehm M. A rational approach to perioperative fluid management. *Anesthesiology*. 2008;**109**(4):723–40.

28. Brandstrup B, Tønnesen H, Beier-Holgersen R, et al. Effects of intravenous fluid restriction on postoperative complications: comparison of two perioperative fluid regimens: a randomized assessor-blinded multicenter trial. *Ann Surg*. 2003;**238**(5):641–8.

29. Lobo DN, Bostock KA, Neal KR, et al. Effect of salt and water balance on recovery of gastrointestinal function after elective colonic resection: a randomised controlled trial. *Lancet*. 2002;**359**(9320):1812–18.

30. Myles PS, Bellomo R, Corcoran T, et al. Restrictive versus liberal fluid therapy for major abdominal surgery. *N Engl J Med*. 2018;**378**(24):2263–74.

31. Suehiro K, Joosten A, Alexander B, Cannesson M. Guiding goal-directed therapy. *Curr Anesthesiol Rep*. 2014;**4** (4):360–75.

32. Hoppe P, Gleibs F, Briesenick L, Joosten A, Saugel B. Estimation of pulse pressure

variation and cardiac output in patients having major abdominal surgery: a comparison between a mobile application for snapshot pulse wave analysis and invasive pulse wave analysis. *J Clin Monit Comput.* 2021;**35**(5):1203–9.

33. Joosten A, Boudart C, Vincent JL, et al. Ability of a new smartphone pulse pressure variation and cardiac output application to predict fluid responsiveness in patients undergoing cardiac surgery. *Anesth Analg.* 2019;**128**(6):1145–51.

34. Desebbe O, Vincent JL, Saugel B, Rinehart J, Joosten A. Pulse pressure variation using a novel smartphone application (Capstesia) versus invasive pulse contour analysis in patients undergoing cardiac surgery: a secondary analysis focusing on clinical decision making. *J Clin Monit Comput.* 2020;**34**(2):379–80.

35. Joosten A, Jacobs A, Desebbe O, et al. Monitoring of pulse pressure variation using a new smartphone application (Capstesia) versus stroke volume variation using an uncalibrated pulse wave analysis monitor: a clinical decision making study during major abdominal surgery. *J Clin Monit Comput.* 2019;**33**(5):787–93.

36. Desebbe O, Joosten A, Suehiro K, et al. A novel mobile phone application for pulse pressure variation monitoring based on feature extraction technology: a method comparison study in a simulated environment. *Anesth Analg.* 2016;**123**(1):105–13.

37. Michard F. Changes in arterial pressure during mechanical ventilation. *Anesthesiology.* 2005;**103**(2):419–28.

38. Coeckelenbergh S, Delaporte A, Ghoundiwal D, et al. Pleth Variability Index versus pulse pressure variation for intraoperative goal-directed fluid therapy in patients undergoing low-to-moderate risk abdominal surgery: a randomized controlled trial. *BMC Anesthesiol.* 2019;**19**(1):34.

39. Fischer MO, Lemoine S, Tavernier B, et al. Individualized fluid management using the Pleth Variability Index: a randomized clinical trial. *Anesthesiology.* 2020;**133**(1):31–40.

40. Cannesson M, Ramsingh D, Rinehart J, et al. Perioperative goal-directed therapy and postoperative outcomes in patients undergoing high-risk abdominal surgery: a historical-prospective, comparative effectiveness study. *Crit Care.* 2015;**19**(1):261.

41. Fischer MO, Fiant AL, Debroczi S, et al. Perioperative non-invasive haemodynamic optimisation using photoplethysmography: a randomised controlled trial and meta-analysis. *Anaesth Crit Care Pain Med.* 2020;**39**(3):421–8.

42. Michard F, Chemla D, Teboul JL. Applicability of pulse pressure variation: how many shades of grey? *Crit Care.* 2015;**19**(1):144.

43. Cannesson M, Le Manach Y, Hofer CK, et al. Assessing the diagnostic accuracy of pulse pressure variations for the prediction of fluid responsiveness: a "gray zone" approach. *Anesthesiology.* 2011;**115**(2):231–41.

44. Messina A, Robba C, Calabrò L, et al. Association between perioperative fluid administration and postoperative outcomes: a 20-year systematic review and a meta-analysis of randomized goal-directed trials in major visceral/noncardiac surgery. *Crit Care.* 2021;**25**(1):43.

45. Cannesson M, Pestel G, Ricks C, Hoeft A, Perel A. Hemodynamic monitoring and management in patients undergoing high risk surgery: a survey among North American and European anesthesiologists. *Crit Care.* 2011;**15**(4):R197.

46. Marik PE, Cavallazzi R. Does the central venous pressure predict fluid responsiveness? An updated meta-analysis and a plea for some common sense. *Crit Care Med* 2013;**41**(7):1774–81.

47. Joosten A, Rinehart J, Cannesson M. Perioperative goal directed therapy: evidence and compliance are two sides of the same coin. *Rev Esp Anestesiol Reanim.* 2015;**62**(4):181–3.

48. Calvo-Vecino JM, Ripollés-Melchor J, Mythen MG, et al. Effect of goal-directed haemodynamic therapy on postoperative complications in low-moderate risk surgical patients: a multicentre randomised controlled trial (FEDORA trial). *Br J Anaesth*. 2018;**120**(4):734–44.

49. De Waal EEC, Frank M, Scheeren TWL, et al. Perioperative goal-directed therapy in high-risk abdominal surgery. A multicenter randomized controlled superiority trial. *J Clin Anesth*. 2021;**75**:110506.

50. Yu J, Che L, Zhu A, Xu L, Huang Y. Goal-directed intraoperative fluid therapy benefits patients undergoing major gynecologic oncology surgery: a controlled before-and-after study. *Front Oncol*. 2022;**12**:833273.

51. Tang W, Qiu Y, Lu H, Xu M, Wu J. Stroke volume variation-guided goal-directed fluid therapy did not significantly reduce the incidence of early postoperative complications in elderly patients undergoing minimally invasive esophagectomy: a randomized controlled trial. *Front Surg*. 2021;**8**:794272.

52. Jessen MK, Vallentin MF, Holmberg MJ, et al. Goal-directed haemodynamic therapy during general anaesthesia for noncardiac surgery: a systematic review and meta-analysis. *Br J Anaesth*. 2022;**128**(3):416–33.

53. Pearse RM, Harrison DA, MacDonald N, et al. Effect of a perioperative, cardiac output-guided hemodynamic therapy algorithm on outcomes following major gastrointestinal surgery: a randomized clinical trial and systematic review. *JAMA*. 2014;**311**(21):2181–90.

54. Lima MF, Mondadori LA, Chibana AY, et al. Outcome impact of hemodynamic and depth of anesthesia monitoring during major cancer surgery: a before-after study. *J Clin Monit Comput*. 2019;**33**(3):365–71.

55. Kouz K, Bergholz A, Diener O, et al. Effect of intraoperative personalized goal-directed hemodynamic management on acute myocardial injury in high-risk patients having major abdominal surgery: a post-hoc secondary analysis of a randomized clinical trial. *J Clin Monit Comput*. 2022;**36**(6):1775–83.

56. Aaen AA, Voldby AW, Storm N, et al. Goal-directed fluid therapy in emergency abdominal surgery: a randomised multicentre trial. *Br J Anaesth*. 2021;**127**(4):521–31.

57. Vincent JL, Joosten A, Saugel B. Hemodynamic monitoring and support. *Crit Care Med*. 2021;**49**(10):1638–50.

58. Michard F. Toward precision hemodynamic management. *Crit Care Med*. 2017;**45**(8):1421–3.

59. Saugel B, Michard F, Scheeren TWL. Goal-directed therapy: hit early and personalize! *J Clin Monit Comput*. 2018;**32**(3):375–7.

60. Saugel B, Vincent JL. Protocolised personalised peri-operative haemodynamic management. *Eur J Anaesthesiol*. 2019;**36**(8):551–4.

61. Futier E, Lefrant JY, Guinot PG, et al. Effect of individualized vs standard blood pressure management strategies on postoperative organ dysfunction among high-risk patients undergoing major surgery: a randomized clinical trial. *JAMA*. 2017;**318**(14):1346–57.

62. Nicklas JY, Diener O, Leistenschneider M, et al. Personalised haemodynamic management targeting baseline cardiac index in high-risk patients undergoing major abdominal surgery: a randomised single-centre clinical trial. *Br J Anaesth*. 2020;**125**(2):122–32.

63. Maheshwari K, Malhotra G, Bao X, et al. Assisted fluid management software guidance for intraoperative fluid administration. *Anesthesiology*. 2021;**135**(2):273–83.

64. Joosten A, Hafiane R, Pustetto M, et al. Practical impact of a decision support for goal-directed fluid therapy on protocol adherence: a clinical implementation study in patients undergoing major abdominal surgery. *J Clin Monit Comput*. 2019;**33**(1):15–24.

65. Joosten A, Coeckelenbergh S, Alexander B, Cannesson M, Rinehart J. Feasibility of computer-assisted vasopressor infusion using continuous non-invasive blood

pressure monitoring in high-risk patients undergoing renal transplant surgery. *Anaesth Crit Care Pain Med.* 2020;**39**(5):623–4.

66. Joosten A, Chirnoaga D, Van der Linden P, et al. Automated closed-loop versus manually controlled norepinephrine infusion in patients undergoing intermediate- to high-risk abdominal surgery: a randomised controlled trial. *Br J Anaesth.* 2021;**126**(1):210–18.

67. Desebbe O, Rinehart J, Van der Linden P, et al. Control of postoperative hypotension using a closed-loop system for norepinephrine infusion in patients after cardiac surgery: a randomized trial. *Anesth Analg.* 2022;**134**(5):964–73.

68. Rinehart J, Cannesson M, Weeraman S, et al. Closed-loop control of vasopressor administration in patients undergoing cardiac revascularization surgery. *J Cardiothorac Vasc Anesth.* 2020;**34**(11):3081–5.

69. Joosten A, Rinehart J, Bardaji A, et al. Anesthetic management using multiple closed-loop systems and delayed neurocognitive recovery: a randomized controlled trial. *Anesthesiology.* 2020;**132**(2):253–66.

70. Coeckelenbergh S, Zaouter C, Alexander B, et al. Automated systems for perioperative goal-directed hemodynamic therapy. *J Anesth.* 2020;**34**(1):104–14.

71. Joosten A, Alexander B, Duranteau J, et al. Feasibility of closed-loop titration of norepinephrine infusion in patients undergoing moderate- and high-risk surgery. *Br J Anaesth.* 2019;**123**(4):430–8.

72. Joosten A, Coeckelenbergh S, Delaporte A, et al. Implementation of closed-loop-assisted intra-operative goal-directed fluid therapy during major abdominal surgery: a case-control study with propensity matching. *Eur J Anaesthesiol.* 2018;**35**(9):650–8.

73. Michard F, Biais M. Predicting fluid responsiveness: time for automation. *Crit Care Med.* 2019;**47**(4):618–20.

Chapter 13

Fluid Responsiveness Assessment

Antonio Messina, Lorenzo Calabrò and Maurizio Cecconi

Introduction

When oxygen delivery doesn't meet a patient's demand, an attempt to increase cardiac output (CO) may be effective to correct the peripheral oxygen debit. When the heart of a patient is preload dependent, fluid administration will increase right ventricular end-diastolic volume (RVEDV) and, according to the Frank–Starling law, stroke volume (SV) and CO. The fluid challenge (FC) is a standardized bolus of fluids (in terms of amount and rate of administration) infused with the purpose of enhancing preload dependency. When FC increases CO above a predefined threshold, the patient is then defined as fluid responsive.

At first, static parameters of preload reserve were developed to assess fluid responsiveness, yet they proved unreliable for this purpose. Dynamic indexes and functional hemodynamic tests (FHT) are effective in predicting fluid responsiveness and, as a consequence, tailoring fluid therapy to avoid inappropriate fluid administration and potentially harmful fluid overload.

This chapter will analyze methods and variables to assess fluid responsiveness in the perioperative setting, how to perform functional hemodynamic tests and how to interpret them considering potential confounding factors and limitations.

Fluid Challenge, Fluid Responsiveness, Fluid Balance and Fluid Optimization: An Integrated View

Postoperative complications occur in a significant proportion of patients undergoing surgery,[1–3] leading to mortality of about 4% in Europe,[4] and having a significant impact on long-term morbidity and, in turn, on health and financial systems.[5,6] Several aspects including preoperative frailty, intraoperative management and events and postoperative care may influence the risk of developing postoperative complications.

Perioperative fluid therapy is a key component of the management of surgical patients and that's why dedicated algorithms and protocols are nowadays included in routine anesthetic care and perioperative care schemes with the aim of balancing the risk of hypovolemia and hypervolemia, which are both associated with worse postoperative outcomes and length of hospital stay.[7–10]

The most effective perioperative overall fluid management is still unclear.[11–14] The Enhanced Recovery After Surgery (ERAS) pathways to support early recovery among patients undergoing major surgery recommend a restrictive approach aiming for the perioperative "zero-balance."[11] In contrast, a recent large randomized-controlled trial (RCT) assigning 2983 patients to either zero-balance or liberal strategy showed comparable disability-free survival outcomes, although the zero-balance approach was associated with a higher rate of acute kidney injury.[15] Moreover, the definitions adopted in the past to define a perioperative fluid approach as restrictive (<1.75 litres per day), balanced (1.75 to 2.75 litres per day) and liberal (>2.75 litres per day) [15] are often overlapped.[16] For all these reasons a moderately positive fluid balance of 1 to 2 litres at the end of surgery is nowadays suggested.[13]

From a different perspective, the so-called perioperative goal-directed therapy (GDT) is based on balancing the increased oxygen demand during surgery by optimizing flow-based hemodynamic parameters.[17–19] Adopting the GDT approach, perioperative overall fluid administration by using repetitive FCs is one of the strategies to achieve a predefined hemodynamic endpoint and not the endpoint itself, irrespective of the final dose needed.

This difference is crucial since the use of a GDT is closely linked to the prediction of fluid responsiveness before administering a FC or to the use of small aliquots of fluids to test for preload dependency. Since the only reason to give fluids should be to increase the SV, the consequent physiological approach to perioperative fluid administration should be based on the integrated use of the FC and FHTs guided by a continuous hemodynamic monitoring.

The Fluid Challenge in the Operating Room

The FC was introduced as a method of identifying those patients likely to benefit from an increase in intravenous volume in order to guide further volume resuscitation.[20] This dynamic test consists of administering an aliquot of fluid over a short period of time.[20,21] The FC is the safest way to administer fluids when the balance between a positive or a negative response is uncertain.[22]

The FC effect is closely linked to two main variables, which are associated with the effect of this test on the heart's ventricles: the amount of fluid administered and the time over which it is given (i.e., the rate of fluid administration). The volume must be sufficient to elicit a stretch in the right ventricular fibres and exploit the Frank–Starling mechanism to increase CO; hence, too little fluid may not result in any significant hemodynamic effect. The minimal dose of FC affecting the final response has been assessed in a recent study on postoperative cardiac patients and defined as at least 4 ml/kg,[23] which is also comparable to the dose of an FC usually adopted in the GDT studies (250 ml).[24]

Moreover, the rate of administration may influence the final FC response. A recent randomized small-sized study was conducted on neurosurgical patients during a period of hemodynamic stability, and it showed that the infusion time of FC administration affects the rate of fluid responsiveness, which shifted from 51.0% after a 4 ml/kg FC was completed within 10 minutes to 28.5% after an FC was completed within 20 minutes.[25] It is intuitive that a very slow rate of infusion would not be sufficient to provide a significant hemo-dynamic effect; moreover, many other variables (i.e., patient's hemodynamic state, sedation, drug infusion, position) may change over a prolonged infusion. Ten minutes is usually the time of infusion adopted in the operating room in clinical practice.[24]

The maximal effect of an FC is typically obtained at the end of the infusion and is assessed by a continuous CO monitoring device or an echocardiographic estimation of CO or its surrogates.[25] A rise of 10–15% from the pre-FC hemodynamic values is commonly considered as positive [20,21,24,26] and the overall effect is dissipated over 5–10 minutes after the infusion.[25,27]

Finally, the FC is a time-dependent hemodynamic test and the time-point of assessment of the fluid responsiveness is a key factor. Since the effect is rapidly dissipated, the evaluation of the FC effect or the response of a FHT to its infusion is affected by the timing and the threshold adopted.[28] In other words, the FC should be standardized to ensure a consistent assessment and a correct interpretation.

Prediction of Fluid Responsiveness: General Principles

If a patient doesn't respond to fluid challenge with a rise in CO, the fluid volume already administered will contribute to patient's fluid overload without any hemodynamic benefit. Prediction of fluid responsiveness means that a hemodynamic pre-FC variable or a FHT is used to determine how likely a patient is to respond to fluid bolus with a significant increase in CO.

The pre-FC variables are usually subdivided into two groups. The static indexes are variables related to baseline volumes and pressures of the cardiovascular system [i.e., central venous pressure (CVP), pulmonary artery occlusion pressure (PAOP), left ventricle end-diastolic pressure (LVEDP), left ventricular end-diastolic area (LVEDA), left ventricular end-diastolic volume (LVEDV), global end-diastolic volume (GEDV)]. The dynamic indexes are those obtained by the interplay between the heart–lung interaction and the volume status [i.e., pulse pressure variation (PPV) and stroke volume variation (SVV)].

A FHT may be defined as a maneuver that affects cardiac function and/or heart–lung interactions with a subsequent hemodynamic response, the extent of which varies between fluid responders and non-responders. These tests rely on physiological heart–lung interactions such as a sudden change in right ventricular preload or afterload altering venous return or in the attempt of increasing SV after the rapid administration of a small aliquot of a predefined FC [29] (Figs. 13.1 and 13.2).

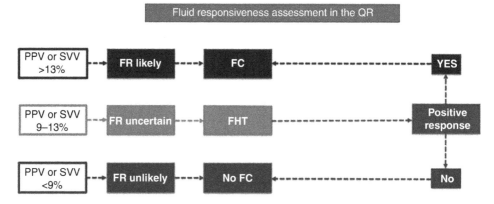

Figure 13.1 In the OR, FHTs can be added to the dynamic indexes evaluation, considering the grey zone reported in the literature (see text). When PPV or SVV values range within the grey zone, it is possible to use the FHTs. A positive response, according to the thresholds reported in the literature for each specific test (see text), suggests fluid responsiveness.
PPV, pulse pressure variation; SVV, stroke volume variation; FR, fluid responsiveness; FC, fluid challenge; SV, stroke volume; FTH, functional hemodynamic test; OR, operating room. A black and white version of this figure will appear in some formats. For the color version, please refer to the plate section.

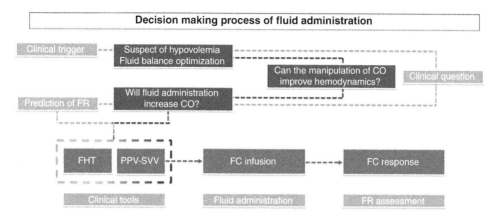

Figure 13.2 In the OR, the decision concerning administering fluids may be triggered by a suspected hypovolemia or by the need to achieve a predefined overall fluid balance. The following step is to assess whether the manipulation of the CO may improve these outcomes, since the only reason to give fluids is to increase it. The prediction of fluid responsiveness is, hence, the final question regarding the preload-dependency of the patient, which can be addressed by the use of dynamic indexes of fluid responsiveness or with the use of a functional hemodynamic test.
PPV, pulse pressure variation; SVV, stroke volume variation; FR, fluid responsiveness; FC, fluid challenge; CO, cardiac output; FTH, functional hemodynamic test; OR, operating room. A black and white version of this figure will appear in some formats. For the color version, please refer to the plate section.

Static Markers of Fluid Responsiveness

Static markers of cardiac preload status were historically considered as the gold standard to guide fluid therapy. The CVP is still frequently used in Europe to asses fluid responsiveness, especially in the intensive care unit (ICU) setting.[30] The general physiological misunderstanding regarding the CVP (and all the other static parameters) is based on the false relationship between baseline values and the changes in SV after FC administration. Very low and high values of CVP may be, in fact, associated with a likely or unlikely response to fluid administration; however, it is not possible to correlate the entire range of CVP values to a predefined SV response. For instance, it has been demonstrated that more than 80% of patients with a CVP <5 responded to fluids, even though 40% to 50% of patients with a high CVP were also fluid responders.[31]

It is generally inappropriate to use filling pressure as an index for filling volume and more importantly as an index for the future reaction of increased preload, because of the non-linear relationship between these variables. Static CVP measurement has no correlation to fluid responsiveness and should not be used for this purpose.[32,33] The same rationale can be applied to the PAOP, which physiologically has the same role as CVP for the left ventricle.[34] Conversely, a dynamic evaluation of the CVP during FC is more informative, since an increase in the right ventricular filling pressure during fluid administration is related to no significant increase in the CO.[21]

GEDV and intrathoracic blood volume (ITBV) are two static markers of preload provided by pulse contour analysis devices (PiCCO™ and VolumeView™). They have been incorporated successfully into a number of optimization protocols as discussed earlier and are superior to the CVP at identifying the fluid-responsive patient.[20] Extravascular lung water (EVLW) reflects the amount of pulmonary interstitial fluid. It does not correlate well with oxygenation or chest radiograph lung opacification but reflects the severity of illness and length of ventilation. Reducing the ITBV to normal levels may reduce the EVLW. These values do not reliably predict the fluid-responsive state and are unable to identify patients who will benefit from fluid therapy. This is because the relationship between cardiac reserve, vascular reserve and contractility is too complex to be adequately represented by one cardiac measurement.[20]

Dynamic Markers of Fluid Responsiveness

Periodic and fixed changes in intrathoracic pressures generated by mechanical ventilation affect right ventricular preload and afterload. During the inspiratory phase, positive pressure affects the right heart preload, reducing ventricular filling. Reducing right ventricular SV reduces left ventricular filling, and subsequently a decrease in left ventricular SV is seen 2–3 seconds later, during the expiratory phase. This delay is due to pulmonary flow transit time, and the extent of the SV changes is related to the volume status of the patient, being limited or absent in an euvolemic state and increased in preload-dependent patients.[26,35]

The pulse pressure variation is the dynamic measurement of pulse pressure (i.e., the difference between systolic and diastolic pressure) changes cyclically related to the changes in intrathoracic and alveolar pressure during controlled mechanical ventilation. Values above 13% or below 9% are highly predictive of fluid responsiveness or non-responsiveness, respectively.[24,36] The beat-by-beat analysis of the SVV is calculated starting from the SV estimation provided by the arterial pulse contour analysis, and then its changes over time. The monitoring device automatically samples the highest and lowest stroke volume registered over a period of 10–30 seconds and calculates the percentage change. Approximately the same cut-offs adopted for the PPV may be applied to SVV use in the operating room.[26]

Dynamic indexes are certainly overall much more reliable than static indexes in predicting fluid responsiveness, but they are limited by several variables that should be recognized to avoid misinterpretation of the data. Most of the validity criteria of PPV and SVV (Table 13.1) are usually present in surgical patients. However, some of them may significantly impact the reliability of these indexes.

The degree of CO variation is proportional to the tidal volume used. If tidal volume is reduced, the degree of intrathoracic pressure change is not sufficient to produce a significant hemodynamic effect.[37] Validation studies of PPV and SVV were conducted with a tidal volume of 8–12 ml/kg; however, intraoperative lung-protective ventilation strategy is associated with a better outcome [38] and is now suggested as standard ventilation in the operating room.[39] Recent data confirm that a protective ventilation strategy limits the use of baseline PPV and SVV in the assessment of the volume status in either prone or supine surgical patients, even if all other validity criteria are respected.[40–42]

The relationship between intrathoracic positive pressure intermittent rise and CO variation holds true only when the thoracic cavity is closed. Thoracotomy during cardiac or thoracic surgery alters the prerequisites for heart–lung interaction to be predictable, to such an extent that no conclusion can be drawn on fluid-responsiveness by looking at SVV and PPV in this case.[43]

Patients with arrhythmias present with elevated stroke volume variability because of the altered cardiac rhythm. In this case, elevated SVV and PPV are independent from patient preload reserve status and cannot be used for fluid management.

Last, patients affected by right-ventricular dysfunction are more sensitive to changes in intrathoracic pressure, due to the reduced ventricular contractile function.[44] SVV and

Table 13.1 Studies adopting a functional hemodynamic test to assess fluid responsiveness in surgical patients

Studies	Functional hemodynamic test	Parameter	AUC (95% CI)	Sensitivity (%)	Specificity (%)	Y	+PV	-PV	+LR	-LR	Threshold	GZ high	GZ low	Pt In GZ (%)
Guinot et al. [58]	EEOT: ventilation interrupted for 15 seconds	DELTA SV (%)	0.78 (0.63–0.89)	82	71	NA	85	67	2.87	0.25	2.3	NA	NA	NA
Biais et al. [53]	EEOT: ventilation interrupted for 30 seconds	DELTA SV (%)	0.91 (0.81–1.0)	100	81	0.81	84	100	NA	NA	5	8	4	17
Biais et al. [50]	Mini-FC: 100 ml – 120 seconds	DELTA SV (%)	0.95 (0.90–0.99)	93	85	0.78	NA	NA	NA	NA	6	7	4	19
Messina et al. [42]	Mini – FC: 100 ml – 60 seconds	DELTA SVI (%)	0.95 (0.88–0.98)	98	85	0.83	NA	NA	NA	NA	5	NA	NA	57.3
Messina et al. [42]	V_TC	DELTA SVV (%)	0.93 (0.80–0.98)	79	95	0.75	NA	NA	NA	NA	12.1	20	8	20
Messina et al. [42]	V_TC during prone position	DELTA SVV (%)	0.96 (0.89–1.02)	95	95	0.92	NA	NA	NA	NA	8	11	3	2.5

Table 13.1 (cont.)

Studies	Functional hemodynamic test	Parameter	AUC (95% CI)	Sensitivity (%)	Specificity (%)	Y	+PV	-PV	+LR	-LR	Threshold	GZ high	GZ low	Pt In GZ (%)
Guinot et al. [49]	Mini-FC: 100 ml – 60 seconds	DELTA SV (%)	0.93 (0.84–0.97)	89	89	NA	83	93	8.18	0.12	7	8	3	14
Biais et al. [57]	LRM: 30 cm H_2O / 30 seconds	DELTA SV (%)	0.96 (0.81–0.99)	88	92	NA	NA	NA	NA	NA	30	−22	−37	36
De Broca et al. [22]	LRM: 25 cm H_2O / 25 seconds	DELTA SV (%)	0.95 (0.91–0.99)	92	96	0.92	100	89	NA	NA	16	−15	−17	8

The area under the receiving operating characteristics (ROC) curve (AUC) of each study is reported as median (25th – 75th interquartile) or mean (± standard deviation), as stated in the original article. NA, data not available; SV, stroke volume; SVI, stroke volume index; SVV, stroke volume variation; EEOT, end-expiratory occlusion test; V_TC, tidal volume challenge; LRM, lung recruitment maneuver; PEEP, positive end-expiratory pressure; FC, fluid challenge; Y, Youden index; +PV, positive predictive value; –PV, negative predictive value; +LR, positive likelihood ratio; –LR, negative likelihood ratio; GZ, grey zone; Pt, patients.

PPV may often be elevated as a sign of the inability of the right ventricle to cope with intermittent increase in afterload due to positive pressure inspiration.

For all these reasons, PPV and SVV evaluation should be integrated into an algorithm of intraoperative hemodynamic management (see Fig. 13.1).

Finally, the use of PPV and SVV may overcome the simplistic evaluation of preload dependency of a patient for each FC infused in the operating room. In fact, the optimization of PPV and SVV by adopting a specific GDT based on these parameters (i.e., below a predefined threshold, usually ranging from 9% to 12%) decreases postsurgical morbidity, the rate of infectious, cardiac and abdominal complications, as well as ICU length of stay.[45] From a physiological point of view, maximizing SV by adopting a GDT approach should minimize dynamic parameters values and, accordingly, a strategy based on PPV or SVV optimization should produce the same beneficial effect, as demonstrated.[45]

Functional Hemodynamic Test in the Operating Room

The Mini-Fluid Challenge

The mini-FC is based on the assessment of SV response to the quick infusion of a small aliquot of fluids (usually 100 ml over 1 min or less) to predict the final response to the whole FC.[46,47] This test has been originally used in critically ill patients [46] by using transthoracic echocardiography and showing that a velocity time integral increase $\geq 10\%$ predicted fluid responsiveness with a sensitivity and specificity of 95% and 78%, respectively. The lowest and the fastest infusion of the mini-FC was tested by Wu et al.,[48] showing a sensitivity and specificity of 74% and 95% for a velocity time integral increase $\geq 9\%$, after an infusion of 50 ml in 10 seconds.

Very few studies have investigated the role of mini-FC in predicting fluid responsiveness in surgical patients. In spontaneously breathing patients undergoing spinal anesthesia, Guinot et al. showed that SV changes after the mini-FC predicted fluid responsiveness with an area under the receiver operating characteristic curve (AUC) of 0.93 [95% confidence interval (95% CI) 0.8 to 0.97, $P < 0.001$]. The cut-off was 7% and a grey zone ranging between 3% and 8%.[49] In mechanically ventilated patients undergoing neurosurgery, Biais et al. found that the changes in stroke volume index induced by 100 ml greater than 6% (grey zone between 4% and 7%) predicted fluid responsiveness with a sensitivity of 93% (95% CI, 77% to 99%) and a specificity of 85% (95% CI, 73 to 93%).[50] More recently, in the only multicentric trial available in the literature in elective patients who underwent laparotomy, Messina et al. showed an AUC of the changes in SV index after mini-FC of 0.95 (0.88–0.98) [sensitivity 98.0% (89.5–99.6) and specificity 86.8% (75.1–93.4)] for a cut-off value of 4% of increase.[42]

The mini-FC use is limited by the reliability of the hemodynamic tool used to define the small changes of the SV discriminating fluid responsiveness. In fact, during the mini-FC the SV physiologically changes during the inspiratory efforts of the patients (if spontaneously breathing) or the insufflation of mechanical ventilation. These fluctuations may impact on the final assessment of the SV change related to the mini-FC infusion. As shown by Messina et al., the least significant change (i.e., the smallest difference between successive SV measurements that can be considered to be a real change and not attributable to chance) is a critical issue of the hemodynamic tool used to assess the effect of the mini-FC.[42]

To overcome this limitation, it has been also demonstrated that a decrease in PPV (−4%) and SVV (−3%) after the mini-FC accurately predicts fluid responsiveness.[51] Combining these two signals (the SV increase and PPV/SVV reduction) may enhance the overall reliability of the test.

The End-Expiratory Occlusion Test

As previously discussed, the intermittent rise in intrathoracic pressure during inspiration in mechanically ventilated patients causes a transient reduction in venous return. It is possible to take advantage of this effect by holding the inspiratory insufflation for seconds (15–30 seconds) by using an end-expiratory pause. The consequent increase in the CO can be used to discriminate fluid responsiveness. After being successfully adopted in critically ill patients in different clinical setting,[52] the end-expiratory occlusion test (EEOT) has also been recently used in surgical patients.

A first metanalysis showed an overall high sensitivity and specificity [pooled AUC of 0.96 (95% CI 0.92–1.00); pooled sensitivity and specificity of 0.86 (95%CI 0.74–0.94) and 0.91 (95% CI 0.85–0.95) respectively, with a best threshold of 5% (4.0–8.0%) of increase in SV or its surrogates. A second metanalysis, showed an AUC of 0.91 (0.86–0.94) with the best threshold of CO increase at 5.1 ± 0.2%.[29,52] Previous conflicting results of the EEOT when performed during a protective ventilation [40,53] were not confirmed by the meta-nalysis of Gavelli et al.[52] However, the reliability of the EEOT was limited during prone position (irrespective to the tidal volume used) [41] and in patients with laparotomy.[42] Finally, the type of hemodynamic monitoring adopted seems to impact the EEOT performance.[54]

The Tidal Volume Challenge

Originally adopted in critically ill patients,[55] this FHT consists of a 1-minute time rise of the tidal volume from 6 to at least 8 ml/kg, which may correct baseline PPV and SVV to values discriminating fluid responsiveness. The most important advantage of this test is that it can be used without continuous hemodynamic monitoring.

In fact, since protective ventilation causes false negative values of the dynamic indexes, raising tidal volume (V_T) and intrathoracic pressure should increase PPV and SVV to a different extent in responders versus non-responders. In the first investigation of Myatra et al.,[55] PVV and SVV increases of 3.5% and 2.5%, respectively, were associated with very high sensitivity and specificity.[55] More recently, the tidal volume challenge has been successfully used in supine [40] and prone neurosurgical patients.[41] In the first setting, a 13.3% increase in PPV after tidal volume challenge (V_TC) predicted fluid responsiveness with a sensitivity of 94.7% and a specificity of 76.1% while a 12.1% increase in SVV after V_TC predicted fluid responsiveness with a sensitivity of 78.9% and a specificity of 95.2%. In prone patients, the change in PPV after the tidal volume challenge application predicted fluid responsiveness with an area under the curve of 0.96 (95% CI 0.87–1.00), showing a sensitivity of 95.2% and a specificity of 94.7%, using a cut-off increase of 12.2%. The change in SVV predicted fluid responsiveness with an area under the curve of 0.96 (95% CI 0.89–1.00) showing a sensitivity of 95.2% and a specificity of 94.7%, using a cut-off increase of 8.0%.

This FHT has been also used during robot-assisted laparoscopic surgery, improving the reliability of dynamic preload indexes.[56]

Lung Recruitment Maneuver or SIGH

Protective ventilation and low compliance may limit validity of the previously described test. Lung recruitment maneuver is an accepted method to reopen a partially collapsed lung by transiently raising intrathoracic pressure to 30–35 cm H_2O for 30 seconds during a mandatory inspiration, usually in pressure-controlled modality. Due to the transient nature of the pressure rise, the deleterious effect of high transpulmonary pressure on lung parenchyma is limited. Very few studies investigated this FHT in the operating room. Biais et al. showed that a reduction in SV of 30% successfully discriminated fluid responsiveness, after a maneuver of 30 seconds applying 30 cm H_2O.[57] In the De Broca et al. study, this threshold was reduced to 16%, after a maneuver of 25 seconds applying 25 cm H_2O.[22] Since mean arterial pressure is often expected to drop during the maneuver without a significant correlation with change in CO, a reliable continuous CO monitoring device is always warranted.

Conclusions

The assessment of fluid responsiveness is a key and challenging evaluation conducted in the operating room. Coupling the response to each aliquot of fluid administered to the overall fluid balance and to the optimization of predefined hemodynamic variables is a valuable strategy to tailor fluid therapy and to avoid inappropriate fluid administration and potentially harmful fluid overload. The fluid challenge (FC) is a standardized bolus of fluids that is infused to enhance preload dependency. Fluid responsiveness should be assessed by considering pre-FC dynamic indexes (PPV and SVV) and/or by using FHTs. The interpretation of these tools is based on specific thresholds of hemodynamic changes identifying fluid responsiveness (often very small) and on the comprehension of potential confounding factors and limitations.

References

1. Jhanji S, Thomas B, Ely A, et al. Mortality and utilisation of critical care resources amongst high-risk surgical patients in a large NHS trust. *Anaesthesia.* 2008;**63**(7):695–700.

2. Thompson JS, Baxter BT, Allison JG, et al. Temporal patterns of postoperative complications. *Arch Surg.* 2003;**138**(6):596–602.

3. Tevis SE, Kennedy GD. Postoperative complications and implications on patient-centered outcomes. *J Surg Res.* 2013;**181**(1):106–13.

4. Pearse RM, Moreno RP, Bauer P, et al. Mortality after surgery in Europe: a 7 day cohort study. *Lancet.* 2012;**380**(9847):1059–65.

5. Khuri SF, Henderson WG, DePalma RG, et al., Participants in the VANSQIP. Determinants of long-term survival after major surgery and the adverse effect of postoperative complications. *Ann Surg.* 2005;**242**(3):326–41.

6. Healy MA, Mullard AJ, Campbell DA Jr, Dimick JB. Hospital and payer costs associated with surgical complications. *JAMA Surg.* 2016;**151**(9):823–30.

7. Thacker JK, Mountford WK, Ernst FR, Krukas MR, Mythen MM. Perioperative fluid utilization variability and association with outcomes: considerations for enhanced recovery efforts in sample US surgical populations. *Ann Surg.* 2016;**263**(3):502–10.

8. Navarro LH, Bloomstone JA, Auler JO, Jr, et al. Perioperative fluid therapy: a statement from the International Fluid Optimization Group. *Perioper Med (London).* 2015;**4**:3.

9. Loftus TJ, Stelton S, Efaw BW, Bloomstone J. A system-wide enhanced recovery program focusing on two key process steps reduces complications and readmissions in patients undergoing bowel surgery. *J Healthc Qual.* 2017;**39**(3):129–35.

10. Miller TE, Mythen M, Shaw AD, et al. Association between perioperative fluid management and patient outcomes: a multicentre retrospective study. *Br J Anaesth.* 2021;**126**(3):720–9.

11. Gustafsson UO, Scott MJ, Schwenk W, et al. Guidelines for perioperative care in elective colonic surgery: enhanced Recovery After Surgery (ERAS((R))) Society recommendations. *World J Surg.* 2013;**37**(2):259–84.

12. Myles PS, Bellomo R, Corcoran T, et al. Restrictive versus liberal fluid therapy for major abdominal surgery. *N Engl J Med.* 2018;**378**(24):2263–74.

13. Miller TE, Myles PS. Perioperative fluid therapy for major surgery. *Anesthesiology.* 2019;**130**(5):825–32.

14. Wrzosek A, Jakowicka-Wordliczek J, Zajaczkowska R, et al. Perioperative restrictive versus goal-directed fluid therapy for adults undergoing major non-cardiac surgery. *Cochrane Database Syst Rev.* 2019;**12**:CD012767.

15. Myles PS, Bellomo R, Corcoran T, et al. Restrictive versus liberal fluid therapy for major abdominal surgery. *N Engl J Med.* 2018;**378**(24):2263–74.

16. Messina A, Robba C, Calabro L, Zambelli D, et al. Perioperative liberal versus restrictive fluid strategies and postoperative outcomes: a systematic review and metanalysis on randomised-controlled trials in major abdominal elective surgery. *Crit Care.* 2021;**25**(1):205.

17. Cecconi M, Corredor C, Arulkumaran N, et al. Clinical review: goal-directed therapy-what is the evidence in surgical patients? The effect on different risk groups. *Crit Care.* 2013;**17**(2):209.

18. Kaufmann T, Saugel B, Scheeren TWL. Perioperative goal-directed therapy – what is the evidence? *Best Pract Res Clin Anaesthesiol.* 2019;**33**(2):179–87.

19. Messina A, Robba C, Calabrò L, et al. Association between perioperative fluid administration and postoperative outcomes: a 20-year systematic review and a meta-analysis of randomized goal-directed trials in major visceral/noncardiac surgery. *Crit Care.* 2021;**25**(1):43.

20. Cecconi M, Parsons AK, Rhodes A. What is a fluid challenge? *Curr Opin Crit Care.* 2011;**17**(3):290–5.

21. Vincent JL, Cecconi M, De Backer D. The fluid challenge. *Crit Care.* 2020;**24**(1):703.

22. De Broca B, Garnier J, Fischer MO, et al. Stroke volume changes induced by a recruitment maneuver predict fluid responsiveness in patients with protective ventilation in the operating theater. *Medicine (Baltimore).* 2016;**95**(28):e4259.

23. Aya HD, Rhodes A, Chis Ster I, et al. Hemodynamic effect of different doses of fluids for a fluid challenge: a quasi-randomized controlled study. *Crit Care Med.* 2017;**45**(2):e161–e168.

24. Messina A, Pelaia C, Bruni A, et al. Fluid challenge during anesthesia: a systematic review and meta-analysis. *Anesth Analg.* 2018;**127**(6):1353–64.

25. Aya HD, Ster IC, Fletcher N, Grounds RM, Rhodes A, Cecconi M. Pharmacodynamic analysis of a fluid challenge. *Critical Care Med.* 2016;**44**(5):880–91.

26. Pinsky MR. Functional hemodynamic monitoring. *Crit Care Clin.* 2015;**31**(1):89–111.

27. Messina A, Palandri C, De Rosa S, et al. Pharmacodynamic analysis of a fluid challenge with 4 ml kg (–1) over 10 or 20 min: a multicenter cross-over randomized clinical trial. *J Clin Monit Comput.* 2021.;**36**(4):1193–1203.

28. Messina A, Sotgiu G, Saderi L, et al. Does the definition of fluid responsiveness affect passive leg raising reliability? A methodological ancillary analysis from a multicentric study. *Minerva Anestesiol.* 2021;**88**(4):272–81.

29. Messina A, Dell'Anna A, Baggiani M, et al. Functional hemodynamic tests: a systematic review and a metanalysis on the reliability of the end-expiratory occlusion test and of the mini-fluid challenge in predicting fluid responsiveness. *Crit Care.* 2019;**23**(1):264.

30. Cecconi M, Hofer C, Teboul JL, et al. Fluid challenges in intensive care: the FENICE study: a global inception cohort study. *Intensive Care Med.* 2015;**41**(9):1529–37.

31. Heenen S, De Backer D, Vincent JL. How can the response to volume expansion in patients with spontaneous respiratory movements be predicted? *Crit Care.* 2006;**10**(4):R102.

32. Marik PE, Cavallazzi R. Does the central venous pressure predict fluid responsiveness? An updated meta-analysis and a plea for some common sense. *Crit. Care Med.*2013; **41**(7):1774–81.

33. Bentzer P, Griesdale DE, Boyd J, et al. Will this hemodynamically unstable patient respond to a bolus of intravenous fluids? *JAMA.* 2016;**316**(12):1298–1309.

34. Osman D, Ridel C, Ray P, et al. Cardiac filling pressures are not appropriate to predict hemodynamic response to volume challenge. *Crit Care Med.* 2007;**35**(1):64–8.

35. Pinsky MR. Heart lung interactions during mechanical ventilation. *Curr Opin Crit Care.* 2012;**18**(3):256–60.

36. Cannesson M, Le Manach Y, Hofer CK, et al. Assessing the diagnostic accuracy of pulse pressure variations for the prediction of fluid responsiveness: a "gray zone" approach. *Anesthesiology.* 2011;**115**(2):231–41.

37. De Backer D, Heenen S, Piagnerelli M, Koch M, Vincent JL. Pulse pressure variations to predict fluid responsiveness: influence of tidal volume. *Intensive Care Med.* 2005;**31**(4):517–23.

38. Futier E, Constantin JM, Paugam-Burtz C, et al. A trial of intraoperative low-tidal-volume ventilation in abdominal surgery. *N Engl J Med.* 2013;**369**(5):428–37.

39. Eikermann M, Kurth T. Apply protective mechanical ventilation in the operating room in an individualized approach to perioperative respiratory care. *Anesthesiology.* 2015;**123**(1):12–14.

40. Messina A, Montagnini C, Cammarota G, et al. Tidal volume challenge to predict fluid responsiveness in the operating room: an observational study. *Eur J Anaesthesiol.* 2019;**36**(8):583–91.

41. Messina A, Montagnini C, Cammarota G, et al. Assessment of fluid responsiveness in prone neurosurgical patients undergoing protective ventilation: role of dynamic indices, tidal volume challenge, and end-expiratory occlusion test. *Anesth Analg.* 2020;**130**(3):752–61.

42. Messina A, Lionetti G, Foti L, et al. Mini fluid chAllenge aNd End-expiratory occlusion test to assess flUid responsiVEness in the opeRating room (MANEUVER study): a multicentre cohort study. *Eur J Anaesthesiol /*2021;**38**(4):422–31.

43. Piccioni F, Bernasconi F, Tramontano GTA, Langer M. A systematic review of pulse pressure variation and stroke volume variation to predict fluid responsiveness during cardiac and thoracic surgery. *J Clin Monit Comput.* 2017;**31**(4):677–84.

44. Michard F, Richards G, Biais M, Lopes M, Auler JO. Using pulse pressure variation or stroke volume variation to diagnose right ventricular failure? *Crit Care.* 2010;**14**(6):451; author reply 451.

45. Benes J, Giglio M, Brienza N, Michard F. The effects of goal-directed fluid therapy based on dynamic parameters on post-surgical outcome: a meta-analysis of randomized controlled trials. *Crit Care.* 2014;**18**(5):584.

46. Muller L, Toumi M, Bousquet PJ, et al. An increase in aortic blood flow after an infusion of 100 ml colloid over 1 minute can predict fluid responsiveness: the mini-fluid challenge study. *Anesthesiology.* 2011;**115**(3):541–7.

47. Lee CT, Lee TS, Chiu CT, et al. Mini-fluid challenge test predicts stroke volume and arterial pressure fluid responsiveness during spine surgery in prone position:

A STARD-compliant diagnostic accuracy study. *Medicine (Baltimore).* 2020;**99**(6): e19031.

48. Wu Y, Zhou S, Zhou Z, Liu B. A 10-second fluid challenge guided by transthoracic echocardiography can predict fluid responsiveness. *CritCare.* 2014;**18**(3):R108.

49. Guinot PG, Bernard E, Defrancq F, et al. Mini-fluid challenge predicts fluid responsiveness during spontaneous breathing under spinal anaesthesia: an observational study. *Eur J Anaesthesiol.* 2016;**32**(9):645–9.

50. Biais M, de Courson H, Lanchon R, et al. Mini-fluid challenge of 100 ml of crystalloid predicts fluid responsiveness in the operating room. *Anesthesiology.* 2017 [**127**(3):450–6.

51. Mallat J, Meddour M, Durville E, et al. Decrease in pulse pressure and stroke volume variations after mini-fluid challenge accurately predicts fluid responsiveness. *Br J Anaesth.* 2015;**115** (3):449–56.

52. Gavelli F, Shi R, Teboul JL, Azzolina D, Monnet X. The end-expiratory occlusion test for detecting preload responsiveness: a systematic review and meta-analysis. *Ann Intensive Care.* 2020;**10**(1):65.

53. Biais M, Larghi M, Henriot J, et al. End-expiratory occlusion test predicts fluid responsiveness in patients with protective ventilation in the operating room. *Anesth Analg.* 2017;**125**(6):1889–5.

54. Monnet X, Teboul JL. End-expiratory occlusion test: please use the appropriate tools! *Br J Anaesth.* 2015;**114**(1):166–167.

55. Myatra SN, Monnet X, Teboul JL. Use of "tidal volume challenge" to improve the reliability of pulse pressure variation. *Crit Care.* 2017;**21**(1):60.

56. Jun JH, Chung RK, Baik HJ, et al. The tidal volume challenge improves the reliability of dynamic preload indices during robot-assisted laparoscopic surgery in the Trendelenburg position with lung-protective ventilation. *BMC Anesthesiol.* 2019;**19**(1):142.

57. Biais M, Lanchon R, Sesay M, et al. Changes in stroke volume induced by lung recruitment maneuver predict fluid responsiveness in mechanically ventilated patients in the operating room. *Anesthesiology.* 2017;**126**(2):260–7.

58. Guinot PG, Godart J, de Broca B, et al. End-expiratory occlusion manoeuvre does not accurately predict fluid responsiveness in the operating theatre. *Br J Anaesth.* 2014;**112**(6):1050–4.

Intra-Abdominal Surgery

Birgitte Brandstrup

Background

Hypovolemia may lead to postoperative complications, circulatory collapse, and death. However, fluid overload may lead to oedema formation, especially in the skin, gut, and lungs, postoperative complications, and death.[1–10] For these reasons it is important to get the correct fluid balance.[11,12]

The controversy in the literature has primarily been what fluid to give in which volumes. "Fixed volume regimens" have been maligned and fluid therapy guided by a physiological goal praised. The different goals in mind may be hemodynamic (stroke volume, pulse pressure variation, among others), biochemical (oxygen tension, lactate concentration, among others), or fluid balance and body weight changes.

Proponents have argued rigorously about which goal is best. Most likely, the answer is neither one nor the other, but some combination of them.

Perioperative intravenous fluid therapy has several goals:

1. To correct preoperative fluid, electrolyte, and blood imbalances (hypovolemia, dehydration, anaemia, hypokalaemia, etc.).
2. To meet basal fluid and electrolyte requirements.
3. To replace intraoperative and later postoperative fluid, electrolyte, and blood losses.
4. To maintain physiological parameters within an acceptable normal range.

Moreover, all the above must be done with minimal risk for the patient in terms of side effects in relation to intravenous fluid, electrolytes, and blood.

Correct Preoperative Fluid and Electrolyte Imbalances

It is best to correct fluid and electrolyte imbalances preoperatively. This is possible in elective surgical conditions; however, in emergency surgical situations, one must balance the patient's risk by postponing the surgery against the risk of anaesthesia and surgery in the presence of the imbalance. In these circumstances, it may be necessary to start the correction of the condition intraoperatively.

How to correct preoperative dehydration and/or electrolyte disturbances is beyond the scope of this chapter. However, as a rule of thumb, imbalances are usually developed over a long period, and preoperative correction is best done slowly and orally.

Basic Fluid and Electrolyte Needs

The basic needs in patients undergoing surgery differ from the normal condition in three aspects:

1. The patient is told to fast.
2. The patient is undergoing a trauma, causing the release of stress hormones including aldosterone, resulting in salt and water retention.
3. The patient is artificially ventilated with 100% moist air.

Normal insensible perspiration is the body's only loss of pure water, and is approximately:

10 ml/kg/day or 0.4 ml/kg/h of pure water.

About 2/3 of the volume comes from the skin and 1/3 from the respiratory tract.

Thus, a patient on mechanical ventilation with 100% moist air has a reduced fluid loss from the respiratory tract of 1/3 and the Insensible perspiration on a ventilator is:

6.7 ml/kg/day or 0.275 ml/kg/h of pure water.

If the patient is not on a ventilator, increasing body temperature (fever) increases the respiratory frequency and thereby the insensible perspiration. The extra fluid lost with fever is, however, very small.

Sensible perspiration is visible sweat. It consists of salt and water and is always hypotonic (lower salt concentration than in the extracellular fluid). Exercise and increasing environmental temperature increase the sensible perspiration. The volume is difficult to measure in clinical practice, but is small for elective surgical patients. It may be large in patients with visible sweat in emergency surgical conditions (sepsis, shock).

Diuresis is approximately 1 litre per day for a healthy person with a normal body weight, food, and fluid intake or:

Urinary output of 0.5–1.0 ml/kg/h is recommended.

The accompanying box outlines the daily requirements for normal fluid and electrolyte losses.

Fluid and Electrolyte Requirements in a Healthy Person with a Body Weight at 70–80 kg

- Potassium: 60–100 mmol.
- Sodium: 60–150 mmol (= 4–9 g), depending on physical activity and temperature.
- Glucose: 850 mmol (= 150 g) (for the basal metabolism of the brain).
- Water: 2–3 litres, or a normal volume of approximately 1–1.5 ml/kg/h.

Hence, 2–3 litres of Na-K-glucose accommodate the normal daily requirements (containing Na 40 mmol, K 20 mmol, and glucose 50 mmol in 1 litre of water).

Diuresis in Elderly Patients

Patients may not have a sufficient diuresis with normal volumes of urine. To evaluate the sufficiency of the diuresis for the individual patient, it is necessary to know their osmotic load and the ability of the kidneys to concentrate the urine.

The glomerular filtration rate (GFR) in young healthy adults is approximately 140 ml/min/1.73 m^2 but decreases after the age of 40 by about 8 ml/min/1.73 m^2 for every 10 years. [13] Elderly patients have a lower muscle mass, and thus a lower production of creatinine.

Because of this, the creatinine concentration may remain normal despite a low GFR.[13,14] Moreover, a significant decrease in the ability to concentrate the urine has been demonstrated with age.[15]

For young healthy male volunteers, the urinary osmolality is the following:

- Following an overnight fast (thirst), osmolality is 500–950 mosm/kg.[16,17]
- Following 24 hours of thirst, osmolality increases to about 1100 mosm/kg.[17]
- Following 4 days of thirst, it reaches a maximum of 1420 mosm/kg urine.[18]

In elderly healthy male volunteers (67–75 years of age) the ability to concentrate the urine is the following:

- Following an overnight fast (thirst), the ability to concentrate urine is about 700 mosm/kg.
- Following 24 hours of thirst, it is about 950 mosm/kg urine.

These findings are significantly lower in the elderly than in the young.[17]

- For frail elderly, the maximal ability to concentrate urine may be even less.[14]
- In an 80-year-old person, the urinary osmolality following 12 hours of thirst can be as low as 400–600 mosm/kg urine.[15]

Moreover, in the elderly volunteers plasma sodium increased significantly compared with volunteers 20–31 years of age. Even so, the elderly did not drink as much water as the young, and the plasma sodium and plasma osmolality stayed elevated for more than five days. The corresponding numbers for woman are completely unknown.

Sodium excretion can represent only a small fraction of the total urine osmolarity.

The ability to excrete sodium was measured in healthy young male volunteers, given a datary salt load (tablets) up to 32 g/day.

- The excretion of sodium reached a max of 300 mmol/l urine.[19] Therefore, drinking seawater, for example, is a bad idea, even if stranded on a lifeboat after a shipwreck. The salt concentration of seawater is about 600 mmol/l (higher close to the equator, lower close to the poles), and with a maximal ability to excrete 300 mmol of sodium in 1 litre of urine (if young and male), drinking seawater would supply the body with salt instead of water. See the accompanying Example.

Example

An 80 kg patient is administered 2 litres of saline 0.9% as the only fluid.

Two litres of saline contain 308 mmol of sodium and chloride in 2 litres of water.

Approximately 800 ml of the water will evaporate as insensible perspiration, leaving 1200 ml to excrete the 308 mmol of sodium and chloride given with the infusion.

This means that the demand on the kidneys' sodium excretion is close to the maximal concentration ability in a young healthy person. It may very well exceed the kidneys' concentration ability in an elderly or sick person.

The hormonal stress response after surgery tends to preserve salt and water in the body. [20,21]

Oedema formations in surgical patients should not be understood as over-hydration (hydra = water) because something with osmotic capacity has to keep the water in the body, and that something is sodium. More correctly, postoperative oedema formation is "over salting," and giving water to help excrete the salt in combination with giving furosemide (that promotes natriuresis) will help reduce the oedema.

Lactated or acetated Ringer's solution has a lower chloride content, but the sodium content is 140 mmol per litre, not much different from that of normal saline.

Because the fluid is slightly hypotonic (in the cell metabolism, lactate is degraded into CO_2 and water), the kidneys are supplied with slightly more water to excrete the salts.

In addition, it is important to know, that without a sufficient water intake, all colloids will form a gel in the tubuli of the kidneys and thereby impose kidney injury.

Fluid Therapy during Preoperative Fasting

Elective surgical patients are allowed to eat until 6 hours before surgery and to drink clear fluids until 2 hours before surgery without increasing the risk of aspiration to the lungs.[22]

However, the volume of clear fluid allowed is inconsistent. In the European Society of Anaesthesiologists (ESA) [22] guideline, a maximal volume is not suggested, and practise varies from 500 ml to "no limit."

In order to arrive well hydrated to the operating room and lessen the need for intravenous fluid therapy, the patients should be encouraged to eat and drink before elective surgery.

In elective surgical patients, the fluid and electrolyte loss during fast will be normal, and if intravenous fluid supplementation is called for, a fluid replacing normal losses is the logical choice: K-Na-glucose or glucose 5%.

Several trials have shown that sugar-containing fluids given preoperatively (orally or intravenously) increases well-being, reduces hunger and thirst, improves muscle strength, and decreases the postoperative insulin resistance in colorectal surgical patients.[23–25]

No evidence exists, however, that treatment with preoperative sugar, containing fluid has effects on postoperative complications, length of stay, or mortality.

Intraoperative Fluid and Blood Loss

Surgery does not increase the normal fluid and electrolyte losses, but results in an evaporative loss from the open abdomen, which approximately equals the reduced water loss from the lungs because the patient is ventilated with moist air (3.3 ml/kg/day or 0.14 ml/kg/h).

In addition, the patient may have pathological losses of blood or ascites.

The perspiration from the open abdomen is small, and depends on the size of the incision and the exteriorization of the viscera:[26]

- In a small incision without exteriorization of the viscera (e.g., open appendectomy), the evaporation is 2.1 ml/h.
- In a medium incision and partly exposure of the viscera (e.g., open cholecystectomy), the evaporation is 8.0 ml/h.
- in a large incision with total exteriorized viscera, the evaporation is 32.2 ml/h.

Note: the unit in the list is ml/h NOT ml/kg/h.

This loss is reduced by 50% after 20 minutes,[26] and by keeping the viscera in a plastic bag, the loss is reduced by approximately 87%.[27]

The magnitude of the evaporative fluid loss during **laparoscopic surgery** is entirely unknown. It is often assumed small, but may in fact be larger than the loss in open surgery because the insufflated air is dry, the entire visceral surfaces as well as the inside of the abdominal wall is exposed, and the air is replaced an unknown number of times during the surgery.

The Loss to Third Space

Previously, we believed that the surgical trauma per se caused a redistribution of the body fluids, so that a large volume of extracellular fluid became unavailable for regeneration of lost plasma. Therefore, large volumes of intravenous "extracellular fluid" were given during surgery. We called this loss "a functional loss of extracellular fluid" or "a loss to third space." A critical review of the studies giving birth to this theory show, however, that the trials finding this "loss to third space" are flawed, and newer and better trials using correct methods do not find this illogical loss.[28] We have therefore abandoned the entire concept.

Manipulation of the intestines and the surgical trauma do cause cell damage and a modest oedema formation.

From experimental studies, we know that the formation of a small bowel anastomosis increases the water content in the tissue surrounding the anastomosis by 5–10%.[29] If the same occurs in humans and the anastomosis has a weight similar to a stoma removed by the reversal of the Hartmann's procedure (50 g),[30] the amount of fluid "lost to the traumatized tissue" is about 2.5–5 g or 2.5–5 ml.

Intravenous fluid therapy increases this oedema formation and destabilizes the bowel anastomosis: If 15 ml/kg/h is given, the water content more than doubles to 10–20% [29] and the stability of the anastomosis decreases (the anastomosis bursts at less pressure) [5] while the inflammation around the anastomosis increases.[3]

This is supported by the findings of Jacob et al.,[31] who describe how fluid overload destroys the endothelial glycocalyx and causes inflammation and escape of fluid to the interstitial space.

Exudation and Blood Loss

In open surgery, fluid can "ooze" from the wound and the intestines. Often this fluid is lost in the surgical dressings, and its magnitude is based on an estimate. In abdominal surgery with exteriorized viscera, the surgeon can wrap the viscera in a plastic bag, and the fluid loss is thus measured more accurately. The exudation contains albumin, and manipulation of the intestines increases the albumin content.

Unless the patient is bleeding profusely or is having an occult blood loss (e.g., to the intestines from a bleeding ulcer), we can measure blood loss rather accurately from the content in suction bottles and the weight change of the dressings.

To Maintain Physiological Parameters within an Acceptable Normal Range

Epidural Analgesia

The use of epidurals blocks the sensory as well as the sympathetic fibres in the affected area of the spinal cord, leading to a decrease in heart rate (for high blocks) and a dilation of the vascular tree, and thus a decrease in arterial blood pressure.

Early trials showed that a fluid bolus of 500 ml of colloid or 1000 ml of crystalloid could counteract this drop in blood pressure. However, randomized clinical trials could not confirm these results. On the contrary, they show that intravenous fluid is ineffective in the treatment of the blood pressure drop caused by epidural dilation, and the cardiac output remains largely unchanged.[32–34]

Goal-Directed Fluid Therapy

Different goals have been used in goal-directed fluid therapy (GDT) trials, and which goals are accepted for a trial to be called "goal directed" vary between the reviews published.

1. The original trials introduced a *pressure-controlled* regimen (blood pressure, central vein pressure).[35]
2. In most cases, the accepted goals refer to "optimization" using the stroke volume (SV) or stroke volume variation (SVV), and can be seen as *flow-controlled* fluid therapy.
3. The goal of "zero fluid balance" (restricted fluid therapy) has been included in the goal-directed fluid therapy family,[36] and can be seen as *balance-controlled* therapy.
4. Others have introduced *biochemical-controlled* therapy with goals such as lactate or central venous oxygen tension.

Most likely, using a combination of the goals is the best approach.

From here forward, GDT refers to number 2 in the foregoing list: giving hydroxy ethyl starch (HES) or gelatin to near maximal SV.

Many trials have tested the effect of GDT against a standard fluid regimen during abdominal surgical procedures, and the results have been divagating. Some of the trials have shown a benefit of the GDT,[37–42] but not all.[43–46] Colloid was used for increasing the stroke volume, and in all the referred trials, it was given on top of a liberal fluid regimen. Moreover, only few trials measured the intravenous fluid volumes given postoperatively, and the few trials that did, measured only for the rest of the day of surgery.[37,41,44,46]

It is interesting that large volumes of crystalloid were given alongside the stroke volume optimization with colloid. This may be interpreted two ways: Either the crystalloid was given as pure fluid overload and left the circulation almost immediately (as crystalloid fluids do when given to normovolemic persons), or crystalloids were unable to increase the SV.

It is also interesting that colloid (including HES) apparently has beneficial effects on outcome in elective bowel surgery, and not the side effects seen in a population of septic patients.[47]

The so-called restricted fluid therapy approach (or zero fluid balance) has been tested against GDT without the fluid overload with crystalloid (GDT on a zero-balance basis) in elective surgery; see Table 14.1.[48–51]

A Cochrane review [52] confirms that GDT is not superior to restricted fluid therapy. This result was found despite the fact that a trial of patients treated with heated intraperitoneal chemotherapy (HIPEC) for peritoneal carcinosis was included. [53] In that trial the so-called restricted group received 8269 litres of intravenous fluid during the surgery versus 5812 litres in the GDT group, making the GDT group restricted. Not surprisingly, the group given the smallest fluid volume had the best outcome. Note that a trial of orthopaedic surgery included in the Cochrane review was excluded from Table 14.1.

Some people have argued that the reason for non-superiority of GDT was the good health of the elective patients included in the trials, and postulated that if more American Society of Anesthesiologists (ASA) levels III–IV patients were included in the trials, the benefits of the GDT "optimization" would be revealed.

To meet this point of view, and because we believed it to be accurate, we did a clinical randomized trial of the sickest abdominal surgical patients: patients with gastrointestinal perforation and bowel obstruction undergoing emergency surgery.

Automatic upper arm cuff

- MBP measurement can be true and precise in acute care settings.
- Performance varies from device model to model.
- SBP is often displayed with a significant error.

- Reliable identification of patients responding to therapy.
- Remarkable ability to detect hypo- and hypertension
  If MBP displayed > 70 mm Hg, hypotension (actual MBP<65 mmHg) is very unlikely)

Beliefs to be (likely) abandoned

- "The upper arm cuff systematically (over-) underestimates BP"
  The direction of the measurement error is often unpredictable!

- "This technique is unreliable during the infusion of a vasopressive drug"
  - *Vasopressive* drugs: impact on the measurement error is uncertain.
  - Caution 1: the intermittent nature of the measurement may delay the detection of hypo - or hypertension related to infusion issues.
  - Caution 2: in the event of an infusion through a peripheral vein of the upper limb, the upper arm cuff is preferably placed at the opposite upper limb.

Cardiac arrhythmia

Consider the average of 3 consecutive measurements.

Obese patients

Place the cuff at the wrist (especially if the upper arm is large and conically shaped).

Contra-indication for placing the cuff at the upper limb

Keep in mind that placing the cuff at the lower leg is associated with a higher degree of measurement error.

Automatic finger cuff

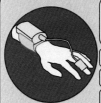

- Measurement error does not fulfil the requirements of the current international standard.
  However, more appropriate assessments are needed for acute care settings.
- Lower measurement error for MBP than SBP or DBP.

Beat-to-beat BP monitoring : earlier detection of hypo-/hypertension.

Trending ability of uncertain performance.

Beware of the limitations of photoplethysmography (vasoconstriction).

The impact of obesity/finger edema and/or cardiac arrhythmia is uncertain.

Displays a reliable estimate of respiratory changes in pulse pressure.

Displays an estimate of cardiac output (not interchangeable with more reliable techniques).

Figure 3.1 Key messages. DBP, diastolic blood pressure; MBP, mean blood pressure; SBP, systolic blood pressure.

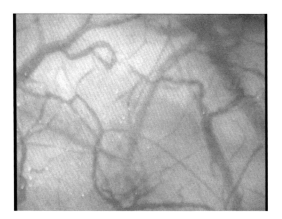

Figure 4.1 Sublingual microcirculation in normal conditions. Photograph of the sublingual microcirculation in a normal individual with septic shock using a sidestream dark field (SDF) imaging device.

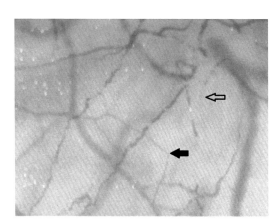

Figure 4.2 Sublingual microcirculation in sepsis. Photograph of the sublingual microcirculation in a patient with septic shock using a sidestream dark field (SDF) imaging device. The solid arrow shows a well-perfused capillary; the empty arrow identifies a stopped flow capillary.

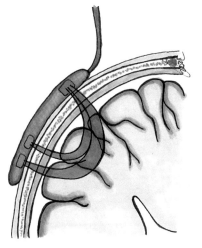

Figure 5.1 Representation of a near infrared spectroscopy sensor with one electrode emitting near infrared light and two electrodes detecting light reflected by the grey matter of the brain.

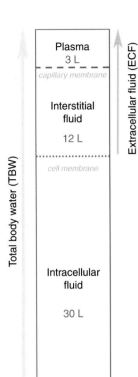

Total body water (TBW)

Extracellular fluid (ECF)

Plasma
3 L

capillary membrane

Interstitial
fluid

12 L

cell membrane

Intracellular
fluid

30 L

Figure 6.1 Schematic drawing of the body fluid compartments.

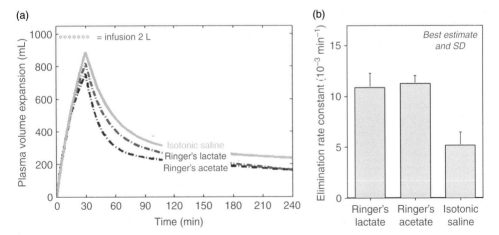

(a)

Plasma volume expansion (mL)

1000 ****** = infusion 2 L

800

600

400

200

0

0   30   60   90   120   150   180   210   240

Time (min)

Isotonic saline
Ringer's lactate
Ringer's acetate

(b)

Elimination rate constant (10^{-3} min^{-1})

*Best estimate
and SD*

15

10

5

0

Ringer's   Ringer's   Isotonic
lactate   acetate   saline

Figure 7.1 (a) Plasma volume expansion from infusion of 2 liters of isotonic saline, Ringer's lactate and Ringer's acetate in 10 healthy volunteers. Each curve is based on the modeled average plasma dilution from experiments performed in 10 male volunteers multiplied by the plasma volume at baseline as estimated by anthropometry. ****** symbolizes the time period when fluid is being infused. (b) The rate of elimination of the three fluids. The half-life is the inverse of the shown elimination rate constant times 0.693. Hence, the half-life is about 60 min for the Ringer's solutions and 130 min for isotonic saline. Recalculations of data from Ref. [5] using a mixed models analytical program (Phoenix NLME).

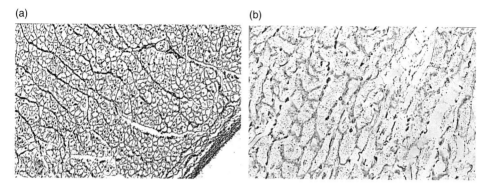

Figure 7.2 (a) Normal cytoarchitecture of a pig´s heart after receiving 150 mL/kg of mannitol 3% over 90 min. Lumina of the vessels are preserved (x 200). (b) Destroyed cytoarchitecture in the subendocardium in a mouse that died after receiving 300 mL/kg of 0.9% saline over 60 min. The reticular fibers are fragmented and degenerated (x 600). Light microscopy with Gordon and Sweet's silver impregnation for reticulum fibers. Photographs were taken during the studies reported in *APMIS* 200;108:487–95, and *J Surg Res* 2001;95:114–25.

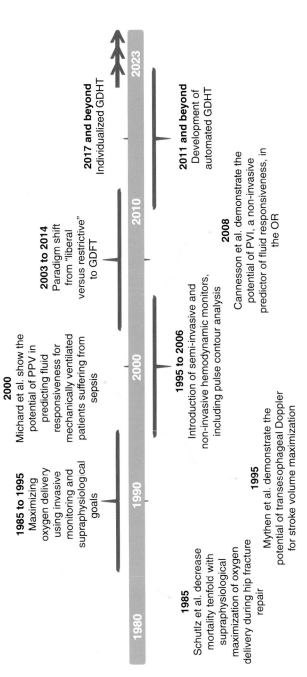

Figure 12.1 Evolution of perioperative goal-directed hemodynamic therapy over time. GDFT, goal-directed fluid therapy; PPV, pulse pressure variation; GDHT, goal-directed hemodynamic therapy; OR, operating room.

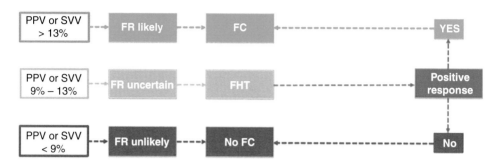

Figure 13.1 In the OR, FHTs can be added to the dynamic indexes evaluation, considering the grey zone reported in the literature (see text). When PPV or SVV values range within the grey zone, it is possible to use the FHTs. A positive response, according to the thresholds reported in the literature for each specific test (see text), suggests fluid responsiveness.
PPV, pulse pressure variation; SVV, stroke volume variation; FR, fluid responsiveness; FC, fluid challenge; SV, stroke volume; FTH, functional hemodynamic test; OR, operating room.

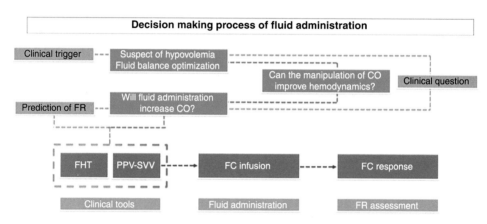

Figure 13.2 In the OR, the decision concerning administering fluids may be triggered by a suspected hypovolemia or by the need to achieve a predefined overall fluid balance. The following step is to assess whether the manipulation of the CO may improve these outcomes, since the only reason to give fluids is to increase it. The prediction of fluid responsiveness is, hence, the final question regarding the preload-dependency of the patient, which can be addressed by the use of dynamic indexes of fluid responsiveness or with the use of a functional hemodynamic test.
PPV, pulse pressure variation; SVV, stroke volume variation; FR, fluid responsiveness; FC, fluid challenge; CO, cardiac output; FTH, functional hemodynamic test; OR, operating room.

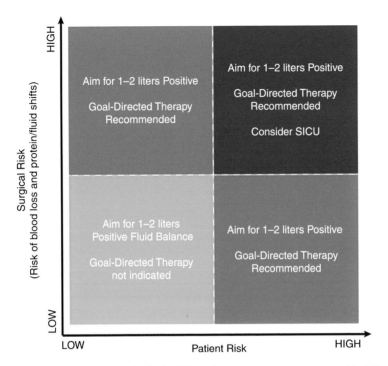

Figure 15.2 [37] The risk-adapted matrix for fluid and hemodynamic management suggested by Miller and Myles [37], the combination of high patient and surgical risk (right upper quarter) should be treated with GDT. Note that the vast majority of the thoracic operations are in this quarter. SICU, surgical intensive care unit.

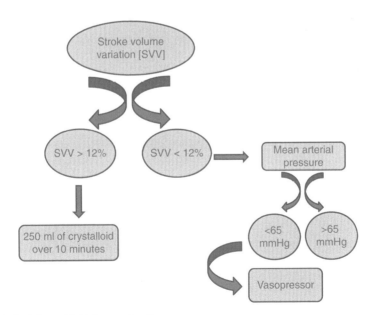

Figure 17.1 Goal-directed fluid therapy algorithm.

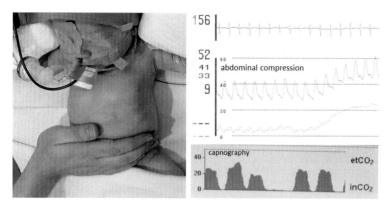

Figure 19.1 Abdominal pressure maneuver as test for fluid responsiveness in small children.

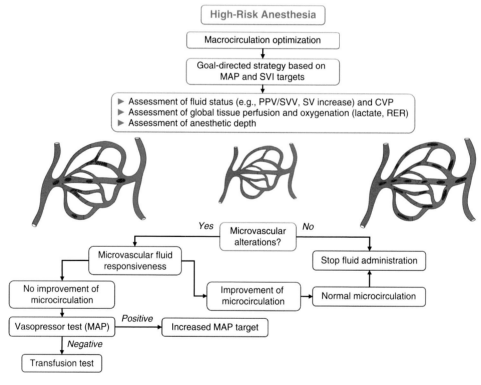

Figure 22.2 Proposed algorithm for assessing and treating hemodynamic instability in high-risk patients requiring invasive monitoring. CVP, central venous pressure; MAP, mean arterial pressure; PPV, pulse pressure variation; SV, stroke volume; SVI, stroke volume index; SVV. stroke volume variation; RER, respiratory exchange ratio.

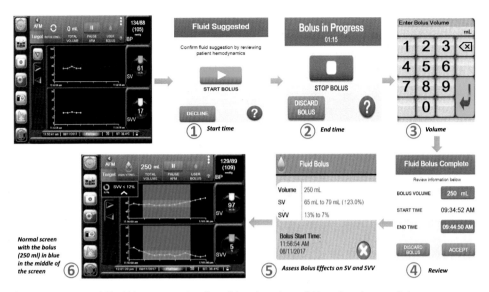

Figure 24.2 Assisted Fluid Management interface. SV, stroke volume; SVV, stroke volume variation.

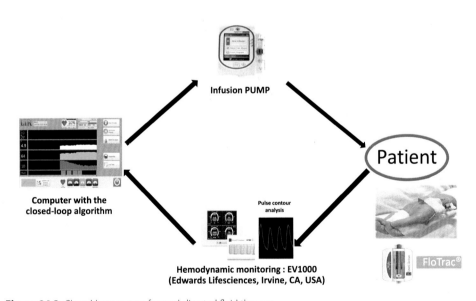

Figure 24.3 Closed-loop system for goal-directed fluid therapy.

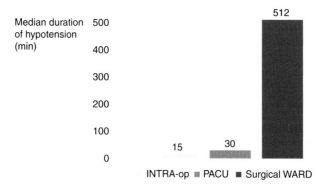

Figure 25.1 Median duration of hypotension during and after surgery in the control group (5001 patients undergoing non-cardiac surgery) of the POISE 2 trial. The median cumulative duration of hypotension exceeded 8 h on surgical wards, whereas it was only 15 min during surgery. Therefore, initiatives to improve patient safety should focus on the early detection and treatment of hypotensive events on the wards. INTRA-op, intraoperative; PACU, postanesthesia care unit.

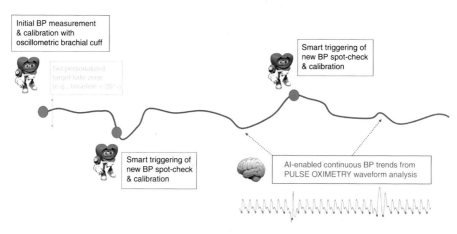

Figure 25.2 Principles of continuous blood pressure monitoring with a machine learning algorithm and a pulse oximeter. Assuming the oscillometric brachial cuff and the pulse oximeter are wireless, mobile and continuous monitoring of blood pressure may become a reality for patients at high risk of clinical deterioration on regular wards. BP, blood pressure.

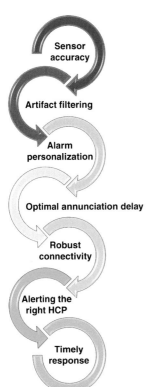

Figure 25.3 The implementation chain for wireless wearables on hospital wards. All links are indispensable for a successful implementation. HCP, healthcare professional.

Sensor accuracy

Artifact filtering

Alarm personalization

Optimal annunciation delay

Robust connectivity

Alerting the right HCP

Timely response

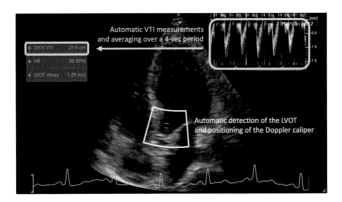

Automatic VTI measurements and averaging over a 4-sec period

+ LVOT VTI   21.9 cm
+ HR   88 BPM
+ LVOT Vmax   1.29 m/s

Automatic detection of the LVOT and positioning of the Doppler caliper

Figure 25.5 Example of machine learning algorithm for the automatic measurement of the sub-aortic velocity time integral (VTI).
First, the algorithm detects the five-chamber apical view and the left ventricular outflow tract (LVOT). A colored trapezoid around the LVOT indicates the quality of the ultrasound image and Doppler signal (green when optimal, yellow when fair, red when not acceptable). There is no need to position the caliper manually in the LVOT. Then, the algorithm automatically measures and averages VTI over a 4-sec period.

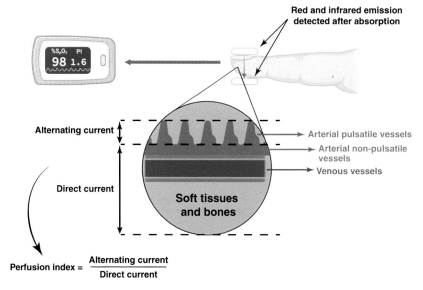

Figure 26.1 Principles of photoplethysmography and PI calculation.

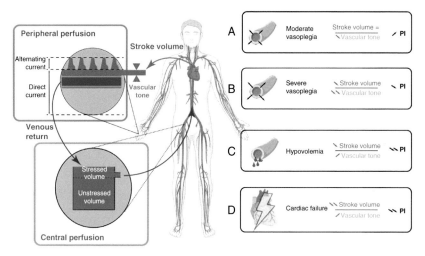

Figure 26.2 Determinants of perfusion index (PI) and typical clinical situations.

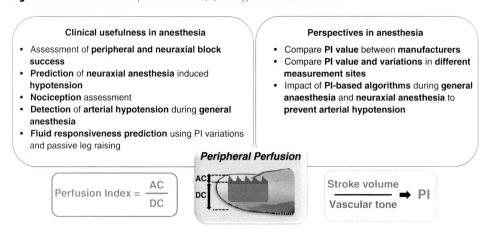

Figure 26.3 Summary of clinical usefulness and perspectives of perfusion index (PI) use in anesthesia.

Table 14.1 Trials of "goal-directed fluid therapy" (GDT) in abdominal surgery versus "restricted fluid therapy." Fluid volumes are in ml

Author	Surgery	No. of patients	Blinding and intervention	Primary outcome	Intervention fluid	Preoperative fluid volume	Intraoperative fluid volume	Postoperative fluid volume	Results
Brandstrup et al. [48] June 2012	Elective laparoscopic or open colectomy	150 in two groups: GDT vs. "restricted"	Observer blinded. Near maximal stroke volume (ODM) (CardiQ®).	Patients with postop. complications	HES 6% (Voluven®)	2 h fasting for fluid. 500 ml saline if no fluid in 6 h.	Coll: 810 (GDT) vs. 475 Total volume 1 877 (GDT) vs. 1 491 (restricted)	Oral fluid in an enhanced recovery protocol. IV-fluid if oliguria, tachycardia or hypotension.	No difference in morbidity or LOS. Mortality: one in each group.
Zhang et al. [51] October 2012	Elective open GI surgery	60 in three groups: 4 ml/kg/h and GDT-Ringer's, 4 ml/kg/h and GDT-HES, and 4 ml/kg/h Ringer's	Observer blinded. Pulse pressure variation (PPV)	LOS	Ringer's lactate and HES 6%	Not given	Total volume: GDT Ringer's: 2 109 vs. GDT colloid: 1 742 vs. Restricted Ringer's 1 260	1.5–2.0 ml/kg/h crystalloid for 3 days. Oral intake not mentioned.	LOS was shortest in GDT colloid group, longest in the GDT Ringer's group. Morbidity: No difference Mortality: None
Srinivasa et al. [50] November 2012	Elective laparoscopic or open colectomy	85 in two groups GDT vs. "restricted"	Observer blinded. Near maximal stroke volume (ODM) (CardiQ®)	Surgical Recovery Score (SRS).	Succinylated gelatin colloid solution Gelatofusine®	13 patients with bowel preparation: 1 000 ml crystalloid	Coll: 591 (GDT) vs. 297 Total volume: 1 997 (GDT) vs. 1 614 (restricted)	Oral fluid in an enhanced recovery protocol. IV-fluid if oliguria, tachycardia, or hypotension.	No difference in SRS, LOS or postoperative morbidity. Mortality: None.
Phan et al. [49] June 2014	Elective colorectal surgery	100 in two groups GDT vs. "restricted"	Near maximal stroke volume (ODM) (CardiQ®)	LOS			Total volume 2 115 (GDT) vs. 1 500 (restricted)	Oral fluid in an enhanced recovery protocol.	No difference in LOS or postoperative morbidity Mortality: None

LOS, length of stay; ODM, oesophageal Doppler monitoring.

However, not even for this group of patients could we show any benefit in outcome for the GDT fluid therapy over restricted fluid therapy. On the contrary, the patients in the restricted group had a shorter length of hospital stay (LOS).[54]

All clinical randomized trials concerning fluid therapy in general have weaknesses.

- They are very difficult to blind. The fluids cause changes in the patient's body weight, the urinary output, and if more than 20% of the extracellular fluid volume is given ($\geq$3 litres for a 75 kg person), a visible subcutaneous oedema is formed.

- LOS as an endpoint has problems. The introduction of fast-track surgery has illustrated that the most important factor for LOS is expectations from the patients and the doctors. They simply stay in hospital as long as they are told.

- Other (perhaps unknown) confounders are difficult to control. This is especially a problem for trials including a small number of patients. Large numbers of patients will equal the confounders between the groups compared. These include:

  ○ surgical traditions including laparoscopic or open surgery, the use of drains, tubes, etc.,

  ○ allowance of the patient to return to oral fluid and food, and

  ○ type of analgesia used postoperatively. For example, postoperative nausea and vomiting (PONV) is highly influenced by the fact that opiates have pronounced PONV side effects.

Preoperative Fluid Therapy in Major Abdominal Surgery

Getting the Balance Right

The downside of fluid overload is well described in Warrillow et al.[55] The authors detail how even in 2010, the patients in their institution on the day of surgery received a median of 4.2 litres intraoperatively and 6.3 litres postoperatively, giving a total of 10.5 litres of intravenous fluid. They reported that 21% of their patients developed pulmonary oedema, 12% had anastomotic leak, and the overall complication rate was 57%, of which 32% was major complications.[55]

Numerous researchers have reported the harm of fluid overload in many different populations.[56–73]

Our trial of restricted fluid therapy [1] published in 2003 emerged from a similar scenario of fluid overload. The result of the trial was clear: fluid overload with saline and the following increase in body weight (in our trial of 4 kg) was harmful. Avoiding fluid overload has almost eliminated postoperative atrial fibrillation, pulmonary congestion, oedema, and acute respiratory distress syndrome (ARDS) in our institution.

Other researchers examined the effect of "restricted or zero-balance" fluid volumes, for patients undergoing gastrointestinal,[4,8,74–77] urologic,[10] pulmonary, [78] cardiac,[79] vascular,[6] and mixed [80] surgical procedures, as well as for surgical patients in the intensive care unit,[81] and the results were unanimous: there is a downside to fluid overload. The number of patients included in the studies varies between 20 [4] and 1000.[78,81]

Myles et al. [82] published the largest trial ($N = 3000$) to date of "restricted versus liberal fluid therapy." The primary outcome was one-year disability-free survival. They found no difference between the groups in the primary outcome, but more patients had renal failures in the restricted group. However, in the restricted group no protocol existed of giving fluid in the case of postoperative oliguria. It is very likely that the restricted regimen was too restricted and therefore caused harm. The trial has several limitations,[12] and the best fluid strategy might in fact be a volume in-between the two treatment arms. With this interpretation, the Myles trial fits the rest of the literature.

Varadhan and Lobo [11] demonstrated beautifully how the different trials and the given fluid volumes can fit a U-shaped curve, with too little fluid on one side and too much on the other.

Recently we have shown for the first time how postoperative complications actually fit a U-shaped curve when plotted against given fluid volume, and that the optimal fluid volume (the volume with fewest complications) differs for different complications.[83] We found a balance of no more than +2 litres was the optimum, even in emergency gastrointestinal surgery. These finding fully agree with our early trials of restricted fluid therapy: in the first [1] we allowed a 1 kg body weight increase and in the second [48] a 2 kg body weight increase.

How to Implement Restricted (No More than +1–2 Litres) Fluid Therapy

Restricted fluid therapy is based on the principle that fluid lost should be replaced with a fluid that resembles the loss in quantity and quality.

Fasting: Ask the patient if they had anything to drink recently and give 80 ml/fasting hour. You can give a Ringer's solution or a glucose-containing fluid.

Note: Glucose has contraindications in a woman giving birth.

Epidural preloading: We do not preload. If you want a fluid "running," think of it as replacement of fasting deficit or as an early replacement of expected blood loss.

Insensible perspiration and the evaporation from open surgical wounds: This should be a maximum of 35 + 32 ml/h. Medical water is enough to replace these losses, and they need no consideration unless the surgery becomes long lasting.

Emptying of pathological fluid: If ascites are emptied, we do not replace them, but note it in the fluid chart intraoperatively. Observation: Postoperative regeneration of such fluid may cause hypovolaemia.

Blood loss and exudation: we replace blood loss with Ringer's solution in the relation 1:2–3, and monitor the hemoglobin (Hb). Red blood cells are given to keep Hb > 4.5 in young healthy patients, and >5.6 in elderly patients with cardiopulmonary diagnosis. Table 14.3 shows the recommendations.

We treat continuous blood loss according to the following: after 6 portions of erythrocytes are given, then fresh frozen plasma (FFP) is started at a rate of 1:1 erythrocytes:FFP. This means if the patient has received 12 portions of erythrocytes, 6 portions of fresh frozen plasma have been given too, and here we commence the supplementation with thrombocytes (the 12:6 rule).

We treat emergency ongoing bleeding with transfusion packages in the relation:

Erythrocytes 4: Plasma 4: Thrombocytes 1 (e.g., full blood).

Urine: We do not replace intraoperative urinary loss. Other reasons than fluid deficit can cause low diuresis during surgery. If you are certain that the patient does not have hypovolaemia, a small intraoperative diuresis is acceptable.

We can achieve this with a background infusion of no more than 2 ml/kg/h and monitoring of blood loss.

Preoperative Fluid Therapy in Outpatient Surgery

Table 14.2 [84–90] shows the trials of different fluid volumes during outpatient and minor abdominal surgery.

These trials show that approximately 1 litre of fluid IV creates well-being (less PONV) after outpatient surgery.

This finding is logical because the patients included in the trials were told to fast from midnight before surgery, that is, they have a fluid deficit of approximately 1 litre.

A surprising finding was given by Holte et al., [85] who examined the effect of 3 litres versus 1 litre fluid on PONV, postoperative ability to run on a treadmill, and pulmonary function as measured by spirometry. The trial showed that patients receiving 3 litres had less PONV and better exercise performance compared with the patients given 1 litre. This trial has, however, a problem with the doses of postoperative opiates given, with smaller doses given (less pain?) to the patients in the group given most fluid.

Postoperative Fluid Therapy

Trials of postoperative fluid restriction show a less clear result: one trial found improved outcome,[91] one trial found no difference in outcome,[92] and one trial found harm resulting from postoperative fluid restriction,[93] comparing nearly the same volumes between groups, approximately 1.5 litres IV per day versus 2.5 litres IV per day. The reason for these findings is most probably that a fixed volume of fluid does not fit all

Table 14.2 Trials of outpatient abdominal surgery

Loss % of blood volume	Loss in ml (70–80 kg person)	Replacement	Volume
0–20%	0–1 000 ml	Ringer's solution	500–3 000 ml
20–40%	1 000–2 000 ml	Additional human albumin (HA)	1 000 ml
40–80%	2 000–4 000 ml	Additional erythrocytes and HA	3–4 portions of erythrocytes (1 000 ml) 1 000 ml (HA)
Thereafter	For each 500 ml	Additional erythrocytes and fresh frozen plasma (FFP)	1 portion (ca. 300 ml) 1 portion (ca. 250 ml)
		Thrombocytes	Are started following 6 (FFP):12 portions erythrocytes

DW, dextrose in water 5%; CSL, compound sodium lactose (Na:131, K:5, Ca:2, Cl:111, lactate: 29 mmol/l); NS, normal saline 0.9%; LR, lactated Ringer's solution.

Table 14.3 Replacement of blood loss during surgery

Author	Surgery	No. of patients	Blinding	Duration of surgery	Intervention	Fast	Postop oral fluid intake	Results
Keane & Murray [86] 1986	Mixed outpatient surgery	212 in 2 groups	No	18 min	1 000 ml Hartman's solution + 1 000 ml DW vs. No fluid	?	?	Fluid reduces thirst, drowsiness and increases well-being. No effect on nausea.
Spencer [89] 1988	Minor gynecologic surgery	100 in 2 groups	No	8 min	1 l CSL vs. No fluid	?	?	Fluid reduces dizziness and nausea.
Cook et al., [84] 1990	Gynecologic laparoscopy	75 in 3 groups	Yes	20 min	CSL 20 ml/kg vs. CSL + DW 20 ml/kg vs. No fluid	11 –16 h	?	Fluid reduces dizziness and drowsiness. Hospital stay reduced in Dextrose group.
Yogendran et al., [90] 1995	Mixed outpatient surgery	200 in 2 groups	Yes	28 min	Plasmolyte 20 ml/kg (1 215 ml) vs. Plasmolyte 2 ml/kg (164 ml)	8–13 h	?	Fluid reduces thirst, dizziness, and drowsiness. No effect on nausea.
McCaul et al., [88] 2003	Gynecologic laparoscopy	108 in 3 groups	Yes	22 min	CSL 1.5 ml/kg/fasting h (1 115 ml) vs. CSL + DW 1.5 ml/kg/fasting h (1 148 ml) vs. no fluid	11.5 h	?	No significant differences between the groups.

Table 14.3 (cont.)

Author	Surgery	No. of patients	Blinding	Duration of surgery	Intervention	Fast	Postop oral fluid intake	Results
Magner et al. [87] 2004	Gynecologic laparoscopy	141 in 2 groups	Yes	20 min	CSL 30 ml/kg vs. CSL 10 ml/kg	13 h	?	Fluid reduced nausea and vomiting. No effect on dizziness or thirst.
Holte et al. [85] 2004	Laparoscopic cholecystectomy	48 in 2 groups	Yes	68 min	LR 15 ml/kg (998 ml) vs. 40 ml/kg (2 928 ml)	2 h	Mean 600 ml	Fluid reduces thirst, nausea, dizziness, drowsiness, improves well-being, pulmonary function and shorten hospital stay.

patients. Some patients drink sufficient amounts and do not need IV replacement, while other patients have postoperative pathological fluid losses exceeding 1.5 litres, making the fixed replacement too little in volume and possibly incorrect in electrolyte composition.

Mixing these trials with the trials of intra- and immediate postoperative (24 h) trials in a meta-analysis adds to the confusion and not the clarification of the subject.[94]

The idea of the original "restricted regimen" [48] was to replace any fluid loss with a fluid of the same volume and similar electrolyte composition as the loss. This means that the patients were given a hypotonic fluid postoperatively to cover their daily needs for water, sodium, potassium, and glucose, and that pathological fluid losses were replaced with a fluid with a similar electrolyte content as the loss.

Urinary output was kept at 1–0.5 ml/kg/hour, and patients with oliguria or hypotension were examined and the reason treated: if the reason was hypovolemia, the patient was given additional IV-crystalloid; if the reason was epidural analgesia overdosing, the dose was reduced or a pressor was given; if the reason was dehydration, additional water or IV-glucose was given. The patients had a permitted body weight increase of maximum 1 [1]–2 [48] kg, and feeding commenced 2 hours postoperatively. Today, we allow patients to eat after surgery as soon as the risk of aspiration is minimal. Modern enhanced recovery after surgery programs (ERAS programs) are based on the above body of evidence, and current recommendations of fluid therapy in ERAS programs call for zero fluid balance with no more than 2–2.5 kg body weight gain.[95,96]

ERAS programs especially for elderly people exist and are highly recommended.[97]

The ERAS-programs call for patients to continue a physiological treatment regimen on the surgical ward. This includes sufficient treatment of pain with primarily non-opioid analgesics, early enteral nutrition, early mobilization, and minimizing or avoiding the use of urinary catheters and surgical drains.

Both fluid chart as well as body weight are needed to provide a logical fluid and electrolyte therapy.[98] The fluid chart indicates the type of fluid lost (the quality), and the body weight is needed for the monitoring of the quantity of fluid lost, that is, the fluid balance. It is therefore necessary to measure the body weight of the patient in the morning before the operation to ensure the recording of a fluid chart, and to continue to measure the body weight every morning postoperatively on the same scale.

Blood samples for control of electrolyte status (Na, K, Hb, creatinine) should be measured daily as long as the patient does not eat a sufficient diet.

Blood pressure decrease for any reason including the use of epidurals or other drugs will cause a decrease in urinary output, because the glomerular filtration rate is pressure dependant. In patients without a stenosis in the renal artery, a mean arterial pressure above 60 mmHg will be sufficient for the maintenance of GFR and thereby urine production.

Blood pressure drops caused by epidurals are best treated with pressor substances; however, pressor substances are not recommended for use in the surgical ward and epidural hypotension is better treated with a reduction in the dose of epidural analgesia or interruption of habitual anti-hypertensive medication.

If hypovolemia is suspected, a fluid bolus may be given and the effect observed.

We recommend that patients are allowed to drink and eat freely postoperatively, and intravenous fluid therapy may be indicated if the oral intake is insufficient, the patient has paralytic ileus, or a complication has occurred.

Recommendations

- Normal as well as pathological fluid losses should be replaced with a fluid resembling the loss in quantity and quality (electrolyte composition).
- Elective surgical patients are allowed to eat until 6 hours and drink up to 2 hours before surgery without increasing the risk of fluid aspiration.
- Preoperative administration of sugar-containing fluids (orally or intravenously) improves postoperative well-being and muscle strength and lessens the postoperative insulin resistance. It does not, however, reduce the number of patients with wound or other complications, length of stay, or mortality.
- Surgery does not increase the normal fluid and electrolyte losses, but causes perspiration from the abdominal wound that approximately equals the decreased water loss from the lungs because of ventilation with moist air.
- It is not possible to treat a decrease in blood pressure caused by the use of epidural analgesia with fluid.
- The goal of no more than +2 litre fluid balance (formerly called "restrictive") reduces postoperative complications and the risk of death in major abdominal surgery. The goal of zero balance in combination with a goal of near maximum stroke volume provides equally good outcome.
- During outpatient surgical procedures, the well-being of the patient is improved by giving approximately 1 litre of fluid. The role of glucose-containing fluid in this setting may be beneficial but evidence is sparse.
- "Postoperative restricted fluid therapy" allowing the patients to drink no more than 1500 ml/day is not recommended. The patients should be allowed to eat and drink freely.
- Fluid chart is insufficient to monitor the fluid balance; body weight measurement is mandatory.

References

1. Brandstrup B, Tønnesen H, Beier-Holgersen R, et al. Effects of intravenous fluid restriction on postoperative complications: comparison of two perioperative fluid regimens. A randomized assessor blinded multi centre trial. *Ann Surg.* 2003;**238**:641–48.

2. de Aguilar-Nascimento JE, Diniz BN, do Carmo AV, et al. Clinical benefits after the implementation of a protocol of restricted perioperative intravenous crystalloid fluids in major abdominal operations. *World J Surg.* 2009;**33**:925–30.

3. Kulemann B, Timme S, Sifert G, et al. Intraoperative crystalloid overload leads to substantial inflammatory infiltration of intestinal anastomosis – a histomorphological analysis. *Surgery.* 2013;**154**:596–603.

4. Lobo DN, Bostock KA, Neal KR, et al. Effect of salt and water balance on recovery of gastrointestinal function after elective colonic resection: a randomised controlled trial. *Lancet.* 2002;**359**:1812–18.

5. Marjanovic G, Villain C, Juettner E et al. Impact of different crystalloid volume fluid regimens on intestinal anastomotic stability. *Ann Surg.* 2009;**249**:181–5.

6. McArdle GT, McAuley DF, McKinley A et al. Preliminary results of a prospective randomized trial of restrictive versus standard fluid regime in elective open abdominal aortic aneurysm repair. *Ann Surg.* 2009;**250**:28–34.

7. Neal JM, Wilcox RT, Allen HW, Low DE. Near-total esophagectomy: the influence of standardized multimodal management and

intraoperative fluid restriction. *Reg Anest Pain Med.* 2003;**28**: 328–34.

8. Nisanevich V, Felsenstein I, Almogy G, et al. Effect of intraoperative fluid management on outcome after intra-abdominal surgery. *Anesthesiology.* 2005;**103**:25–32.

9. The National Heart LaBIARDSACTN, Weidemann HP, Wheeler AP, et al. Comparison of two fluid-management strategies in acute lung injury. *N Engl J Med.* 2006;**354**:2564–75.

10. Wuethrich PY, Burchard FC, Thalmann GN, et al. Restrictive deferred hydration combined with preemptive norepinephrine infusion during radical cystectomy reduces postoperative complications and hospitalization time: a randomized clinical trial. *Aneshsiology.* 2014;**120**:365–77.

11. Varadhan KK, Lobo DN. A meta-analysis of randomised controlled trials of intravenous fluid therapy in major elective open abdominal surgery: getting the balance right. *Proct Nutr Soc.* 2010;**69**:488–98.

12. Brandstrup B. Finding the right balance. *N Engl J Med.* 2018;**378**:2335–6.

13. Weinstein JR, Anderson S. The aging kidney: physiological changes. *Adv Chronic Kidney Dis.* 2010;**17**:302–7.

14. Beck LH. Perioperative renal, fluid and electrolyte management. *Clin Geriatric Med.* 1990;**6**:557–69.

15. Rowe JW, Shock NW, DeFonzo RA. The influence of age on the renal responce to water deprivation in man. *Nephron.* 1976;**17**:270–8.

16. Drummer C, Gerzer R, Heer M, et al. Effect of an acute saline infusion on fluid and electrolyte metabolism in humans. *Am J Physiol.* 1992;**262**:F744–F754.

17. Phillips PA, Rolls BJ, Ledingham JGG, et al. Reduced thirst after water deprivation in healthy elderly men. *N Engl J Med.* 1984;**311**:753–9.

18. Gamble JL. The Harvey Lectures, Series XLIII, 1946–1947: physiological information gained from studies on the life raft ration. *Nutr Rev.* 1989;**47**:199–201.

19. Prough IC, Baker EM. Maximum physiological concentration of sodium in human urine. *J Appl Physiol.* 1959;**14**:1036–8.

20. Blichert-Toft M, Christensen V, Engquist A, et al. Influence of age on the endocrine-metabolic response to surgery. *Ann Surg.* 1979;**190**:761–70.

21. Kudoh A, Ishihara H, Matsuki A. Renin-aldosterone system and atrial natriuretic peptide during anesthesia in orthopedic patients over 80 years of age. *J Clin Anesth.* 1999;**11**:101–7.

22. Rekommendationer for præoperativ faste. www.dasaim.dk, May 2014.

23. Henriksen MG. Effects of preoperative oral carbohydrates and peptides on postoperative endocrine response, mobilization, nutrition and muscle function in abdominal surgery. *Acta Anesthesiol Scand.* 2003;**47**:191–9.

24. Ljungqvist O, Thorell A, Gutniak M, et al. Glucose infusion instead of preoperative fasting reduces postoperative insulin resistance. *J Am Coll Surg.* 1994;**178**:329–36.

25. Nygren J, Soop M, Thorell A, et al. Preoperative oral carbohydrates and postoperative insulin resistance. *Clin Nutr.* 1999;**18**:117–20.

26. Lamke LO, Nielsson GE, Reithner HL. Water loss by evaporation from the abdominal cavity during surgery. *Acta Chir Scand.* 1977;**143**:279–84.

27. Roe CF. Effect of bowel exposure on body temperature during surgical operations. *Am J Surg.* 1971;**122**:13–15.

28. Brandstrup B, Svendsen C, Engquist A. Hemorrhage and operation cause a contraction of the extra cellular space needing replacement – evidence and implications? A systematic review. *Surgery.* 2006;**139**:419–32.

29. Chan STF, Kapadia CR, Johnson AW, et al. Extracellular fluid volume expansion and third space sequestration at the site of small bowel anastomoses. *Br J Surg.* 1983;**70**:36–9.

30. Brandstrup B. *Restricted Intravenous Fluid Therapy in Colorectal Surgery: Results of*

a Clinical Randomised Multi Centre Trial. 2003. Doctoral thesis, University of Copenhagen.

31. Jacob M, Chappel D, Rehm M. The third space – fact or fiction? *Best Prac Res Clin Anaesth.* 2009;**23**:145–57.

32. Kinsella SM, Pirlet M, Mills MS, et al. Randomized study of intravenous fluid preload before epidural analgesia during labour. *Br J Anaesth.* 2000;**85**:311–13.

33. Kubli M, Shennan AH, Seed PT, et al. A randomised controlled trial of fluid pre-loading before low dose epidural analgesia for labour. *Int J Obstet Anesth.* 2003;**12**:256–60.

34. Nishimura N, Kajimoto Y, Kabe T, et al. The effect of volume loading during epidural analgesia. *Resuscitation.* 1985;**13**:31–9.

35. Rivers E, Nguyen B, Havstad S, et al. Early goal-directed therapy in the treatment of severe sepsis and septic shock. *N Engl J Med.* 2001;**345**:1368–77.

36. Navarro LH, Bloomstone JA, Auler JO Jr, et al. Perioperative fluid therapy: a statement from the international Fluid Optimization Group. *Periop Med (London).* 2015;**4**:1–20.

37. Benes J, Chytra I, Altmann P, et al. Intraoperative fluid optimization using stroke volume variation in high risk surgical patients: results of prospective randomized study. *Crit Care.* 2010;**14**:1–15.

38. Gan TJ, Soppitt A, Maroof M, et al. Goal-directed intraoperative fluid administration reduces length of hospital stay after major surgery. *Anesthesiology.* 2002;**97**:820–6.

39. Lopes MR, Olivera MA, Pereira VOS, et al. Goal-directed fluid management based on pulse pressure variation monitoring during high-risk surgery: a pilot randomized controlled trial. *Crit Care.* 2007;**11**:R100.

40. Mayer J, Boldt J, Mengistu AM, et al. Goal-directed intraoperative therapy based on autocalibrated arterial pressure waveform analysis reduces hospital stay in high-risk

surgical patients: a randomized, controlled trial. *Crit Care.* 2010;**14**:1–9.

41. Salzwedel C, Puig J, Carstens A, et al. Perioperative goal-directed hemodynamic therapy based on radial arterial pulse pressure variation and continous cardiac index trending reduces postoperative complications: a multi-center, prospective, randomized study. *Crit Care.* 2013;**17**:1–11.

42. Wakeling HG, McFall MR, Jenkins CS, et al. Intraoperative oesophageal doppler guided fluid management shortens postoperative hospital stay after major bowel surgery. *Br J Anaesth.* 2005;**95**:634–42.

43. Buettner M, Schummer W, Huetttemann E, et al. Influence of systolic-pressure-variation-guided intraoperative fluid management on organ function and oxygen transport. *Br J Anaesth.* 2008;**101**:194–9.

44. Challand C, Struthers R, Sneyd JR, et al. Randomized controlled trial of intraoperative goal-directed fluid therapy in aerobically fit and unfit patients having major colorectal surgery. *Br J Anaesth.* 2012;**108**:53–62.

45. Conway DH, Mayall R, Abdul-Latif MS, et al. Randomised controlled trial investigating the influence of intravenous fluid titration using oesophageal Doppler monitoring during bowel surgery. *Anaesthesia.* 2002;**57**:845–9.

46. Forget P, Lois F, de Kock M. Goal-directed fluid management based on the pulse oximeter-derived Pleth variability index reduces lactate levels and improves fluid management. *Anesth Analg.* 2010;**111**:910–14.

47. Perner A, Haase N, Guttormsen AB, et al. Hydroxyethyl starch 130/0.42 versus Ringer's acetate in severe sepsis. *N Engl J Med.* 2012;**367**:124–34.

48. Brandstrup B, Svendsen PE, Rasmussen M, et al. Which goal for fluid therapy during colorectal surgery is followed by the best outcome: near maximal stroke volume or zero fluid balance? A clinical randomized

double blinded multi centre trial. *Euro J Anaesth*. 2010;**27**:4.

49. Phan TD, D'Sousa B, Rattray MJ, et al. A randomised controlled trial of fluid restriction compared to oesophageal Doppler-guided goal-directed fluid therapy in elective major colorectal surgery within an Enhanced Recovery After Surgery program. *Anaesth Intensive Care*. 2014;**42**:752–60.

50. Srinivasa S, Taylor MH, Singh PP, et al. Randomized clinical trial of goal-directed fluid therapy within an enhanced recovery protocol for elective colectomy. *Br J Anaesth*. 2013;**100**:66–74.

51. Zheng H, Guo H, Ye J, et al. Goal-directed fluid therapy in gastrointestinal surgery in older coronary heart disease patients: Randomized trial. *World J Surg*, 2013;**37**:2820–9.

52. Wrzosek A, Jakowicka-Wordliczek J, Zajaczkowska R, et al. Perioperative restrictive versus goal-directed fluid therapy for adults undergoing major non-cardiac surgery. *Cochrane Database Syst Rev*. 2019;**12**:CD012767.

53. Colantonio L, Claroni C, Fabrizi L, et al. A randomized trial of goal directed vs. standard fluid therapy in cytoreductive surgery with hyperthermic intraperitoneal chemotherapy. *J Gastrointest Surg*. 2015;**19**:722–9.

54. Aaen AA, Voldby AW, Storm N, et al. Goal-directed fluid therapy in emergency abdominal surgery: a randomised multicentre trial. *Br J Anaesth*. 2021;**127**:521–31.

55. Warrillow SJ, Weinberg L, Parker F, et al. Perioperative fluid prescription, complications and outcomes in major elective open gastrointestinal surgery. *Anaesth Intensive Care*. 2010;**38**:259–65.

56. Walsh SR, Walsh CJ. Intravenous fluid-associated morbidity in postoperative patients. *Ann R Coll Surg Engl*. 2005;**87**:126–30.

57. Kalus JS, Caron MF, White CM, et al. Impact on fluid balance on incidence of atrial fibrillation after cardiothoracic surgery. *Am J Cardiol*. 2004;**94**:1423–5.

58. Hübner M, Schäfer M, Demartines N, et al. Impact of restrictive intravenous fluid replacement and combined epidural analgesia on perioperative volume balance and renal function within a Fast Track program. *J Surg Res*. 2012;**173**:68–74.

59. Ettinger KS, Arce K, Lohse CM, et al. Higher perioperative fluid administration is associated with increased rates of complications following head and neck microvascular reconstruction with fibular free flaps. *Microsurgery*. 2017;**37**:128–36.

60. Bjerregaard LS, Møller-Sørensen H, Hansen KL, et al. Using clinical parameters to guide fluid therapy in high-risk thoracic surgery. A retrospective, observational study. *BMC Anesthesiol*. 2015;**15**:91–8.

61. Elofson KA, Eiferman DS, Porter K, et al. Impact on late fluid balance on clinical outcomes in the critical ill surgical and trauma population. *J Crit Care*. 2015;**30**:1338–43.

62. Jurt J, Hübner M, Pache B, et al. Respiratory complications after colorectal surgery: avoidable or fate? *World J Surg*. 2018;**42**:2708–14.

63. Askild D, Segelman J, Gedda C, et al. The impact of perioperative fluid therapy on short-term outcomes and 5-year survival among patients undergoing colorectal cancer surgery – a prospective cohort study within an ERAS protocol. *Eur J Surg Oncol*. 2017;**43**:1433–9.

64. Nielsson L, Wodlin NB, Kjølhede P. Risk factors for postoperative complications after fast-track abdominal hysterectomy. *Aust N Zealand J Obst Gyn*. 2012;**52**:113–20.

65. Duke MD, Guirdy C, Guice J, et al. Restrictive fluid resuscitation in combination with damage control resuscitation: time for adaption. *J Trauma Acute Care Surg*. 2012;**73**:674–8.

66. Minambres E, Rodrigo E, Ballesteros MA, et al. Impact of restrictive fluid balance focused to increase lung procurement on renal function after kidney transplantation. *Nephrol Dial Transplant*. 2010;**25**:2352–6.

67. Weinberg L, Wong D, Karalapilli D, et al. The impact of fluid intervention on

complications and length of hospital stay after pancreaticoduodenectomy (Whipple's procedure). *BMC Anesthesiol.* 2014;**14**:35–43.

68. Møller AM, Pedersen T, Svendsen P-E, et al. Perioperative risk factors in elective pneumonectomy: the impact of excess fluid balance. *Eur J Anaesthes,* 2002;**19**:57–62.

69. Parquin F, Marchal M, Mehiri S, et al. Post-pneumonectomy pulmonary edema: analysis and risk factors. *Eur J Cardiothorac Surg.* 1996;**10**:929–33.

70. Patel RL, Townsend ER, Fountain SW. Elective pneumonectomy: factors associated with morbidity and operative mortality. *Ann Thorac Surg.* 1992;**54**:88.

71. Turnage WS, Lunn JJ. Postpneumonectomy pulmonary edema. A retrospective analysis of associated variables. *Chest.* 1993;**103**:1646–50.

72. Verheijen-Breemhaar L, Bogaard JM, van den Berg B, et al. Post-pneumonectomy pulmonary edema. *Thorax.* 1998;**43**:323–6.

73. Zeldin RA, Normandin D, Landtwing D, et al. Postpneumonectomy pulmonary edema. *J Thorac Cardiovasc Surg.* 1984;**87**:359–65.

74. Abraham-Nordling M, Hjern F, Pollack J, et al. Randomized clinical trial of fluid restriction in colorectal surgery. *Br J Surg.* 2012;**99**:186–91.

75. Gao T, Li N, Zhang J, et al. Restricted intravenous fluid regimen reduces the rate of postoperative complications and alters immunological activity of elderly patients operated for abdominal cancer: a randomized prospective clinical trial. *World J Surg.* 2012;**36**:993–1002.

76. Lobo SM, Lobo FR, Polachini CA, et al. Prospective, randomized trial comparing fluids and doputamine optimization of oxygen delivery in high-risk surgical patients. *Crit Care.* 2006;**10**:R72.

77. Wenkui Y, Ning L, Jianfeng G, et al. Restricted peri-operative fluid administration adjusted by serum lactate level improved outcome after major elective surgery for gastrointestinal malignancy. *Surgery.* 2010;**147**:542–52.

78. National Heart and Blood Institute Acute Respiratory Distress Syndrome (ARDS) Clinical Trials Network. Comparison of two fluid management strategies in acute lung injury. *N Engl J Med.* 2006;**354**:2564–75.

79. Bhaskaran K, Arumugam G, Kumar PV. A prospective randomized comparison study on effect of perioperative use of chloride liberal intravenous fluids versus chloride restricted intravenous fluids on postoperative acute kidney injury in patients undergoing off-pump coronary artery bypass grafting surgeries. *Ann Card Anaesth.* 2018;**21**:413–18.

80. Lobo SM, Ronchi LS, Oliveira NE, et al. Restrictive strategy of intraoperative fluid maintenance during optimization of oxygen delivery decreases major complications after high-risk surgery. *Crit Care.* 2011;**15**:R226.

81. Stewart RM, Park PK, Hunt JP, et al. less is more: improved outcomes in surgical patients with conservative fluid administration and central venous catheter monitoring. *J Am Coll Surg.* 2009;**208**:725–37.

82. Myles PS, Bellomo R, Corcoran T, et al. Restrictive versus liberal fluid therapy for major abdominal surgery. *N Engl J Med.* 2018;**378**:2263–74.

83. Voldby AW, Aaen AA, Loprete R, et al. Perioperative fluid administration and complications in emergency gastrointestinal surgery – an observational study. *Periop Med (London).* 2022;**11**:9.

84. Cook R, Anderson S, Riseborough M, et al. Intravenous fluid load and recovery. A double-blind comparison in gynaecological patients who had day-case laparoscopy. *Anaesthesia.* 1990;**45**:826–30.

85. Holte K, Klarskov B, Christensen DS, et al. Liberal versus restrictive fluid administration to improve recovery after laparoscopic cholecystectomy. A randomized, double-blind study. *Ann Surg.* 2004;**240**:892–9.

86. Keane PW, Murray PF. Intravenous fluids in minor surgery. Their effect on recovery from anaesthesia. *Anaesthesia.* 1986;**41**:635–7.

87. Magner JJ, McCaul C, Carton E, et al. Effect of intraoperative intravenous crystalloid infusion on postoperative nausea and vomiting after gynaecological laparoscopy: comparison of 30 and 10 ml/kg (−1). *Br J Anaesth*. 2004;**93**:381–5.

88. McCaul C, Moran C, O'Cronin D, et al. Intravenous fluid loading with or without supplementary dextrose does not prevent nausea, vomiting and pain after laparoscopy. *Can J Anaesth*. 2003;**5**:440–4.

89. Spencer EM. Intravenous fluids in minor gynaecological surgery. Their effect on postoperative morbidity. *Anaesthesia*. 1988;**43**:1050–1.

90. Yogendran S, Asokumar B, Cheng DC, et al. A prospective randomized double-blinded study of the effect of intravenous fluid therapy on adverse outcomes on outpatient surgery. *Anesth Analg*. 1995;**80**:682–6.

91. Gonzalez-Fajardo JA, Mengibar L, Brizuela JA, et al. Effect of postoperative restrictive fluid therapy in the recovery of patients with abdominal vascular surgery. *Eur J Vasc Endovasc Surg*. 2009;**37**:538–43.

92. MacCay G, Fearon K, McConnachie A, et al. Randomized clinical trial of the effect of postoperative intravenous fluid restriction on recovery after elective colorectal surgery. *Br J Surg*. 2006;**93**:1469–74.

93. Vermeulen H, Hofland J, Legemate DA, et al. Intravenous fluid restriction after major abdominal surgery: a randomized blinded clinical trial. *Trials*. 2009;**7**:10–50.

94. Boland MR, Noorani A, Varty K, et al. Perioperative fluid restriction in major abdominal surgery: systematic review and meta-analysis of randomized clinical trials. *World J Surg*. 2013;**37**:1193–202.

95. Feldheiser A, Aziz O, Baldini G, et al. Enhanced recovery after surgery (ERAS) in gastrointestinal surgery, part 2: consensus statement for anaesthesia practice. *Acta Anesthesiol Scand*. 2016;**60**:289–334.

96. Ljungqvist O, Scott M, Fearon KC. Enhanced recovery after surgery: a review. *JAMA Surg*. 2017;**152**:292.

97. Montroni I, Ugolini G, Saur, et al. Personalized management of elderly patients with rectal cancer: expert recommendations of the European Society of Surgical Geriatric Oncology, and American College of Surgeons Comission on Cancer. *Eur J Surg Oncol*. 2018;**44**:1685–702.

98. Tulstrup J, Brandstrup B. Clinical assessment of fluid balance is incomplete for colorectal surgical patients. *Scand J Surg*. 2014;**104**:161–8.

Chapter 15

Fluid and Hemodynamic Monitoring in Pulmonary Surgery

Mert Şentürk, Achmet Ali, Zerrin Sungur
and Emre Sertaç Bingül

Introduction

"Fluid therapy" can be considered as one of most "famous" challenges of the perioperative care of thoracic surgery. On one hand, in spite of hundreds of studies, there is still no "evidence-based" suggestion that can be applied in the specific conditions of thoracic anesthesia; on the other hand, these specific conditions make it harder to evaluate possible suggestions in an objective way. Moreover, some "myths" from the previous century can still cause confusions, making the problem more challenging. This chapter will focus on these specific challenges of fluid management and hemodynamic monitoring in thoracic surgery.

A Confusing Question: "Restrictive" versus "Liberal"?

In 1984, Zeldin et al. first defined postpneumonectomy pulmonary edema (PPPE), reporting that there is a correlation between the amount of perioperative fluid and postoperative edema.[1] However, this study was associated with some concerns: First, the amount of administered fluid (>37 mL/kg intraoperatively and 24 h postoperatively) is far above of the current possible (even more than the most "liberal") regimens. Second, the study was performed in 10 patients with edema, which makes the study very difficult to repeat with current sample size assumptions. Moreover, some other findings [e.g., low pulmonary capillary wedge pressure (PCWP), "exudate" as edema fluid] are contrary to the assumption of the relationship between the edema and volume administration. As a pioneer study showing a link between the fluid administration and postoperative complications, this article [1] exceeds its scientific contribution and has inevitably supported some "urban myths."

As a matter of fact, in the past decades, numerous comparative ("liberal" vs. "restrictive") or observational studies have confirmed the effects of the intraoperative amount of the fluid on postoperative complications: As examples, Alam et al. reported that for every 500-mL increase in perioperative fluids, the odds ratio (OR) of developing acute lung injury after lung resection was 1.17;[2] Arslantas et al. have reported in the retrospective analysis of 139 patients that intraoperative infusion rate of fluids exceeding 6 mL/kg/h was associated with more frequent postoperative pulmonary complications (PPCs).[3] Recently, the analysis of the German Thorax Registry in 376 patients undergoing lung resection via video-assisted thoracoscopic surgery (VATS) have confirmed that the intraoperative amount of crystalloid fluids exceeding 6 mL/kg/h was one of the four independent risk factors [among preoperative forced expiratory volume (FEV1), preoperative PaO_2 and duration of surgery] that can lead to PPCs.[4,5] This relationship has also been shown in esophagectomies ("non-pulmonary thoracic surgery"): In a recent study, increased intraoperative fluid administration (median: 11.92 mL/kg/h) was found to be associated with worse PPCs, specifically acute respiratory distress syndrome (ARDS).[6]

Unfortunately, there are some common problems in studies regarding fluid management in thoracic surgery:[7]

- The vast majority of these studies are retrospective and can avoid a classical "chicken-egg" question only in a limited manner, if any: In a single-center study, why has the same anesthesiologist given different amounts of fluids to different patients? Was it the amount of fluid that has made the patient sicker, or was it the sicker patient who required (?) higher amounts of fluid? In spite of hundreds of studies and guidelines, there is still a large variation in the fluid management in daily practice: At the Johns Hopkins Hospital, over a 4-year period, the median crystalloid volume that was infused during lung surgery was 11.3 mL/kg/h with large variations between anesthesiologists.[8]
- Even the definitions of "liberal" and "restrictive" regimens differ essentially among different studies: this leads further to heterogeneous and unreliable results of meta-analyses, as the amount of fluid in the "restrictive" group in one study can exceed the amount given to the "liberal" groups in another.
- The cliché of "lungs do not have a third space" has somehow gained popularity as a possible explanation of why the fluid management in thoracic operations should be "restrictive" compared with other operations. "Third fluid compartment" was probably a physician's description of some decades ago, in an attempt to explain the destiny of the huge amounts of volume needed in clinical cases such as major trauma and burns with trauma-induced capillary injuries. Today, we know that not only the lung but any other organ in the body does not have this "mythic space" either: 1) the neuroendocrine stress response always leads to fluid retention and peripheral vasoconstriction; and 2) capillary lesions causing fluid exudation are transient and limited to the operative site in the absence of sepsis.[9,10]

Changing evidence is changing the approach to the historical question of liberal versus restrictive. Recent trends in major abdominal (not thoracic!) operations have begun to favor a more liberal strategy. A recent meta-analysis of 18 studies in major abdominal (no thoracic!) surgery has found no difference in the occurrence of severe postoperative complications and mortality between the two regimens, and the liberal approach was associated with even lower overall renal major events.[11] In the RELIEF study, a restrictive fluid regimen was associated with a higher rate of acute kidney injury (AKI; 8.6% in the restrictive vs. 5.0% in the liberal fluid group, $p < 0.001$), and was not associated with a higher rate of disability-free survival.[12] As underlined, these studies cover only the abdominal operations and cannot be extrapolated to thoracic surgery.

Changing evidence is also changing the definitions of perioperative renal problems: In the past decades, new definitions of "acute kidney injury," created by the RIFLE and AKIN studies, have been introduced. One of the important differences of these new approaches is that changes of creatinine values are taken into consideration (instead of its absolute value as in the historical definition), achieving a more precise and predictive evaluation of changes in renal functions. Indeed, the incidence of postoperative AKI after thoracic operations is much higher than predicted earlier (an incidence of 5.9% [13] to 10% [14]). Although it has been shown that hypovolemia can lead to renal complications, we have to underline that some of these studies have found either a weak or no correlation between intraoperative fluid restriction and postoperative AKI. Matot et al. have reported that In patients undergoing VATS, intraoperative urinary output and postoperative renal function are not affected by administration of fluids in the range of 2 to 8 mL/kg·h^{-1}, and Ahn et al. have shown that crystalloid restriction ($\leq$3mL·kg·h^{-1}) was unrelated to AKI, regardless of preoperative renal functions.[15,16] However, it is conspicuous that the paradigm has changed: One can see that in these studies that the amounts of fluids even in the most "liberal" groups are not to be compared with earlier studies.

As a matter of fact, new evidence has shown that "dry" anesthesia and postanesthesia care can potentially lead to greater occurrence of hypovolemia, hypoperfusion, and organ damage:[17] "the more, the worse" does not mean "the less, the better."[18]

Can the Terms "Moderate" and "Normovolemia" Help to Resolve the Confusion?

More recent studies have chosen to examine the effects of "moderate" regimens in comparison with both liberal and restrictive strategies. In two studies, a predefined "moderate" fluid infusion was found superior in terms of postoperative pulmonary complications when compared to "restrictive" and "liberal" fluid therapy groups that are within the studies. [19,20] It can be concretely argued that as both restrictive and liberal intraoperative fluid administration are related with adverse effects on postoperative outcomes, a "moderate" fluid regimen achieving "normovolemia" should also be the strategy of choice in the daily practice of thoracic surgery. Yet, the definitions of "moderate" and "normovolemia" are also not clear and may differ among different studies.[19,20] The defined thresholds in different (though similar) studies are based completely on the collected data of the patient population and have almost no scientific background.[21] The classical V-shaped curve of normovolemia would be appropriate in the majority of thoracic operations [22] (Fig. 15.1a), but there is no "magic number" for normovolemia;[9] the turning point of the curve can differ not only in different patients, but also in different conditions (e.g., preoperative fluid status), in different operations (e.g., VATS vs. open thoracotomy), and in different organs (e.g., kidney vs. lung) (Fig. 15.1b).[7,9] Therefore, a more concrete definition than just "moderate" is required, and defining a "goal" appears to be more appropriate.[23] But before defining the "goal," the physiology of fluid balance, the changes in this physiology under clinical conditions, and specific differences in pulmonary tissue should be clearly understood.

Physiology and Pathophysiology of Fluid Balance

Classical Starling Principle: Distribution of body water within compartments is well known: About 60% of body mass is water; approximately two-thirds distributed within the cells, and one-third in the extracellular space [interstitial space (ISS, 15%) and intravascular space (IVS, 5%)]. The IVS further includes the "stressed" volume that contributes to the venous return flow via the pressure gradient between venous system and the right atrium, and the remaining "unstressed volume." The balance between the compartments is determined by the classical Starling principle: opposite hydrostatic and colloid osmotic pressure gradients, the permeability of the cells, and the lymphatic clearance capacity. The maintenance of the balance between the compartment is maintained with the regulation of the renin–angiotensin–aldosterone (RAS), antidiuretic, and atrial natriuretic hormone

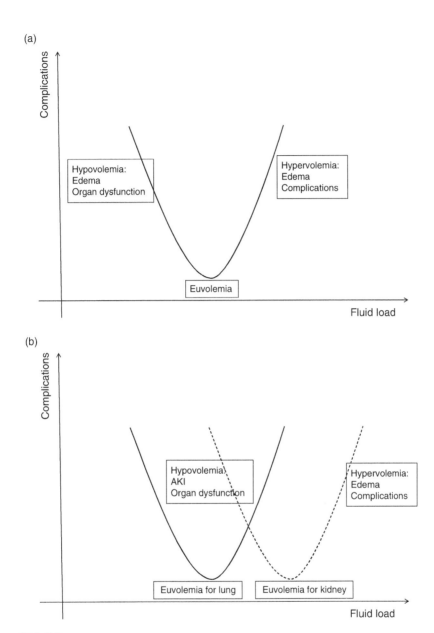

Figure 15.1 [7,9]
(a) Relationship between morbidity and volume load. "Moderate" approach aims at euvolemia, avoiding hypo- and hypervolemia. (b) It is not easy to define the euvolemic state: Dashed line can present different scenarios:
  i. One size does not fit all: The optimal volume can be different in different patients.
  ii. It can also differ between different conditions of the same patients (e.g., differences in preoperative fasting time can shift the curve between the solid and dashed lines).
  iii. It can be speculated that optimal volume status can be different in different organs [e.g., optimal volume for lungs (solid line) can be less than for one of the kidneys].
  iv. "Optimal volume" of open thoracotomy (dashed line) and VATS (solid line) is different.
    AKI, acute kidney injury.

systems. The components of this balance also explain the difference between the behaviors of different types of external fluids: Solutions with glucose are distributed within the whole system including the intracellular component, crystalloids like saline within only extracellular system (ISS + IVS), while colloids remain in IVS. Theoretically (just "theoretically"!), the so-called volume effect (i.e., the effective portion of the administered fluid remaining within the IVS) can be considered as approximately 7–10% for glucose 5%, 25–30% for saline, and 100% for colloids.

Endothelial Glycocalyx Layer (EGL) and the Revised Starling Principle: The EGL, a gel-like layer of glycosaminoglycans, glycoproteins, and proteoglycans in which various active compounds are embedded, plays a pivotal role in transcapillary fluid movements, in modulating the inflammatory response, and in promoting tissue blood flow.[24] As an integral structural and functional part of the IVS, it has changed the paradigm of the classical Starling rule. In the "revised" Starling principle, the role of the colloid osmotic pressure gradient is considered negligible, and the hydrostatic pressure gradient becomes the only component, whereby lymphatic clearance and recycling into the systemic circulation prevent the accumulation of fluids in the ISS.[25]

The role of EGL in balance of fluid distribution can help to answer some questions of clinical practice: The amount and the type of the administered fluid is not the only reason for edema formation. An injury of the EGL can also lead to impaired balance of fluid distribution. Trauma, shock, inflammation, ischemia-reperfusion injury and –not at least – sepsis can all harm the EGL, resulting in capillary fluid leakage and interstitial edema.[9,26] In clinical settings, hypoalbuminemia, hyperglycemia, rapid infusion of large volumes of acidic crystalloids, and the induction of hypervolemia with IV colloids have been shown to be harmful to the EGL and consequently facilitate the interstitial edema.[27]

In the lungs, there are some differences in the components affecting the balance of fluid distribution. First, in addition to "tight junctions" of the epithelial cells ensuring a seal to maintain the balance of permeability, there are additional mechanisms in the lungs to keep the alveoli "dry" by continuous extrusion of sodium, chloride, and water towards the interstitial space.[28] The capacity of thoracic and pulmonary lymphatic flow can increase up to 6- to 7-fold, so that despite a drastic decrease in plasma oncotic pressure "pulmonary edema would still be prevented".[29] These findings seem to reveal that the formation of a pulmonary edema appears to be more difficult than tissue edema. But things change, if there are multiple "hits," which are cumulatively strong enough to exceed the threshold of the protective mechanisms.

Multiple Hit Phenomenon: The clinical consequence of the "revised" Starling principle and the role of EGL in fluid management in daily practice is that there are numerous possible reasons for an EGL damage, which can lead to a pulmonary edema and (postoperative) lung injury.[30] Factors that may be not deleterious enough to cause an injury by themselves can contribute to postoperative complications when similar other "hits" are present. For instance, it is interesting that a non-protective ventilation (e.g., unnecessary high tidal volumes) can contribute to an inflammatory response (also via the injury to EGL) during a surgical manipulation, which alone would probably be not hazardous to lungs. This "multiple hit phenomenon" should make us wonder whether the incredibly high tidal volumes in Zeldin's study [1] could also be a reason for PPPE, and not only the high volumes of fluid.

Therefore, in defining the goal of a so-called goal-directed therapy during thoracic operations, protection of EGL and the multiple hit phenomenon should also be taken into consideration.

Goal-Directed Therapy: Its Controversies and Challenges in Thoracic Operations

During surgical stress, restoration and maintenance of oxygen delivery (DO_2) by normalizing gas exchange and circulatory flow are inevitable goals to support the cellular oxygen consumption (VO_2).[31] From this point of view, the principal difference of "goal-directed therapy" (GDT) and "moderate" (or "restrictive" or "zero-balance") strategies is that GDT aims to achieve specific hemodynamic endpoints rather than a predetermined fluid strategy, targeting a balance between systemic oxygen delivery and the – increased – oxygen demand of the tissue and involves optimization of cardiac preload, afterload, and contractility.[32,33] For particular reasons, discussed in what follows, the majority of the studies examining the possible benefits of GDT are focused on major abdominal surgery and not on thoracic operations. As a result, current and reliable reviews are also based on studies performed in abdominal surgery; some extrapolation can be made for the possible effects (and limitations) in thoracic surgery.

1. **Normovolemia**: There are four indications for fluid administration: resuscitation, maintenance, replacement, and nutrition, or a combination. In anesthetized surgical patients, the administration of fluids (and cardiovascular drugs) should compensate on one hand the loss of body fluid, and on the other hand the changes in intravascular volume and fluid shifts to interstitial space due to anesthesia-induced vasorelaxation and inhibition of the sympatho-adrenal activity.[34] Under general anesthesia with/without thoracic epidural anesthesia, hypovolemia can be diagnosed by decreased arterial pressure, stroke volume, and cardiac output. But how can the anesthetist decide whether a hypotension or decreased cardiac output is due to a hypovolemia or a decreased pump function of the heart or a vasodilation? Hypovolemia is associated with an increase in pulse pressure variation (PPV) and/or stroke volume variation (SVV) in mechanically ventilated patients.[35] Unfortunately, PPV and SVV require an intact cardiopulmonary interaction and, therefore, the evaluation in thoracic surgery (open or VATS) is unreliable and limited.

   "Fluid responsiveness" is defined as a 10% or greater increase in stroke volume (SV) as a response to an increase in preload, and can also be used as a diagnostic tool in the setting of surgery, including thoracic operations. It can be evaluated either by "fluid challenge" (with typically 250 mL colloid, but a mini-fluid challenge with less crystalloid can also be effective [36]) or by "passive leg raising," wherein approximately 300 mL of venous blood returning into the right atrium should mimic an external fluid challenge.[37] However, some important points regarding fluid challenge should be kept in mind:

   a. The test relies on the physiological basis of the Frank–Starling curve, of which the y-axis is the stroke volume, which is not a routine monitoring of daily practice. Arterial pressure is not equivalent to or a surrogate of stroke volume.[38] Obviously, one can use this test also to observe the change in arterial pressure instead of stroke volume, but this empiric approach would no longer be based on Frank–Starling.

b. In some patients, the steep part of the slope of the curve (i.e., the part indicating fluid responsiveness) may not be steep enough to show an increase in SV (although the patient is actually fluid responsive).

c. Finally, "fluid responsiveness" does not mean necessarily that the patient is hypovolemic; other factors such as a decrease in venous tone with increased venous capacity can lead to "fluid responsiveness." As stated by Takala, "giving volume to fluid responders as long as they respond should not become the iatrogenic syndrome of the decade."[39]

2. **Addition of inotropic or vasoactive agents**: A meta-analysis has shown that trials that relied solely on the administration of fluids (goal-directed fluid therapy) for hemodynamic optimization without the use of vasoactive drugs has also shown a significant reduction in the risk of PPCs,[40] but the general approach (and the sense of GDT) relies on the addition of catecholamines to improve the outcome. Here, the question arises whether to prefer an inotrope or a vasopressor:

a. "Optimizing the cardiac output (CO)" (previously "maximizing") inspires the use of inotropes. One of the first large, multicenter trials of GDT, OPTIMISE, used an inotrope (dopamine) to optimize the CO, but was not able to report a statistically significant difference in complications.[41] However, in anesthesia, and particularly in thoracic anesthesia, a hypotension after correction to normovolemia is very rarely caused by a decrease in inotropy; the common cause is vasodilation (effects of anesthetic drugs and/or thoracic epidural anesthesia). The question remains why an inotrope should be – inappropriately – applied only for the sake of an increase in CO.

b. For an appropriate tissue oxygenation, all "flow," "volume," and "pressure" are crucial, and although related to each other, none of them can be considered as a surrogate of the other.[38] A series of studies from the Outcomes Research Institute have shown that even a short duration of hypotension (mean blood pressure <65 mmHg) is associated with myocardial and kidney complications.[42,43] For most organ systems, mean arterial pressure (MAP) is the inflow pressure [44] [where central venous pressure (CVP) acts as outflow pressure (mean perfusion pressure = MAP – CVP)].[45]

The authors agree with the comment of Hu and Lim [46] that "in contrast to intensive care unit settings, in the operating room, vasopressors do not need to indicate hypotension: it appears to be a smart approach to apply some 'prophylactic' low-dose vasopressor infusions to counteract vasodilation after ensuring adequate volume and anesthetic depth. Correcting SVR early may curtail downstream hypotension and excessive volume administration."[46] Two important conclusions can be made:

i. Monitoring of depth of anesthesia (DoA) should be considered a part of fluid and hemodynamic monitoring during general anesthesia.

ii. It should be underlined that the recommendation for vasopressor is "after ensuring adequate volume" and "to avoid excessive volume administration." The limit between "adequate" and "excessive" remains, again, as a challenge to be solved individually: a titration, based not only on the objective information obtained from monitoring, but also on the clinical skills of the anesthesiologist.

3. **Monitoring of GDT:** Monitoring of fluid responsiveness and GDT is even more challenging in thoracic operations. Static variables such as CVP [and also pulmonary artery occlusion pressure (PAOP)] have been shown to be unreliable to predict the fluid responsiveness in many studies and meta-analyses.[47,48] Perhaps the only possible scientific application of CVP in patients undergoing thoracic surgery would be in pulmonary hypertension (PH). In PH patients (an important subgroup of patients undergoing thoracic surgery), if left ventricular (LV) function is preserved, the right ventricle is independently subjected to pressure and volume overload, and CVP monitoring can be useful to assess those changes in right ventricular (RV) preload, RV filling pressure, and global RV performance, with or without changes in volume status.[49] However, the authors of this chapter also belong to the large group of anesthesiologists who are aware of the low level of reliability of CVP but still use it, albeit always keeping its limitations in mind. Considering that "dynamic variables" also have a limited informative value in "open-thorax" cases, CVP can help (just help) as a follow-up parameter; a decrease in CVP compared with pre-incisional values can be associated with fluid responsiveness.

"Dynamic variables" have been shown to be reliable, at least in patients undergoing abdominal surgery. How far these findings can be extrapolated to thoracic surgery (where the data of "cardiopulmonary interaction" are changed exclusively) remains a question. Examples of dynamic variables include mainly PPV, SVV, and several other less invasive surrogates, such as pulse contour analysis and volume-clamp photo-plethysmography.[50,51] SVV is induced by changes due to positive pressure of mech-anical ventilation and relies on an intact cardiopulmonary interaction. Generally, it is considered that PPV >13% implies fluid responsiveness, while PPV <10% indicates fluid unresponsiveness;[52] the area between 9–13% remains as a grey zone with a decreased sensitivity and specificity.[53]

Oesophageal Doppler monitor (ODM) can also be used as a monitor of fluid responsiveness. Its probe uses Doppler ultrasound to measure the velocity of blood flow in the adjacent descending aorta. The blood flow in the descending aorta is correlated to CO.[54] However, except for scientific purposes, it does not appear to be realistic to use this probe in every thoracic operation.

There are some conditions in which PPV and SVV are less reliable (if any) (Table 15.1).[55] Among them, open chest is the most important one to limit the use of dynamic variables in thoracic anesthesia. From this point of view, video-assisted thor-acoscopic surgery also raises similar concerns. Moreover, hypoxic pulmonary vasocon-striction in the not-ventilated lung and the increased pulmonary shunt might also influence the heart–lung interaction. Compared with the studies examining GDT in abdominal surgery, those performed in thoracic surgery are few and report controversial results.[56–63] On the one hand, Mukai et al. [58] have reported that intraoperative GDT [in which the "goal" was stroke volume variation <8%, plus systolic blood pressure (BP) maintained >90 mm Hg, using colloids and vasopressors as necessary] might reduce major morbidity and mortality, and shorten hospital stay, after transthoracic esopha-gectomy: an interesting study with "extremely" significant results compared with similar studies. On the other hand, Miñana et al. have shown that the values of the dynamic parameters of volume response (SVV ≥ 8% and PPV ≥ 10%) do not "distinguish" against responder patients and non-responders during open lung resection surgery.[60]

Table 15.1 Conditions in which pulse pressure variation is less reliable

Initials		False positive	False negative
L	Low HR/RR ratio (extreme bradycardia or high-frequency ventilation)		X
I	Irregular heart beats	X	
M	Mechanical ventilation with low tidal volume		X
I	Increased abdominal pressure (pneumoperitoneum)	X	
T	Thorax open		X
S	Spontaneous breathing	X	X

HR, heart rate; RR, respiratory rate.

Overall, it can be argued that thoracic surgery is a limitation, but not a contraindication of dynamic measurements: Dynamic variables can be used considering their limitations. PPV and SVV threshold values are probably lower in one-lung ventilation than in two-lung ventilation. Regarding Piccioni et al., given the great heterogeneity found among studies, any conclusion must be cautious. Dynamic indices still need to be studied under open-chest circumstances and, moreover, it is necessary to evaluate their usefulness in real clinical practice.[64]

A connection of a thermodilution catheter to a SVV/PPV monitor [transpulmonary thermodilution (TPTD)] can estimate extravascular lung water (EVLW), which is a measure of pulmonary edema, and pulmonary vascular permeability, which is a measure of pulmonary capillary leakage.[65,66] This approach can help both to prevent an excessive fluid load leading to an increase of vascular permeability and to detect other approaches than fluid management (e.g., non-protective ventilation [66]) that can cause pulmonary edema.

4. **Evidence of benefits of GDT:** Numerous meta-analyses and several studies have reported a beneficial effect of GDT reducing postoperative complications and length of hospital stay.[32,67,68] However, there are two important concerns:

   a. Evidence of benefits of GDT in abdominal surgery is controversial: clinical heterogeneity in the trials was found too large to perform a meta-analysis on all trials.[69] Some meta-analyses showing the benefits of GDT also declare a "low" evidence level because of heterogeneity.[68]

   b. The vast majority of studies in the meta-analyses have been performed in abdominal surgery; studies examining "GDT and thoracic anesthesia" are scarce: Among the 59 studies included in a 2018 meta-analysis, there were only two studies performed in thoracic anesthesia.[68]

5. **Possible methods to overcome the limitations of monitoring methods using dynamic variables:** Functional hemodynamic tests have been developed for situations where dynamic indices cannot be used.[70] The purpose of these tests is to create an instant and minimal change in preload while monitoring the changes in hemodynamic parameters

and to use these data to predict fluid responsiveness. Except for the recruitment maneuver challenge, no functional hemodynamic test has been studied in patients undergoing thoracic surgery. These tests are briefly described below.

a. Mini-Fluid Challenge (MFC): This test is based on evaluating the change in stroke volume subsequent to the administration of 100 mL of fluid to the patient. The most important feature of this test is that it does not require any cardiopulmonary interactions. Ali et al. studied MFC in patients with low respiratory system compliance and revealed that fluid responsiveness is predicted with 96.7% accuracy when a cut-off value of >5.8% is used for the increase in stroke volume after MFC. [71] There is no study conducted under one-lung ventilation.

b. Tidal Volume Challenge (TVC): This test is based on causing a reduction in preload by temporarily increasing the tidal volume. Messina et al. reported that a >12.2% increase in PPV subsequent to TVC could predict fluid responsiveness with a 94.7% accuracy. In the study, the tidal volume was increased to 8 mL/kg during the maneuver in patients who were ventilated with 6 mL/kg.[72] There is no study conducted under one-lung ventilation.

c. Short-Time Low PEEP Challenge (SLPC): This test is based on the evaluation of the hemodynamic changes that occur as a result of increasing the PEEP value of the patient by 5 cm H_2O. Ali et al. reported that a >14.2% reduction in stroke volume subsequent to SLPC could predict fluid responsiveness with 94.4% accuracy in patients ventilated with protective ventilation.[73] There is no study conducted under one-lung ventilation.

d. Recruitment Maneuver Challenge (RMC): Use of recruitment maneuvers is recommended as part of the protective ventilation strategy. Therefore, using this maneuver for predicting fluid responsiveness claimed to be rational. Kimura et al. applied continuous positive pressure of 30 cm H_2O for 30 seconds to the patients undergoing one-lung ventilation. They found that a >23.7% reduction in stroke volume subsequent to the maneuver can predict fluid responsiveness with 84% accuracy.[74] Nevertheless, this test raises some concerns. First, fluid responsive patients are expected to become severely hypotensive with such an intrathoracic pressure. Second, diversion of blood flow to the non-dependent lung is also expected and can result with desaturation.

6. **Timing of fluid commencement:** The same amount of the same type of fluid can lead to a different outcome, if administered with the wrong timing.[37] The approach of "four D's and the four phases of fluid therapy" in septic shock should also be implemented to anesthesia settings: Four D's: drug, duration, dosing, and de-escalation; and four phases: resuscitation, optimization, stabilization, and evacuation.[75] In phases when capillary pressure (or transendothelial pressure difference) is low, as in hypovolemia or during hypotension (e.g., after induction and anesthesia), the behavior of crystalloid infusions is similar to albumin or plasma substitutes: they all remain intravascular; that is, the "volume effect" of a crystalloid would differ depending on whether the patient is hypovolemic or not. From this point of view, a "prehydration" has no sense and can be hazardous; and the longer the delay in fluid administration, the more microcirculatory hypoperfusion and subsequent organ damage related to ischaemia-reperfusion

injury: If "in time," the volume effect of a crystalloid can increase to 100% when the arterial pressure has dropped.[76]

Similarly, the speed of the infusion also plays an important role: A rapid infusion of fluids (especially saline) can cause an injury to the fragile structure of the glycocalyx layer, leading to a state of global increased permeability syndrome (GIPS).[25]

Choice of Fluids: Crystalloid versus Colloid and Saline versus Balanced

As underlined earlier, if the patient is hypovolemic (relative hypovolemia as a result of vasodilation also being included), crystalloids have a much higher volume effect than previously believed. Moreover, it has been shown that colloid administration during thoracic surgery is associated with an increased risk of postoperative acute kidney injury.[16] These two facts lead us to the conclusion that there is a very limited (if any) indication of colloids in thoracic operations. It has been considered that the colloids would potentially remove water from the lungs and into the intravascular compartment. Some studies confirm the assumption that colloids can obtain an increased cardiac output, increased colloid osmotic pressure with less volumes compared with crystalloids in cardiac and vascular surgery.[77] However, today it appears that a rational approach is to limit the use of colloids [especially hydroxyl ethyl starch (HES)] only to resuscitation of hyperacute hypovolemic states (e.g., massive, abrupt hypovolemia), if at all.

Normal saline as resuscitation fluid is associated with a risk of hypernatremic hyperchloremic metabolic acidosis, acute kidney injury, and death. Although it does not contain potassium, it will result in a higher increase in potassium levels in patients with renal impairment compared with a balanced solution (lactated Ringer's) containing potassium, because of the concomitant metabolic acidosis due to a decreased strong ion difference (SID).[78]

Should GDT Be a Perioperative Approach of Thoracic Surgery?

"Absence of evidence is not evidence of absence." Although the evidence of GDT in thoracic operations is limited, it is in any case a more objective approach than those that are empiric and associated with several potential benefits:

1. Regarding the risk-adapted matrix for fluid and hemodynamic management suggested by Miller and Myles,[37] the combination of high patient and surgical risk should be treated with GDT (Fig. 15.2). Meanwhile, the vast majority of the patients undergoing thoracic operations are considered part of the high-risk group: regarding the ARISCAT score, thoracic operations count per se for a risk score of 24, whereby a risk score of >26 is considered intermediate [so if the patient is older than 60 years of age (risk score 3), she/he would be automatically in the intermediate-risk group].[79] This implies that the majority of the patients deserve GDT.
2. GDT can obtain objective information about the timing of fluid application and can help in the decision of when to start, when to stop, and how fast the infusion should be.
3. One of the most important concerns about fluid application in thoracic anesthesia is pulmonary edema: TPTD can assess EVLW and pulmonary vascular permeability.

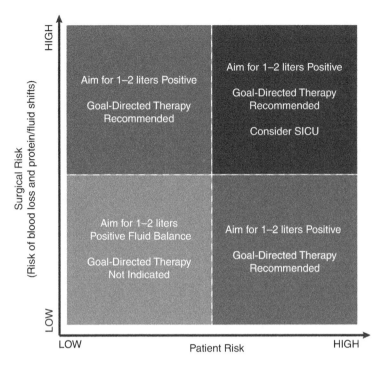

Figure 15.2 [37]
The risk-adapted matrix for fluid and hemodynamic management suggested by Miller and Myles [37], the combination of high patient and surgical risk (right upper quarter) should be treated with GDT. Note that the vast majority of the thoracic operations are in this quarter. SICU, surgical intensive care unit. A black and white version of this figure will appear in some formats. For the color version, please refer to the plate section.

4. To answer several questions regarding the addition of vasoactive agents (e.g., Is it indicated? If yes, an inotrope and/or vasopressor? Timing? Dosage? Timing of escalation?), implementation of a GDT-protocol can be a rational approach to achieve an "objective and individualized" indication and avoid a subjective decision.

Considering the rather new principles such as "multiple hit phenomenon" and "protection of glycocalyx," we now know that an "enhanced outcome" is a composite result of several parameters, including appropriate fluid management. With this point of view, we can understand why in older studies "hypervolemia" was found to be a major cause of postoperative complications. In newer studies, the effect of administered volume is not as important as in the older ones.[32] Not only are the amounts of volumes of fluid given comparable with recent studies, there are also several other factors (e.g., non-protective ventilation, non-protective surgery, inappropriate analgesia), which would interfere in the outcome and exaggerate the differences between the groups. In other words, - protective ventilation, minimal invasive surgery, and goal-directed fluid therapy all work in synergy to achieve an improvement of postoperative outcome (Fig. 15.3).[7]

Enhanced Recovery After Surgery (ERAS) aims to combine different strategies. In contrast to some previous ERAS–thoracic recommendations,[80] the recent and most sophisticated recommendation of ESTS and ERAS® societies suggested that "very restrictive or liberal fluid regimes should be avoided in favor of euvolemia."[81]

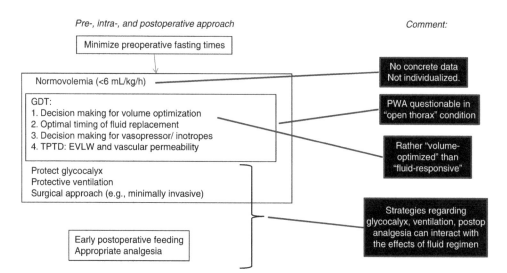

Figure 15.3 [7]
A possible strategy (with low evidence) including GDT as a part of a general approach to improve the postoperative outcome. Note that:
i. some concerns regarding different steps are highlighted on the right
ii. several conditions (e.g., setting of ventilation, perioperative analgesia, protection of glycocalyx) can affect the outcome related to fluid management. TPTD, transpulmonary thermodilution; EVLW: extravascular lung water.

New Aspects and Conclusion

It should be borne in mind that the reputation of "restricted fluid in thoracic anesthesia" is far more overrated than its evidence suggests. GDT has changed the point of view of fluid management and hemodynamic monitoring,[82] albeit in thoracic anesthesia, this change is limited compared with other disciplines. In any case, there is an obvious strong relationship between the "PERIoperative" hemodynamic stability and postoperative outcome. To achieve this stability, appropriate fluid management and hemodynamic monitoring are crucial.

Technology helps and will help us to define the "goal" of GDT more concretely; and serves us with new pathways to achieve this goal. New key phrases like "big data," "automated closed loop," and "computer-assisted individualization" are the recent advances in hemodynamic monitoring.[83,84] Most promising, information from a "big data bank" and several other parameters are used as early warning systems to predict hypotension before it occurs.[85,86] A closed-loop vasopressor controller has been found to be significantly more effective to prevent hypotensive periods in patients undergoing intermediate- to high-risk abdominal surgery.[83] As this method is not dependent on cardiopulmonary interaction, current results from studies performed in other types of surgeries can be extrapolated to thoracic operations, too. However, studies in thoracic (pulmonary and non-pulmonary) operations are lacking.

Appropriate fluid management was, is, and will remain an important element of perioperative care. Although we now know that it is not just the amount of intraoperative fluid (Peter Slinger's quote regarding PPE: "With intravenous fluids, we can make it worse, but we do not cause it"[87]), concrete evidence is still missing in thoracic operations. Technological improvements will help to achieve a more rational, practical approach based on more scientific evidence.

References

1. R.A. Zeldin, D. Normandin, D. Landtwing, et al. Postpneumonectomy pulmonary edema. *J Thorac Cardiovasc Surg.* 1984;**87**:359–65.

2. N. Alam, B.J. Park, A. Wilton, et al. Incidence and risk factors for lung injury after lung cancer resection. *Ann Thorac Surg.* 2007;**84**:1085–91.

3. M.K. Arslantas, H.V. Kara, B.B. Tuncer, et al. Effect of the amount of intraoperative fluid administration on postoperative pulmonary complications following anatomic lung resections. *J Thorac Cardiovasc Surg.* 2015;**149**:314–20.

4. Working Group of the German Thorax Registry. Risk factors for post-operative pulmonary complications in lung cancer patients after video-assisted thoracoscopic lung resection: results of the German Thorax Registry. *Acta Anaesthesiol Scand.* 2019;**63**:1009–18.

5. K. Kaufmann, S. Heinrich. Minimizing postoperative pulmonary complications in thoracic surgery patients *Curr Opin Anesthesiol.* 2021;**34**:13–19.

6. R.S. D'Souza, C.R. Sims, N. Andrijasevic, et al. pulmonary complications in esophagectomy based on intraoperative fluid rate: a single-center study. *J Cardiothorac Vasc Anesth.* 2021;**35**:2952–60.

7. M. Şentürk, E.S. Bingül, Ö. Turhan. Should fluid management in thoracic surgery be goal directed? *Curr Opin Anaesthesiol.* 2022;**35**:89–95.

8. Y. Kim, F. Gani, G. Spolverato, et al. Variation in crystalloid administration: an analysis of 6248 patients undergoing major elective surgery. *J Surg Res.* 2016;**203**:368-77.

9. M. Licker, A. Hagerman, B. Bedat, et al. Restricted, optimized or liberal fluid strategy in thoracic surgery: a narrative review. *Saudi J Anaesth.* 2021;**15**:324–34.

10. M. Sentürk, M.O. Sungur, Z. Sungur. Fluid management in thoracic anesthesia. *Minerva Anestesiol.* 2017;**83**:652–9.

11. A. Messina, C. Robba, L. Calabrò, et al. Perioperative liberal versus restrictive fluid strategies and postoperative outcomes: a systematic review and metanalysis on randomised-controlled trials in major abdominal elective surgery. *Crit Care.* 2021;**25**:205.

12. P.S. Myles, R. Bellomo, T. Corcoran, et al. Restrictive versus liberal fluid therapy for major abdominal surgery. *N Engl J Med.* 2018;**378**:2263–74.

13. S. Ishikawa, D.E. Griesdale, J. Lohser. Acute kidney injury after lung resection surgery: incidence and perioperative risk factors. *Anesth Analg.* 2012;**114**:1256–62.

14. D. Cardinale, N. Cosentino, M. Moltrasio, et al. Acute kidney injury after lung cancer surgery: incidence and clinical relevance, predictors, and role of N-terminal pro B-type natriuretic peptide. *Lung Cancer.* 2018;**123**:155–9.

15. I. Matot, E. Dery, Y. Bulgov, et al. Fluid management during video-assisted thoracoscopic surgery for lung resection: a randomized, controlled trial of effects on urinary output and postoperative renal function. *J Thorac Cardiovasc Surg.* 2013;**146**:461–6.

16. H.J. Ahn, J.A. Kim, A.R. Lee, et al. The risk of acute kidney injury from fluid restriction and hydroxyethyl starch in thoracic surgery. *Anesth Analg.* 2016;**122**:186–93.

17. S. Romagnoli, Z. Ricci. Postoperative acute kidney injury. *Minerva Anestesiol.* 2015;**81**:684–96.

18. S. Assaad, W. Popescu, A. Perrino. Fluid management in thoracic surgery. *Curr Opin Anesthesiol.* 2013, **26**:31–9.

19. J.A. Kim, H.J. Ahn, A.R. Oh, et al. Restrictive intraoperative fluid management was associated with higher incidence of composite complications compared to less restrictive strategies in open thoracotomy: a retrospective cohort study. *Sci Rep.* 2020;**10**:8449.

20. Y. Wu, R. Yang, J. Xu, et al. Effects of intraoperative fluid management on

postoperative outcomes after lobectomy. *Ann Thorac Surg.* 2019;**107**:1663–9.

21. A.M. Budacan, B. Naidu. Fluid management in the thoracic surgical patient: where is the balance? *J Thorac Dis.* 2019;**11**(6):2205–7.

22. M. Doherty, D.J. Buggy. Intraoperative fluids: how much is too much? *Br J Anaesth.* 2012;**109**:69–79.

23. H.F. Batirel. Fluid administration during lung resection: what is the optimum? *J Thorac Dis.* 2019;**11**(5):1746–8.

24. S. Weinbaum, L.M. Cancel, B.M. Fu, et al. The glycocalyx and its role in vascular physiology and vascular related diseases. *Cardiovasc Eng Technol.* 2021;**12**:37–71.

25. T.E. Woodcock, T.M. Woodcock. Revised Starling equation and the glycocalyx model of transvascular fluid exchange: an improved paradigm for prescribing intravenous fluid therapy. *Br J Anaesth.* 2012;**108**:384–94.

26. R. Uchimido, E.P. Schmidt, N.I. Shapiro. The glycocalyx: a novel diagnostic and therapeutic target in sepsis. *Crit Care.* 2019;**23**:16.

27. D. Chappell, D. Bruegger, J. Potzel, et al. Hypervolemia increases release of atrial natriuretic peptide and shedding of the endothelial glycocalyx. *Crit Care.* 2014;**18**:538.

28. S. Simmons, L. Erfinanda, C. Bartz, et al. Novel mechanisms regulating endothelial barrier function in the pulmonary microcirculation. *J Physiol.* 2019;**597**:997–1021.

29. C.K. Zarins, C.L. Rice, R.M. Peters, et al. Lymph and pulmonary response to isobaric reduction in plasma oncotic pressure in baboons. *Circ Res.*1978;**43**:925–30.

30. V. Manou Stathopoulou, M. Korbonits, G. L. Ackland. Redefining the perioperative stress response: a narrative review. *Br J Anaesth.* 2019;**123**:570–83.

31. J. Lohser, P. Slinger. Lung injury after one-lung ventilation: a review of the pathophysiologic mechanisms affecting the ventilated and the collapsed lung. *Anesth Analg.* 2015;**121**:302–18.

32. A. Messina, C. Robba, L. Calabrò, et al. Association between perioperative fluid administration and postoperative outcomes: a 20-year systematic review and a meta-analysis of randomized goal-directed trials in major visceral/noncardiac surgery. *Crit Care.* 2021;**25**:43.

33. T. Kaufmann, B. Saugel, T.W.L. Scheeren. Perioperative goal-directed therapy – what is the evidence? *Best Pract Res Clin Anaesthesiol.* 2019;**33**:179–87.

34. S. Feng, S. Yang, W. Xiao, et al. Effects of perioperative goal-directed fluid therapy combined with the application of alpha-1 adrenergic agonists on postoperative outcomes: a systematic review and meta-analysis. *BMC Anesthesiol.* 2018;**18**:113.

35. A. Messina, C. Pelaia, A. Bruni, et al. Fluid challenge during anesthesia: a systematic review and meta-analysis. *Anesth Analg.* 2018;**127**:1353–64.

36. A. Messina, G. Lionett, L. Foti. Mini fluid chAllenge aNd End-expiratory occlusion test to assess flUid responsiVEness in the opeRating room (MANEUVER study): a multicentre cohort study *Eur J Anaesthesiol.* 2021;**38**:422–31.

37. T.E. Miller, P.S. Myles. Perioperative fluid therapy for major surgery. *Anesthesiology.* 2019;**130**:825–32.

38. K. Kouz, A. Bergholz, L.M. Timmermann, et al. The relation between mean arterial pressure and cardiac index in major abdominal surgery patients: a prospective observational cohort study. *Anesth Analg.* 2022;**134**:322–9.

39. J. Takala. Volume responsive, but does the patient need volume? *Intensive Care Med.* 2016;**42**:1461–3.

40. P.M. Odor, S. Bampoe, D. Gilhooly, et al. Perioperative interventions for prevention of postoperative pulmonary complications: systematic review and meta-analysis. *BMJ.* 2020;**368**:m540.

41. OPTIMISE Study Group. Effect of a perioperative, cardiac output-guided

hemodynamic therapy algorithm on outcomes following major gastrointestinal surgery: a randomized clinical trial and systematic review. *JAMA.* 2014;**311**:2181–90.

42. M. Walsh, P.J. Devereaux, A.X. Garg, et al. Relationship between intraoperative mean arterial pressure and clinical outcomes after noncardiac surgery: toward an empirical definition of hypotension. *Anesthesiology.* 2013;**119**:507–15.

43. V. Salmasi, K. Maheshwari, D. Yang, et al. Relationship between intraoperative hypotension, defined by either reduction from baseline or absolute thresholds, and acute kidney and myocardial injury after noncardiac surgery: a retrospective cohort analysis. *Anesthesiology.* 2017;**126**:47–65.

44. B. Saugel, D.I. Sessler. Perioperative blood pressure management. *Anesthesiology.* 2021;**134**:250–61.

45. M. Ostermann, A. Hall, S. Crichton. Low mean perfusion pressure is a risk factor for progression of acute kidney injury in critically ill patients – a retrospective analysis. *BMC Nephrol.* 2017;**18**:151.

46. Y. Hu, A. Lim. MAP 65 – is it enough? *Curr Opin Anaesthesiol.* 2022;**35**:242–7.

47. P. Bentzer, D.E. Griesdale, J. Boyd J, et al. Will this hemodynamically unstable patient respond to a bolus of intravenous fluids? *JAMA.* 2016;**316**:1298–309.

48. P.E. Marik, R. Cavallazzi. Does the central venous pressure predict fluid responsiveness? An updated meta-analysis and a plea for some common sense. *Crit Care Med.* 2013;**41**:1774–81.

49. L.C. Price, G. Martinez, A. Brame, et al. Perioperative management of patients with pulmonary hypertension undergoing non-cardiothoracic, non-obstetric surgery: a systematic review and expert consensus statement. *Br J Anaesth.* 2021;**126**:774–90.

50. K. Bartels, R.H. Thiele. Advances in photoplethysmography: beyond arterial oxygen saturation. *Can J Anaesth.* 2015;**6**:1313–28.

51. J. Grensemann. Cardiac output monitoring by pulse contour analysis, the technical basics of less-invasive techniques. *Front Med.* 2018;**5**:64.

52. X. Yang, B. Du. Does pulse pressure variation predict fluid responsiveness in critically ill patients? A systematic review and meta-analysis. *Crit Care.* 2014;**18**:650.

53. M. Cannesson, Y. Le Manach, C.K. Hofer, et al. Assessing the diagnostic accuracy of pulse pressure variations for the prediction of fluid responsiveness: a "gray zone" approach. *Anesthesiology.* 2011;**115**:231–41.

54. K.B. Kaufmann, L. Stien, L. Bogatyreva, et al. Oesophageal Doppler guided goal-directed haemodynamic therapy in thoracic surgery – a single centre randomized parallel-arm trial. *Br J Anaesth.* 2017;**118**:852–61.

55. F. Michard, D. Chemla, J.L. Teboul. Applicability of pulse pressure variation: how many shades of grey? *Crit Care.* 2015;**19**:144.

56. K.B. Kaufmann, L. Stien, L. Bogatyreva, et al. Oesophageal Doppler guided goal-directed haemodynamic therapy in thoracic surgery – a single centre randomized parallel-arm trial. *Br J Anaesth.* 2017;**118**:852–61.

57. H. Bahlmann, I. Halldestam, L. Nilsson. Goal-directed therapy during transthoracic oesophageal resection does not improve outcome: randomised controlled trial. *Eur J Anaesthesiol.* 2019;**36**:153–61.

58. A. Mukai, K. Suehiro, R. Watanabe, et al. Impact of intraoperative goal-directed fluid therapy on major morbidity and mortality after transthoracic oesophagectomy: a multicentre, randomised controlled trial. *Br J Anaesth.* 2020;**145**:953–61.

59. H. Xu, S. Shu, D. Wang, et al. Goal-directed fluid restriction using stroke volume variation and cardiac index during one-lung ventilation: a randomized controlled trial. *J Thorac Dis.* 2017;**9**:2992–3004.

60. A. Miñana, M.J. Parra, J. Carbonell, et al. Validation study of the dynamic parameters of pulse wave in pulmonary resection surgery. *Rev Esp Anestesiol Reanim (Engl Ed).* 2020;**67**:55–62.

61. M. Lema Tome, F.A. De la Gala, P. Piñeiro, et al. Behaviour of stroke volume variation in hemodynamic stable patients during thoracic surgery with one-lung ventilation periods. *Braz J Anesthesiol.* 2018;**68**:225–30.

62. D.M. Jeong, H.J Ahn, H.W. Park, et al. Stroke volume variation and pulse pressure variation are not useful for predicting fluid responsiveness in thoracic surgery. *Anesth Analg.* 2017;**125**:1158–65.

63. C. Sahutoglu, E. Turksal, S. Kocabas, et al. Influence of stroke volume variation on fluid treatment and postoperative complications in thoracic surgery. *Ther Clin Risk Manag.* 2018;**14**:575–81.

64. F. Piccioni, F. Bernascomi, G.T. A. Tramontano, M. Langer. A systematic review of pulse pressure variation and stroke volume variation to predict fluid responsiveness during cardiac and thoracic surgery. *J Clin Monit Comput.* 2017;**31**:677–84.

65. S. Assaad, B. Shelley, A. Perrino. Transpulmonary thermodilution: its role in assessment of lung water and pulmonary edema. *J Cardiothorac Vasc Anesth.* 2017;**31**:1471–80.

66. H. Qutub, M.R. ElTahan, H.A. Mowafi, et al. Effect of tidal volume on extravascular lung water content during one-lung ventilation for video-assisted thoracoscopic surgery: a randomised, controlled trial. *Eur J Anaesthesiol.* 2014;**31**:466–73.

67. F. Michard, M.T. Giglio, N. Brienza. Perioperative goal-directed therapy with uncalibrated pulse contour methods: impact on fluid management and postoperative outcome. *Br J Anaesth.* 2017;**119**:22e30.

68. M.A. Chong, Y. Wang, N.M Berbenetz, et al. Does goal-directed haemodynamic and fluid therapy improve peri-operative outcomes?: a systematic review and meta-analysis. *Eur J Anaesthesiol.* 2018;**35**:469–83.

69. T. Kaufmann, R.P. Clement, T.W. L. Scheeren, et al. Perioperative goal-directed therapy: a systematic review without meta-analysis. *Acta Anaesthesiol Scand.* 2018;**62**:1340–55.

70. J.I. Alvarado Sánchez, W.F. Amaya Zúñiga, M.I. Monge García. Predictors to intravenous fluid responsiveness. *J Intensive Care Med.* 2018;**33**(4):227–40.

71. A. Ali, Y. Dorman, T. Abdullah, et al. Ability of mini-fluid challenge to predict fluid responsiveness in obese patients undergoing surgery in the prone position. *Minerva Anestesiol.* 2019;**85**(9):981–8.

72. A. Messina, C. Montagnini, G. Cammarota, et al. Tidal volume challenge to predict fluid responsiveness in the operating room: an observational study. *Eur J Anaesthesiol.* 2019;**36**(8):583–91.

73. A. Ali, E. Aygun, T. Abdullah, et al. A challenge with 5 cmH2O of positive end-expiratory pressure predicts fluid responsiveness in neurosurgery patients with protective ventilation: an observational study. *Minerva Anestesiol.* 2019;**85**(11):1184–92.

74. A. Kimura, K. Suehiro, T. Juri, et al. Hemodynamic changes via the lung recruitment maneuver can predict fluid responsiveness in stroke volume and arterial pressure during one-lung ventilation. *Anesth Analg.* 2021;**133**(1):44–52.

75. M.L.N.G. Malbrain, N. Van Regenmortel, B. Saugel, et al. Principles of fluid management and stewardship in septic shock: it is time to consider the four D's and the four phases of fluid therapy. *Ann Intensive Care* 2018;**8**:66.

76. R.G. Hahn. Why crystalloids will do the job in the operating room. *Anaesthesiol Intensive Ther.* 2014;**46**(5):342–9.

77. J. Verheij, A. Van Lingen, P. G. Raijmakers, et al. Effect of fluid loading with saline or colloids on pulmonary permeability, oedema and lung injury score after cardiac and major vascular surgery. *Br J Anaesth.* 2006;**96**:21–30.

78. N.M. Yunos, R. Bellomo, C. Hegarty, et al. Association between a chloride-liberal vs chloride-restrictive intravenous fluid administration strategy and kidney injury in critically ill adults. *JAMA.* 2012;**308** (15):1566–72.

79. V. Mazo, S. Sabaté, J. Canet, et al. Prospective external validation of a predictive score for postoperative pulmonary complications. *Anesthesiology.* 2014;**121**:219–31.

80. L.W. Martin, B.M. Sarosiek, M. A. Harrison, et al. Implementing a thoracic enhanced recovery program: lessons learned in the first year. *Ann Thorac Surg.* 2018;**105**:1597–1604.

81. T.J.P. Batchelor, N.J. Rasburn, E. Abdelnour-Berchtold, et al. Guidelines for enhanced recovery after lung surgery: recommendations of the Enhanced Recovery After Surgery (ERAS®) Society and the European Society of Thoracic Surgeons (ESTS). *Eur J Cardiothorac Surg.* 2019;**55**:91–115.

82. J.L. Vincent, A. Joosten, B. Saugel. Hemodynamic monitoring and support. *Crit Care Med.* 2021;**49**:1638–50.

83. A. Joosten, J. Rinehart, P. Van der Linden, et al. Computer-assisted individualized hemodynamic management reduces intraoperative hypotension in intermediate- and high-risk surgery: a randomized controlled trial. *Anesthesiology.* 2021;**135**:258–72.

84. A. Joosten, A. Delaporte, B. Alexander, et al. Automated titration of vasopressor infusion using a closed-loop controller: in vivo feasibility study using a swine model. *Anesthesiology.* 2019;**130** (3):394–403.

85. M. Wijnberge, B.F. Geerts, L. Hol, et al. Effect of a machine learning-derived early warning system for intraoperative hypotension vs standard care on depth and duration of intraoperative hypotension during elective noncardiac surgery: the HYPE Randomized Clinical Trial. *JAMA.* 2020;**323**:1052–60.

86. P. Murabito, M. Astuto, F. Sanfilippo, et al. Proactive management of intraoperative hypotension reduces biomarkers of organ injury and oxidative stress during elective non-cardiac surgery: a pilot randomized controlled trial. *J Clin Med.* 2022;**11**:392.

87. P.D. Slinger. Postpneumonectomy pulmonary edema: good news, bad news. *Anesthesiology.* 2006;**105**:2–5.

Chapter 16

Fluid Management in Cardiac Surgery

Saqib H. Qureshi, Metesh N. Acharya
and Giovanni Mariscalco

Introduction

Optimal fluid balance is crucial in patients undergoing cardiac surgery. Systolic and diastolic left ventricular dysfunction, right ventricular dysfunction, and the presence of valvular heart disease all affect the response to fluid administration. Although dependent on adequate preload, volume overload in the perioperative period can lead to peripheral and pulmonary edema, since the heart cannot adapt easily to elevated filling pressures. Indeed, cardiac surgical patients may receive more than 10 liters of fluid during the intraoperative and postoperative course, whilst alterations in capillary endothelial function arising from cardiopulmonary bypass (CPB) [1–6] also exacerbate volume overload. Concurrently, intravascular volume depletion can contribute to organ dysfunction, such as acute lung and acute kidney injury, by reducing tissue perfusion or by inducing arrhythmias, such as atrial fibrillation. This can increase the duration of intensive care and overall hospital stay with resultant financial implications. The choice of fluid therapy, its indication, and intended target parameters following its use are often non-specific and outcomes are thus variable in clinical practice.[1–5]

This chapter will focus on the ongoing debate regarding whether colloids or crystalloids are superior in cardiac surgical patients and discuss how the supporting evidence should be evaluated. We will consider why novel fluids for intravascular resuscitation are necessary specifically for the cardiac surgical population, whilst also understanding the requirement for well-designed randomized controlled trials to assess the safety and efficacy of existing fluids, such as hydroxyethyl starch (HES), dextrans, gelatins, and balanced and unbalanced crystalloids.

Cardiac Surgery and Vascular Endothelial Alterations

Perioperative hypothermia, CPB-related cytokine storm, ischemia-reperfusion injury and generation of reactive oxygen species, fluctuations in renin–angiotensin responses from myocardial depression, and atrial natriuretic peptide (ANP) release can all affect vascular barrier function. The endothelial glycocalyx, a carbohydrate-rich layer on the luminal surface of the vascular endothelium that helps to maintain blood plasma composition and reduce exudation into tissue spaces, is particularly susceptible to degradation.[6–9] The main components of the endothelial glycocalyx, syndecan-1 and heparan sulfate, are known to be elevated in the plasma of patients with global or regional ischemia,[7,8] with their release being proportional to the duration of intraoperative ischemia. Furthermore, both on- and off-pump coronary artery bypass surgery has been associated with glycocalyx degradation. ANP, IL-6, IL-8, and IL-10 are implicated.[10–14] Plasma-based enzymes such as human heparinase-1 (HPSE-1) are recognized in breakdown of the glycocalyx; their activity is increased in disease states such as sepsis,[14,15] and over-expression of HPSE-1 in transgenic mice leads to the development of early proteinuria and renal failure.

Fluid Therapy and Effect on Endothelial Glycocalyx Layer (EGL)

Rapid crystalloid infusion has been shown to have a detrimental effect on the endothelial glycocalyx layer (EGL), as evidenced by sharp increases in plasma hyaluronic acid, an essential polysaccharide comprising the EGL from which it is presumably cleaved.[16,17] Hyaluronic acid, in combination with other components of the EGL wall including syndecan-1 and heparan sulfate, is also cleaved off by natriuretic peptides. ANP release is stimulated by increased right atrial pressure resulting from large volume fluid resuscitation and right atrial cannulation during cardiac surgery.[18,19] Owing to capillary leak, <5% of crystalloid remains within the intravascular compartment within 3 hours of infusion,[20] leading to interstitial edema, which further compounds myocardial dysfunction.

Revised Starling Equation and Glycocalyx Model Paradigm: Implications for Fluid Therapy

Our view of capillaries as semi-permeable membranes has been revised as our understanding of the glycocalyx has evolved.[21,22] The principle underlying colloid infusion is that capillaries maintain and augment intravascular colloid osmotic pressure (COP) to prevent filtration and thus peripheral edema. However, the revised Starling equation and glycocalyx model paradigm propose that the filtration in systemic capillaries is not regulated by the capillary–interstitial fluid COP difference, but rather by the capillary–subglycocalyx space (πc–πg). Since the latter COP difference is zero and results in a significantly higher difference than that for the original Starling hypothesis (Fig. 16.1), a "no-reabsorption rule" applies. This suggests that even with low mean capillary pressures, fluid transit to the interstitial space continues. Importantly, the administration of colloids will oppose, but not reverse, absorption. Therefore, the reported advantage of colloids in generating a higher COP compared with crystalloids becomes invalid. This is even more pertinent in disease states such as sepsis, where the glycocalyx undergoes progressive degradation.

Types of Resuscitation Fluids

Colloids

Human Albumin Solutions

Albumin contributes 80% of plasma oncotic pressure (25 mmHg) in healthy humans, compared with 19 mmHg in critically ill patients.[23,24] Albumin has a multifactorial role. It is involved in the transport and metabolism of bile acids, eicosanoids, copper, zinc, folate, aquacobalamin, and drugs. It imparts half of the normal anion gap, has significant antioxidant properties, and maintains vascular nitric oxide levels via stable S-nitrosothiol. Human albumin solution (HAS) is produced by the fractionation of blood, which is then heat treated to reduce viral transmission. The Saline versus Albumin Fluid Evaluation (SAFE) study, including 6,997 patients randomized to either albumin or saline, concluded that albumin was not superior to saline when analyzed for 28-day mortality

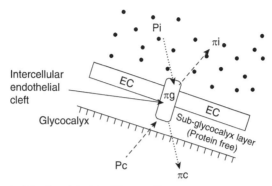

Classical Starling Principle: Filtration Force = (Pc – Pi) – σ(πp – πi)
Revised Starling Principle: Filtration Force = (Pc – Pi) – σ(πp – πg)

Figure 16.1 Two-dimensional glycocalyx–cleft model of capillary fluid exchange: the sub-glycocalyx space is protected and is protein free, forming the basis for the "no-reabsorption rule." The glycocalyx–cleft model identifies glycocalyx as a semipermeable layer. Its underside is subjected to the colloid osmotic pressure of fluid high inside the intercellular cleft rather than interstitial fluid (ISF), with important functional consequences. Pc, plasma capillary hydrostatic pressure; Pi, interstitial hydrostatic pressure; πc, oncotic pressure of plasma; πi, oncotic pressure of interstitial fluid; πg, oncotic pressure of intercellular endothelial cleft; EC, endothelial cell. Derived and modified from Ref. [16].

(relative risk 0.99, 95% confidence interval 0.91–1.09, $p = 0.87$).[25] Thang et al. demonstrated that early exposure to albumin in patients undergoing valve and/or coronary bypass surgery was associated with a reduction in adjusted hospital mortality (odds ratio 0.68, 95% confidence interval 0.48–0.97, $p < 0.05$), albeit with an increase in hospital and intensive care lengths of stay.[26] The FEAST trial evaluating the effects of saline or albumin fluid boluses in the resuscitation of febrile African children as well as the ALBIOS trial, which assessed the influence of albumin compared with crystalloid fluid in adults with severe sepsis or septic shock, have not shown the superiority of albumin over crystalloids.[27–29]

Semi-Synthetic Colloids

Hydroxyethyl Starches (HES)

The high cost of human albumin led to the development of synthetic colloids. Currently, HES are the most commonly used synthetic colloids (Table 16.1). They are produced by hydroxyl substitution of amylopectin obtained from sorghum, maize, or potatoes in the presence of an alkaline catalyst. Residual solvents are removed by ultrafiltration. A high degree of substitution on glucose molecules protects against hydrolysis by non-specific amylases in the blood, although HES is recognized as a foreign substance, leading to its accumulation in the body's reticulo-endothelial system and stored in the liver, spleen, and skin.[30] HES administration alters coagulation and fibrinolysis. The fibrinolytic effect is driven by a reduction in alpha 2-antiplasmin/plasmin interactions manifesting as a reduction in all coagulation parameters, such as clotting time, maximum clot firmness, and alpha-angle. These changes are also observed with platelet dysfunction and depletion of coagulation factors.[31,32] Growing evidence regarding the incidence of mortality and renal failure observed in large randomized controlled trials has put the safety of both traditional and modern HES into speculation. These trials, however, have focused only on

Table 16.1 Pharmacological properties of different HES preparations. Molar substitution and the C2/C6 (i.e., quotient of the numbers of glucose residues hydroxyethylated at positions 2 and 6, respectively) dictate the kinetics of degradation: a higher C2/C6 substitution protects from hydrolysis, thus increasing plasma half-life and potential toxicity

Preparation[a]	Concentration	Trade name	MW (kDa)	Specification range (kDa)	Top fraction[b] (kDa)	Bottom fraction[c] (kDa)	MS	C2/C6 ratio	In vitro COP (mmHg)	Initial volume effect	T$^{1/2}$ alpha (h)	T$^{1/2}$ beta (h)	Clearance (ml/min)
Hetastarch													
HES 450/0.7	6%	Plasmasteril, Hespan	450	150	2 170	19	0.7	4–5	26	100	n/a	300	n/a
HES 670/0.7	6%	Hextend	670	175	2 500	20	0.75	4	n/a	100	6.3	46.4	0.98
Hexastarch													
HES 200/0.62	6%	Elohes	200	25	900	15	0.62	9	25	110	5.08	69.7	1.23
Pentastarch													
HES 70/0.5	6%	Rheohes, Expafusin	70	10	180	7	0.5	3	30	90	n/a	n/a	n/a
HES 200/0.5	10%	HAES-steril, Hemohes	200	50	780	13	0.5	4–5	50–60	145	3.35	30.6	9.24
HES200/0.5	6%	HAES-steril, Hemohes	200	50	780	13	0.5	4–5	30–35	100	n/a	n/a	n/a
HES 200/0.5	3%	HAES-steril, Hemohes	200	50	780	13	0.5	4–5	15–18	60	n/a	n/a	n/a
Tetrastarch (waxy-maize-derived)													
HES 130/0.4	10%	Votuven	130	20	380	15	0.4	9	70–80	200	1.54	12.8	26
HES 130/0.4	6%	Votuven, Volulyte	130	20	380	15	0.4	9	36	100	1.39	12.1	31.4
Tetrastarch (potato-derived)													
HES 130/0.42	10%	Tetraspan	130	15	n/a	n/a	0.42	6	60	150	n/a	n/a	n/a
HES 130/0.42	6%	Vencfundin, Tetraspan, VitaHES	130	15	n/a	n/a	0.42	6	36	100	n/a	12	19

Derived and modified from Ertmer et al. [34]

[a] Data extracted from manufacturer's product information.

[b] Bottom fraction: <10% of molecules are less than the molecular weight defined by bottom fraction.

[c] Top fraction: <10% of molecules exceed the molecular weight defined by bottom fraction.

COP, colloid osmotic pressure; MW, molecular weight; MS, molar substitution; n/a, not applicable or not available; T$^{1/2}$ alpha, distribution half-life; T$^{1/2}$ beta, elimination half-life.

critically ill patients with sepsis, and do not include trauma and cardiac surgical populations.

HES in current use has a reduced concentration (6%) with a molecular weight (MW) of 130 kDa and a substitution of 0.38–0.45. HES with a substitution of 0.5 or 0.6 is denoted as pentastarch or hexastarch, respectively. First-generation HES consist of heta- and hexastarches, whereas pentastarch is second-generation. The latest, third-generation HES, consists of modern tetrastarches (HES 130/0.4 and HES 130/0.42).

Gelatins

These are prepared by hydrolysis of bovine collagen. Succinylated gelatin (Gelofusine™) is produced by enzymatic alterations of the basic gelatin peptide and is presented in isotonic saline. Urea-linked gelatin (Polygeline, Haemaccel™) is produced by thermal degradation of the raw material to small peptides (12 000–15 000 Da) followed by urea cross-linking to produce polymers of around 35 000 Da that are suspended in isotonic sodium chloride with 5.1 mmol/L potassium and 6.25 mmol/L calcium.[33] Concerns have been raised about the association between the use of bovine-derived gelatin (but not pharmaceutically derived), bovine spongiform encephalitis, and Creutzfeldt–Jakob disease.[33,34]

Dextrans

These are biosynthesized from sucrose by *Leuconostoc* bacteria using the enzyme dextran sucrase. This enzyme catalyzes the alpha-1,6-glycosidic linkage of glucose monomers. Dextrans are defined by their MW, with dextran 40 and 70 having MW 40 000 Da and 70000 Da, respectively. Allergic reactions (<0.35%) have been associated with dextrans.[35] Injection of a hapten, dextran 1 before administering dextran solutions has significantly reduced the incidence to <0.0015%.[36] This involves a 20 ml injection of low-MW dextran 1 (1 000 Da) prior to infusion of a dextran volume expander, which leads to inactivation of anti-dextran IgGs in the recipient.

Crystalloids

The most commonly used crystalloid is normal (0.9%) saline with a sodium concentration of 154 mmol/L. The term "normal" was coined by Dutch physiologist Hartog Jacob Hamburger, who in 1882 suggested that blood salt concentration was 0.9% rather than 0.6%.

Normal saline is suspected to induce hyperchloremic metabolic acidosis ($NaCl + H_2O \rightarrow HCl + NaOH$), although the clinical consequences of this are unclear.[37] Administration of large volumes of normal saline may contribute to fluid overload and therefore small-volume resuscitation with hypertonic saline (3%, 5%, or 7%) has been introduced.

Hypertonic Saline

In 1980, de Felippe reported almost miraculous recovery from near-fatal hemorrhagic shock of 11 patients treated with hypertonic saline (HS).[38] Various HS solutions have been employed, ranging in concentration from 0.9% to 30% (Table 16.2). The hyperosmotic and hyperoncotic properties of the HS solutions result in an increased fluid shift ability, providing approximately 750 ml of plasma volume expansion per 1 liter of HS compared with 300 ml plasma volume expansion per 1 liter of crystalloid. Hypertonicity leads to vasodilatation by improving endothelial cell volume, improves cardiac output, and has been

Table 16.2 Physico-chemical properties of various HS solutions

Solution	Osmolarity (mosmol/l)	Sodium concentration (mosmol/l)
0.9% normal saline	308	154
Ringer's lactate	275	130
1.7% saline	291	582
3% saline	1 026	513
7.2% saline/6% HAES (200/0.6)	2 464	1 232
7.5% saline	2 566	1 283
7.5% saline/6% dextran 70	2 568	1 283
10% saline	3 424	1 712
23% saline	8 008	4 004
30% saline	10 000	5 000

Derived from Strandvik [39].

shown to reduce neutrophilic activation.[39] HS solutions have, however, not demonstrated efficacy at reducing intra-cranial pressure, or a survival or outcome benefit following traumatic brain injury.[40]

Physiologically "Balanced" and "Unbalanced" Fluids

Balanced or physiological fluids contain inorganic ions (calcium, potassium, magnesium), molecular glucose, and buffer components such as lactate or bicarbonate and have a lower chloride content to prevent hyperchloremic metabolic acidosis. Current evidence suggests that patients randomized to receive balanced fluids are subject to less coagulopathy (reduced effect in thromboelastography and platelet aggregation),[41] and may have better preservation of renal function, compared with those receiving unbalanced crystalloids.[42]

A typical balanced crystalloid is Hartmann's solution/Ringer's lactate. Balanced colloids are available as 6% HES (Hextend®, Volulyte®). Table 16.3 summarizes the advantages and disadvantages of colloids and crystalloids, whilst Table 16.4 details the compositions of commonly used colloids and crystalloids.

Controversies of Randomized-Controlled Trials Comparing Efficacy of Colloids with Crystalloids

The clinical risks and benefits of crystalloids versus colloids is a subject of significant controversy. One the one hand, randomized-controlled trials (RCTs) such as CHEST indicate that modern colloids such as HES (tetrastarch 130/0.4) may promote acute kidney injury in intensive care patients and increase mortality risk in septic patients.[43,44] On the other hand, a recent analysis by Morath et al. [45] of HES in patients undergoing elective cardiac surgery did not reveal any association between this colloid and the postoperative occurrence of acute kidney injury. Trials such as FIRST, BaSES, and CRISTAL suggest

Table 16.3 Comparative overview of generic advantages and disadvantages of colloids and crystalloids

Solution	Advantages	Disadvantages
Colloids	1. Smaller infused volumes 2. Prolong increase in plasma volumes 3. Less peripheral edema 4. Endothelial protection	1. Renal dysfunction (dextran>HES>albumin) 2. Coagulopathy (older HES>tetrastarch>albumin) 3. Pulmonary edema (capillary leak syndrome) 4. Pruritus (HES, dextran>albumin) 5. Anaphylaxis (dextran>HES>albumin) 6. Greater cost (albumin>other synthetic colloids)
Crystalloids	1. Lower cost 2. Higher glomerular filtration rate 3. Interstitial fluid replacement	1. Short-term increase in intravascular volume 2. Short-term hemodynamic improvement 3. Interstitial fluid accumulation

similar outcomes for colloids and crystalloids.[43,44,46–48] Specifically for crystalloids, recent evidence indicates that whilst normal saline usage may be associated with a greater incidence of hyperchloremic acidosis, the impact on clinical outcomes is comparable to that when using balanced crystalloids.[49–51] Similarly, a recent systematic review examining the effect of colloids versus crystalloids on mortality and blood transfusion or renal replacement therapy (RRT) requirement in critically ill patients found that there was little or no difference in terms of mortality.[52] Starches were thought to slightly increase the need for blood transfusion and RRT, whilst the use of dextran or albumin made little or no difference.

Unfortunately, much of the evidence is confounded by clinical, methodological, or statistical heterogeneity. Careful scrutiny of the CHEST and 6S trials, for example, by adopting a standardized method shows lack of consistency in trial design, indications for colloid use, or maximum administered volume.[53] The recent major trials and their key limitations are highlighted in Table 16.5. Critics have used these and other observations, such as the lack of robust evidence of harm attributable to colloids in the non-critically ill septic population, as bases for their continued support.

An additional consideration is the increased cost of colloid solutions, which has been justified until now by their purported clinical benefits. Furthermore, the publication of RCTs showing harm from colloid administration has resulted in rapid regulatory steps to suspend marketing authorization of these colloids. This has simultaneously increased the downstream risk of widespread crystalloid usage, even in patients with fragile microcirculation and delicate fluid balance, known risk factors for increased morbidity.[54,55]

Safety Outcomes in Cardiac Surgery: An Up-to-Date Review of Randomized-Controlled Trials

A meta-analysis conducted by our group comprising 59 RCTs comparing safety outcomes in 16 889 patients randomized to receive colloid or crystalloids [56] did not demonstrate colloid superiority. Interestingly, no safety concerns, such as renal morbidity related to HES,

Table 16.4 Constituents of commonly used colloids and crystalloids

Variable	Human plasma	4% albumin	10% (200/0.5) HES	6% (450/0.7) HES	6% (130/0.4) HES		6% (130/0.42) HES		4% succinylated modified fluid gelatin	3.5% urea-linked gelatin	0.9% Saline	Compounded sodium lactate	Balanced salt solution
Trade name		Albumex	Hemohes	Hextend	Voluven	Volulyte	Venofundin	Tetraspan	Gelofusine	Haemaccel	Normal saline	Hartmann's or Ringer's lactate	Plasma-Lyte
Colloid source		Human donor	Potato starch	Maize starch	Maize starch	Maize starch	Potato starch	Potato starch	Bovine gelatin	Bovine gelatin			
Osmolarity (mosmol/l)	291	250	308	304	308	286	308	296	274	301	308	280.6	294
Sodium[a]	135–145	148	154	143	154	137	154	140	154	145	154	131	140
Potassium[a]	4.5–5.0	-	-	3.0	-	4	-	4	-	5.1	-	5.4	5
Calcium[a]	2.2–26	-	-	5	-	-	-	2.5	-	6.25	-	2	-
Magnesium[a]	0.8–1	-	-	0.9	-	1.5	-	1	-	-	-	-	3
Chloride[a]	94–111	128	154	124	154	110	154	118	120	145	154	111	98
Acetate[a]	-	-	-	-	-	34	-	24	-	-	-	-	27
Lactate[a]	1–2	-	-	28	-	-	-	-	-	-	-	29	-
Malate[a]	-	-	-	-	-	-	-	5	-	-	-	-	-
Gluconate[a]	-	-	-	-	-	-	-	-	-	-	-	-	23
Bicarbonate[a]	23–37	-	-	-	-	-	-	-	-	-	-	-	-
Octanoate[a]	-	6.4	-	-	-	-	-	-	-	-	-	-	-

Derived from Myburgh et al. [43].

[a] Units of measurement are mmol/l.

Table 16.5 Characteristics and relative risks of various outcomes in RCTs evaluating HES

Trial	VISEP	6S Trial	CHEST	CRYSTMAS	CRISTAL
Number of included patients	537	804	7 000	196	2 857
Disease condition	Severe sepsis	Severe sepsis	ICU admission requiring fluid administration	Severe sepsis	Sepsis, trauma, hypovolemic shock
Starch solution	10% 200/0.5	6% 130/0.42	6% 130/0.4	6% 130/0.4	Any colloid solution
Comparator	Ringer's lactate	Ringer's acetate	Saline	Saline	Isotonic or hypertonic saline, buffered solutions
Renal replacement therapy	1.66[a]	1.35[a]	1.21[a]	1.83	0.93
90-day mortality	1.21	1.17[a]	1.06, 95% CI 0.96, 1.18, $p = 0.26$	1.20	0.92[a]
Limitations	Considerable no. of patients received higher dose than manufacturer recommendation. Study used older HES. Considerable no. of patients in control group received HES	Randomization of 52% of patients after initial stabilization with colloids. Lack of valid resuscitation endpoints or resuscitation protocols. Failure to use pre-specified treatment algorithms. 36% of patients receiving HES had pre-existing renal impairment. No hemodynamic monitoring.	Inclusion of patients after initial stabilization. Lack of valid resuscitation endpoints or resuscitation protocols. Failure to use pre-specified treatment algorithms.	Not powered to assess renal safety. Publication and reporting bias. 68% of patients receiving HES had pre-existing renal impairment.	Trial fluid not blinded. No stratified comparison according to subgroups.

[a] These relative risks differed from 1.00 with statistical significance at the 5% level.
CI, confidence interval.

were reported. Sensitivity analyses were undertaken to sensitize against low-volume studies (<250 patients) and low-quality studies (high risk of selection or performance bias) to evaluate the robustness of evidence. In general, these did not affect the summary estimates of effect.

- **Mortality.** Seven trials comparing colloids versus crystalloids were included. Neither benefit nor harm was seen with either intervention (odds ratio 0.74, 95% confidence interval 0.17–0.32, $p = 0.70$) (Fig. 16.2).
- **Acute kidney injury.** This was analyzed in four studies showing neither benefit nor harm (odds ratio 1.28, 95% confidence interval 0.72–2.26, $p = 0.40$) (Fig. 16.3). No analyses could be performed after exclusion of low-volume studies owing to lack of studies remaining. Exclusion of low-quality studies had no effect on the outcome.
- **Renal replacement therapy.** This was analyzed in two studies showing neither benefit nor harm (odds ratio 1.94, 95% confidence interval 0.20–18.71, $p = 0.57$) (Fig. 16.4). No analyses could be performed after exclusion of low-volume studies owing to lack of studies remaining. Exclusion of low-quality studies had no effect on the outcome.
- **Cerebrovascular accident.** An assessment on four studies was performed. No effect was observed in favor of colloids or crystalloids (odds ratio 1.95, 95% confidence interval 0.52–0.76, $p = 0.32$) (Fig. 16.5). No analyses could be performed after exclusion of low-volume studies owing to lack of studies remaining. Exclusion of low-quality studies had no effect on the outcome.

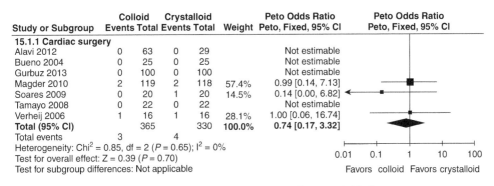

Study or Subgroup	Colloid Events	Total	Crystalloid Events	Total	Weight	Peto Odds Ratio Peto, Fixed, 95% CI
15.1.1 Cardiac surgery						
Alavi 2012	0	63	0	29		Not estimable
Bueno 2004	0	25	0	25		Not estimable
Gurbuz 2013	0	100	0	100		Not estimable
Magder 2010	2	119	2	118	57.4%	0.99 [0.14, 7.13]
Soares 2009	0	20	1	20	14.5%	0.14 [0.00, 6.82]
Tamayo 2008	0	22	0	22		Not estimable
Verheij 2006	1	16	1	16	28.1%	1.00 [0.06, 16.74]
Total (95% CI)		365		330	100.0%	0.74 [0.17, 3.32]
Total events	3		4			

Heterogeneity: Chi² = 0.85, df = 2 (P = 0.65); I² = 0%
Test for overall effect: Z = 0.39 (P = 0.70)
Test for subgroup differences: Not applicable

Favors colloid   Favors crystalloid

Figure 16.2 Comparison: colloid versus crystalloid. Outcome: mortality. From Ref. [56].

Study or Subgroup	Colloid Events	Total	Crystalloid Events	Total	Weight	Peto Odds Ratio Peto, Fixed, 95% CI
15.2.1 Cardiac surgery						
Gurbuz 2013	9	100	6	100	29.5%	1.54 [0.54, 4.39]
Lee 2011	1	53	0	53	2.1%	7.39 [0.15, 372.38]
Magder 2010	19	119	18	118	66.3%	1.06 [0.52, 2.13]
Soares 2009	1	20	0	20	2.1%	7.39 [0.15, 372.38]
Total (95% CI)		292		291	100.0%	1.28 [0.72, 2.26]
Total events	30		24			

Heterogeneity: Chi² = 1.95, df = 3 (P = 0.58); I² = 0%
Test for overall effect: Z = 0.85 (P = 0.40)
Test for subgroup differences: Not applicable

Favors colloid   Favors crystalloid

Figure 16.3 Comparison: colloid versus crystalloid. Outcome: acute kidney injury. From Ref. [56].

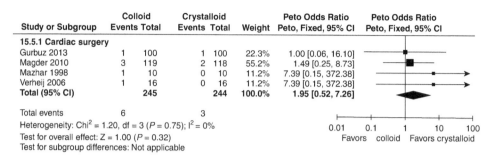

Figure 16.4 Comparison: colloid versus crystalloid. Outcome: renal replacement therapy. From Ref. [56].

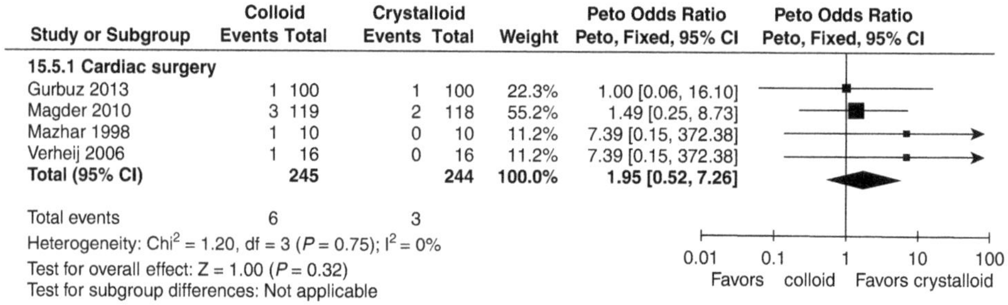

Figure 16.5 Comparison: colloid versus crystalloid. Outcome: cerebrovascular accident. From Ref. [56].

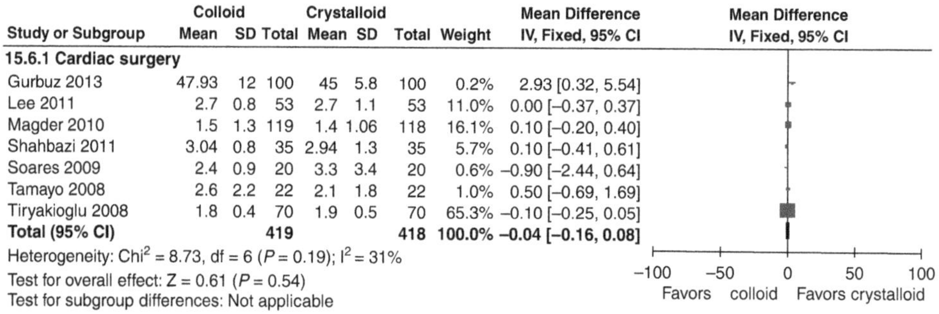

Figure 16.6 Comparison: colloid versus crystalloid. Outcome: ICU length of stay (days). From Ref. [56].

- **Hospital stay.** This was assessed in six studies, showing non-significant effect estimate (mean differences 0.14, 95% confidence interval 0.23–0.52, $p = 0.46$) (Figs. 16.6, 16.7). Significant heterogeneity was observed, however. No analyses could be performed after exclusion of low-volume studies owing to lack of studies remaining. Exclusion of low-quality studies had no effect on the outcome From Ref.

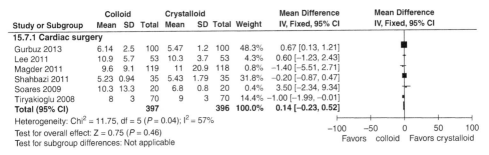

Figure 16.7 Comparison: colloid versus crystalloid. Outcome: hospital length of stay (days). From Ref. [56].

References

1. Mariscalco G, Musumeci F. Fluid management in the cardiothoracic intensive care unit: diuresis–diuretics and hemofiltration. *Curr Opin Anaesthesiol.* 2014;**27**:133–9.

2. Habicher M, Perrino A, Spies CD, et al. Contemporary fluid management in cardiac anesthesia. *J Cardiothorac Vasc Anesth.* 2011;**25**:1141–53.

3. Assaad S, Popescu W, Perrino A. Fluid management in thoracic surgery. *Curr Opin Anaesthesiol.* 2013;**26**:31–9.

4. Bignami E, Guarnieri M, Gemma M. Fluid management in cardiac surgery patients: pitfalls, challenges and solutions. *Minerva Anestesiol.* 2017;**83**:638–51.

5. Romagnoli S, Rizza, A, Ricci Z. Fluid status assessment and management during the perioperative phase in adult cardiac surgery patients. *J Cardiothorac Vasc Anesth.* 2016;**30**:1076–84.

6. Hu Z, Cano I, D'Amore PA. Update on the role of the endothelial glycocalyx in angiogenesis and vascular inflammation. *Front Cell Dev Biol.* 2021;**9**:734276.

7. Rehm M, Bruegger D, Christ F, et al. Shedding of the endothelial glycocalyx in patients undergoing major vascular surgery with global and regional ischemia. *Circulation.* 2007;**116**:1896–906.

8. Passov A, Schramko A, Salminen US, et al. Endothelial glycocalyx during early

reperfusion in patients undergoing cardiac surgery. *PLoS One.* 2021;**16**:e0251747.

9. Dekker NAM, Veerhoek D, Koning NJ, et al. Postoperative microcirculatory perfusion and endothelial glycocalyx shedding following cardiac surgery with cardiopulmonary bypass. *Anaesthesia,* 2019;**74**:609–18.

10. Bruegger D, Jacob M, Rehm M, et al. Atrial natriuretic peptide induces shedding of endothelial glycocalyx in coronary vascular bed of guinea pig hearts. *Am J Physiol Heart Circ Physiol.*2005;**289**:H1993–9.

11. Bruegger D, Schwartz L, Chappell D, et al. Release of atrial natriuretic peptide precedes shedding of the endothelial glycocalyx equally in patients undergoing on- and off-pump coronary artery bypass surgery. *Basic Res Cardiol.* 2011;**106**:1111–21.

12. Chappell D, Hofmann-Kiefer K, Jacob M, et al. TNF-alpha induced shedding of the endothelial glycocalyx is prevented by hydrocortisone and antithrombin. *Basic Res Cardiol.* 2009;**104**:78–89.

13. Jedlicka J, Becker BF, Chappell D. Endothelial glycocalyx. *Crit Care Clin.* 2020;**36**:217–232.

14. Goligorsky MS, Sun D. Glycocalyx in endotoxaemia and sepsis. *Am J Pathol.* 2020;**190**:791–8.

15. Pape T, Hunkemöller AM, Kümpers P, et al. Targeting the "sweet spot" in septic

shock – a perspective on the endothelial glycocalyx regulating proteins heparanse-1 and -2. *Matrix Biol Plus.* 2021;**12**:100095.

16. Berg S, Engman A, Hesselvik JF Laurent TC. Crystalloid infusion increases plasma hyaluronan. *Crit Care Med.* 1994;**22**:1563–7.

17. Milford EM, Reade MC. Resuscitation fluid choices to preserve the endothelial glycocalyx. *Crit Care.* 2019;**23**:77.

18. Ueda S, Nishio K, Akai Y, et al. Prognostic value of increased plasma levels of brain natriuretic peptide in patients with septic shock. *Shock.* 2006;**26**:134–9.

19. Singh H, Ramai D, Patel H, et al. B-type natriuretic peptide: a predictor for mortality, intensive care unit length of stay, and hospital length of stay in patients with resolving sepsis. *Cardiol Res.* 2017;**8**:271–5.

20. Bark BP, Persson J, Grande PO. Importance of the infusion rate for the plasma expanding effect of 5% albumin, 6% HES 130/0.4, 4% gelatin, and 0.9% NaCl in the septic rat. *Crit Care Med.* 2013;**41**:857–66.

21. Erstad BL. The revised starling equation: the debate of albumin versus crystalloids continues. *Ann Pharmacother.* 2020;**54**:921–7.

22. Hahn RG, Dull RO, Zdolsek J. The extended Starling principle needs clinical validation. *Acta Anaesthesiol Scand.* 2020;**64**:884–7.

23. Nicholson JP, Wolmarans MR, Park GR. The role of albumin in critical illness. *Br J Anaesth.* 2000;**85**:599–610.

24. Bihari S, Bannard-Smith J, Bellomo R. Albumin as a drug: its biological effects beyond volume expansion. *Crit Care Resusc.* 2020;**22**:257–65.

25. Finfer S, Bellomo R, Boyce N, et al. A comparison of albumin and saline for fluid resuscitation in the intensive care unit. *N Engl J Med.* 2004;**350**:2247–56.

26. Thang C, Marella P, Kumar A, et al. Early albumin exposure after cardiac surgery. *J Cardiothorac Vasc Anesth.* 2022;**36**:1310–17.

27. Maitland K, Kiguli S, Opoka RO, et al. Mortality after fluid bolus in African children with severe infection. *N Engl J Med* 2011;**364**:2483–95.

28. Levin M, Cunnington AJ, Wilson C, et al. Effects of saline or albumin fluid bolus in resuscitation: evidence from re-analysis of the FEAST trial. *Lancet Respir Med/* 2019;**7**:581–93.

29. Caironi P, Tognoni G, Masson S, et al. Albumin replacement in patients with severe sepsis or septic shock. *N Engl J Med.* 2014;**370**:1412–21.

30. van Rijen EA, Ward JJ, Little RA. Effects of colloidal resuscitation fluids on reticuloendothelial function and resistance to infection after hemorrhage. *Clin Diagn Lab Immunol.* 1998;**5**:543–9.

31. Skhirtladze K, Base EM, Lassnigg A, et al. Comparison of the effects of albumin 5%, hydroxyethyl starch 130/0.4 6%, and Ringer's lactate on blood loss and coagulation after cardiac surgery. *Br J Anaesth.* 2014;**112**:255–64.

32. Nielsen VG. Hydroxyethyl starch enhances fibrinolysis in human plasma by diminishing alpha2-antiplasmin-plasmin interactions. *Blood Coagul Fibrinolysis.* 2007;**18**:647–56.

33. Ertmer C, Rehberg S, Van Aken H, et al. Relevance of non-albumin colloids in intensive care medicine. *Best Pract Res Clin Anaesthesiol.* 2009;**23**:193–212.

34. Tseng CH, Chen TT, Wu MY, et al. Resuscitation fluid types in sepsis, surgical, and trauma patients: a systematic review and sequential network meta-analysis. *Crit Care.* 2020;**24**:693.

35. Hanžek I, Tonković D, Margaretić Piljek N, et al. Allergic reactions to colloid fluids in anesthesia. *Psychiatr Danub.* 2020;**32** (Suppl 4):429–31.

36. Ljungström KG. Dextran 40 therapy made safer by pretreatment with dextran 1. *Plast Reconstr Surg.* 2007;**120**:337–40.

37. Morgan TJ. The idea crystalloid – what is "balanced"? *Curr Opin Crit Care.* 2013;**19**:299–307.

38. De Felippe J, Timoner J, Velasco IT, Lopes OU, Rocha-e-Silva M. Treatment of refractory hypovolaemic shock by 7.5% sodium chloride injections. *Lancet.* 1980;2:1002–4.

39. Strandvik GF. Hypertonic saline in critical care: a review of the literature and guidelines for use in hypotensive states and raised intracranial pressure. *Anaesthesia.* 2009;64:990–1003.

40. Tisherman SA, Schmicker RH, Brase KJ, et al. Detailed description of all deaths in both the shock and traumatic brain injury hypertonic saline trials of the Resuscitation Outcomes Consortium. *Ann Surg.* 2015;261:586–90.

41. Smorenberg A, Ince C, Groeneveld AJ. Dose and type of crystalloid fluid therapy in adult hospitalized patients. *Perioper Med (Lond).* 2013;2:17.

42. Lobo DN, Awad S. Should chloride-rich crystalloids remain the mainstay of fluid resuscitation to prevent "pre-renal" acute kidney injury?: con. *Kidney Int.* 2014;86:1096–1105.

43. Myburgh JA, Finfer S, Bellomo R, et al. Hydroxyethyl starch or saline for fluid resuscitation in intensive care. *N Engl J Med.* 2012;367:1901–11.

44. Perner A, Haase N, Guttormsen AB, et al. Hydroxyethyl starch 130/0.42 versus Ringer's acetate in severe sepsis. *N Engl J Med.* 2012;367:124–34.

45. Morath B, Meid B, Rickmann J, et al. Renal safety of hydroxyethyl starch 130/0.42 after cardiac surgery: a retrospective cohort analysis. *Drug Saf.* 2021;44:1311–21.

46. James MF, Michell WL, Joubert IA, et al. Resuscitation with hydroxyethyl starch improves renal function and lactate clearance in penetrating trauma in a randomized controlled study: the FIRST trial (Fluids in Resuscitation of Severe Trauma). *Br J Anaesth.* 2011;107:693–702.

47. Siegemend M. BaSES trial: Basel Starch Evaluation in Sepsis. ClinicalTrialsgov Identifier NCT00273728. 2013.

48. Annane D, Siami S, Jaber S, et al. Effects of fluid resuscitation with colloids vs. crystalloids on mortality in critically ill patients presenting with hypovolemic shock: the CRISTAL randomized trial. *JAMA.* 2013;310:1809–17.

49. Self WH, Semler MW, Wanderer JP, et al. Balanced crystalloids versus saline in noncritically ill adults. *N Eng J Med.* 2018;378:819–28.

50. Jahangir A, Sahra S, Niazi MRK, et al. Comparison of normal saline solution with low-chloride solutions in renal transplants: a meta-analysis. *Kidney Res Clin Pract.* 2021;40:484–95.

51. Maheswari K, Turan A, Makarova N, et al. Saline versus lactated Ringer's solution: the Saline or Lactated Ringer's (SOLAR) Trial. *Anesthesiology.* 2020;132:614–24.

52. Lewis SR, Pritchard MW, Evans DJ, et al. Colloids versus crystalloids for fluid resuscitation in critically ill people. *Cochrane Database Syst Rev* 2018;8: CD000567.

53. Meybohm P, van Aken H, De Gasperi A, et al. Re-evaluating currently available data and suggestions for planning randomised controlled studies regarding the use of hydroxyethyl starch in critically ill patients – a multidisciplinary statement. *Crit Care.* 2013;17:R166.

54. Heßler M, Arnemann PH, Ertmer C. To use of not to use hydroxyethyl starch in intraoperative care: are we ready to answer the "Gretchen question"? *Curr Opin Anaesthesiol.* 2015;28:370–7.

55. Zarychanski R, Abou-Setta AM, Turgeon AF, et al. Association of hydroxyethyl starch administration with mortality and acute kidney injury in critically ill patients requiring volume resuscitation: a systematic review and meta-analysis. *JAMA.* 2013;309:678–88.

56. Qureshi SH, Rizvi SI, Patel NN, Murphy GJ. Meta-analysis of colloids versus crystalloids in critically ill, trauma and surgical patients. *Br J Surg.* 2016;103:14–26.

Fluid and Hemodynamic Monitoring in Brain Surgery

Indu Kapoor, Charu Mahajan and Hemanshu Prabhakar

Introduction

Neurosurgical patients form a special population that poses challenges to anesthetists and intensivists when it comes to fluid administration. Issues pertaining to elevated intracranial pressure (ICP) and intraoperative blood losses have to be dealt with more compositely. Earlier, it was believed that fluid intake restriction up to 1 liter daily in patients undergoing craniotomy maintained good homeostasis. Larger volumes may result in expansion of the extracellular space and may result in brain edema.[1] It was cautioned that fluid restriction may actually be dangerous in patients receiving hyperoncotic fluids, diuretics and dexamethasone. However, over the years the practice has changed, and it is now believed that restrictive fluid strategy may in fact be dangerous as these neurosurgical patients might be receiving mannitol and diuretics to prevent a rise in ICP and reduce brain edema. The effect of anesthetics may be additive in causing systemic hypotension. Systemic hypotension may compromise the cerebral perfusion pressure (CPP), reduce cerebral oxygenation and produce deleterious intracranial complications. These neurosurgical patients are also not excluded from the controversy of the colloids versus crystalloids.[2] Hemodynamic monitoring for fluid therapy in neurosurgical patients is prudent, as these patients are prone to hypovolemia. Studies have shown that goal-directed fluid therapy (GDFT) in comparison with standard therapy in these patients has positive outcomes with regard to stable intraoperative hemodynamics, good surgical field and postoperative period.

This chapter deals with various neurosurgical situations where fluid administration is vital to the overall management of the patient. While the main focus of the chapter is on the perioperative fluid management and hemodynamic monitoring in different clinical scenarios, it also discusses the therapeutic roles of fluid aimed at reduction of ICP and improving CPP.

General Principles

Crystalloids or colloids along with blood and blood products are routinely used during neurosurgical procedures. It has, in general, become a common practice in neuroanesthesia to avoid fluids that are hypo-osmolar or contain glucose. This is with a view that the free water produced by the hypo-osmolar and glucose-containing solutions results in brain edema. Thus the fluids of choice include 0.9% normal saline and lactated Ringer's solution, both being nearly equiosmolar to the normal plasma. For the purpose of achieving brain relaxation in the intraoperative period, hypertonic fluids such as mannitol and hypertonic saline are frequent used. It is by the virtue of these hypertonic fluids that water is drawn from intracellular and interstitial compartments into the intravascular compartment.

This results in relaxation of the brain and increased compliance. However, it is essential that the blood–brain barrier be intact for the hypertonic fluids to produce their effect on the brain.[3]

In general, sufficient fluids should be administered to neurosurgical patients so as to maintain good cardiac output and hemodynamic stability. It has been accepted that the respiratory variations in the arterial pressure during mechanical ventilation reflect volume status and fluid responsiveness of the patients.[4] These "dynamic" hemodynamic parameters, such as the stroke volume, arterial pulse pressure and the variations during positive pressure mechanical ventilation, have been considered accurate in predicting the volume status by many authors.[5]

Following are some of the situations in neurosurgery where fluid administration requires special considerations.

Supratentorial Tumor Surgery

Administration of fluids in patients undergoing craniotomy for supratentorial surgery is not only for the purpose of replacement but also to provide brain relaxation. Whereas mannitol and hypertonic saline are popular fluids used for providing brain relaxation, normal saline remains the choice of fluid for maintaining the volume status of the patients. There remains a controversy over which fluid to be used for intraoperative brain relaxation, mannitol or hypertonic saline. In a recent meta-analysis the authors found that hypertonic saline significantly reduced the risk of tense brain, but the quality of evidence was low and the findings were from only a limited number of studies.[6] Normal saline remains the fluid of choice to maintain intraoperative volume status. However, amidst the controversy of crystalloid versus colloid of neurosurgical patients, a recent study by Xia and colleagues compared the goal-directed crystalloid and goal-directed colloid therapy in patients undergoing craniotomy.[7] Based on a study conducted on 40 patients, the authors concluded that goal-directed hydroxyethyl starch therapy was not superior to goal-directed lactate Ringer's solution therapy for brain relaxation and cerebral metabolism. The authors found that less fluid was needed to maintain the target stroke volume variation in the colloid group when compared with the crystalloid group.

Subarachnoid Hemorrhage

Fluid management in patients with subarachnoid hemorrhage (SAH) aims to maintain a good fluid balance and correction of hyponatremia, which accompanies the cerebral salt wasting syndrome, often associated with SAH. This also formed the basis of the "triple-H" therapy. The standard triple H-therapy consisted of hypervolemia, hemodilution and hypertension. However, in a recent exploratory analysis on 413 patients enrolled in the CONSCIOUS-1 trial, the authors found that administration of colloid and maintenance of a positive fluid balance during the period of vasospasm after SAH was associated with poor outcome.[8] In a systematic review by Dankbaar and colleagues, the authors concluded that evidence was lacking from controlled studies that supported use of triple-H therapy or any of its components in improving the cerebral blood flow. They also found out from uncontrolled studies that "hypertension" was possibly the most effective component of triple-H therapy in increasing cerebral blood flow.[9]

Considering the fluid of choice in these patients, a pilot study demonstrated that balanced solutions reduce the incidence of hyperchloremic acidosis, associated with administration of chloride-rich solutions, when the latter was compared in patients with severe brain injury.[10] Similar findings have also been reported by Lehmann and colleagues, who found that in the management of patients with SAH, saline-based fluids resulted in a greater number of patients with hyperchloremic acidosis, hyperosmolality and positive fluid balance when compared with balanced solutions.[11] As evidence is accumulating in favor of balanced solutions in comparison with normal saline, it is still too early for any conclusive statement to be made in support of any type of fluid to be recommended for patients with SAH.

Pituitary Surgery

Surgical procedures related to the pituitary pose challenges in terms of fluid and electrolyte imbalance, which may be frequently related. Diabetes insipidus (DI), during both the intraoperative and postoperative periods, may be observed. Fluid balance needs close monitoring to avoid complications and disabling electrolyte imbalance and to avoid fluid overload. Syndrome of inappropriate antidiuretic hormone secretion (SIADH) is another postoperative complication associated with pituitary surgery.[12] The management of these syndromes is beyond the scope of this chapter; however, it cannot be overemphasized that fluid and electrolyte disturbances occur during the treatment of patients with pituitary tumors. Half normal saline and 5% dextrose are fluids of choice in cases of DI, whereas in cases of SIADH, fluid restriction is the most appropriate treatment. A comparative tabulation of these two conditions is given in Table 17.1. It is important to check serum osmolality frequently to guide the administration of amount and type of fluid.

Traumatic Brain Injury

The major work in the field of fluid management related to neurosurgery is probably carried out in the group of patients suffering from traumatic brain injury. The need for early restoration of intravascular fluid status and maintenance of hemodynamics predicts the outcome of these patients by preventing secondary injuries to the brain. Euvolemia is the mainstay in managing head-injured patients. Hypovolemia must be avoided as must fluid overload, because it can worsen cerebral edema. Choice of fluid is always a controversy in

Table 17.1 Salient differential features between diabetes insipidus (DI) and syndrome of inappropriate antidiuretic hormone secretion (SIADH)

Clinical parameters	DI	SIADH
Urine output	>30 ml/kg/hr	Decreased
Fluid balance (Intravascular)	Reduced	Neutral or slightly positive
Serum osmolality	Increased	Decreased
Serum Na^+ concentration	Increased	Decreased
Urine osmolality	Decreased	Increased (>100 mOsm/kg)
Urinary Na^+ concentration	<15 mEq/l	>20 mEq/l
Fluid replacement	Half normal saline or 5% dextrose	Fluid restriction

patients with traumatic brain injury (TBI). Many studies have been done in which the authors have tried to prove superiority of one fluid over another. In the popular study by the Saline versus Albumin Fluid Evaluation (SAFE) investigators, the authors found that higher rates of mortality were associated with use of albumin as resuscitating fluid when compared with saline.[13] Small-volume fluid resuscitation with hypertonic saline had been actively popularized earlier and success was reported even in pediatric patients.[14] Soon these fluids, hypertonic saline and colloids, fell into controversy, and the debate continues. Discussing the types of fluids used for resuscitation in traumatic brain injury, Van Aken and colleagues have rightly described in their article that it is the osmolality of an infusion solution rather than the colloid osmotic pressure that represents the key determinant in the pathogenesis of cerebral edema formation.[15] In a systematic review on the use of crystalloids versus colloids in prehospital fluid management in TBI, Tan and colleagues found that none was superior to the other.[16] In general, hypotonic fluids and glucose-containing fluids have to be avoided during management of patients with TBI. It is suggested to maintain the iso-osmolality (using fluid having osmolality around 300 mOsm/l) when administering large amounts of fluid for resuscitation. Patients with TBI have multisystemic injuries, which make them prone for hypervolemia. Fluid resuscitation should not be avoided in these patients for fear of developing brain edema. Isotonic, glucose-free crystalloid solution should be used for resuscitation both in the pre-hospital setting and in the emergency department while the patient receives primary treatment for TBI.

Spine Surgery

Surgeries on the spine may be extensive, involving many sections of the vertebral column, especially when instrumentation is planned. Massive blood loss and blood transfusions may be expected. It is important to maintain adequate fluid status without producing fluid overload, which may lead to venous congestion and at the same time compromising the blood flow and oxygenation of the spinal cord.[17] A study revealed that there was a correlation between the total amount of fluid administered and length of hospital stay and pulmonary complications.[18] With an increase of 1000 ml of crystalloids, the odds of pulmonary complications increased by 30%.

Hemodynamic Monitoring

To achieve an optimal fluid balance, it is prudent to avoid both over-hydration and excessive restriction. There are several monitoring modalities available to guide peri-operative fluid therapy. Various common clinical indices such as mean arterial pressure (MAP), central venous pressure (CVP), urine output (UO), capillary refill, cold extremities and blood lactate levels can be used to guide the fluid therapy in a neurosurgical patient. Traditionally CVP has been used to monitor fluid therapy in patients undergoing major surgery or in the intensive care unit (ICU).[19] It is believed that low CVP reflects low intravascular volume and high CVP denotes fluid overload. It is based on the assumption that CVP is a good indicator of right ventricular (RV) preload, and because RV stroke volume determines left ventricular filling (LV) filling, the CVP is assumed to be an indirect measure of LV preload.[20] There are number of factors, such as intrathoracic pressure, venous tone, RV and LV compliance, that can directly affect the CVP and RV end-diastolic volume. In a systematic review of more than 24 studies, authors tried to determine the relationship between CVP and blood volume and the ability of CVP to predict fluid responsiveness. However, they found a very poor relationship between CVP and blood volume as well as the inability of CVP to predict the hemodynamic response to a fluid challenge.[21] Several studies show CVP as a static parameter is a poor predictors of fluid responsiveness.[21,22] Hence CVP should not be used as a sole indicator to make clinical decisions regarding fluid management.

Goal-directed fluid therapy (GDFT) on the basis of the dynamic parameters such as stroke volume variation (SVV) and pulse pressure variation (PPV) proved feasible and beneficial [23–25] (Fig. 17.1). Transesophageal echocardiography (TEE) can be used during the intraoperative period to provide continuous dynamic parameters to manage fluid therapy, and SVV can be measured centrally by TEE.[26] This method of SVV measurement is operator dependent and invasive. The less invasive transthoracic echocardiography can be used intraoperatively but it is not often convenient to use. While PPV is obtained directly from the peripheral arterial pressure waveform, SVV can be peripherally derived from this arterial pressure waveform. SVV as well as PPV have been found to be far better predictors than static indicators.[27,28] However, there are also several limitations with dynamic parameters. SVV is found to be inaccurate in patients who are on pressure support ventilation.[29] PVV is found to be unreliable as a predictor of fluid responsiveness in case of tidal volumes <8 ml/kg.[30] Irregular heart rhythm such as atrial fibrillation can also influence the SVV and PPV.

Although there is paucity of data, a meta-analysis comparing GDFT and restrictive fluid therapy in major non-cardiac surgeries concluded that the mortality was slightly lower in the GDFT group, and there were no differences between the two groups in the complication rate and length of hospital stay.[31] In high-risk patients undergoing brain surgery for intracranial tumor, abscess or aneurysms, intraoperative GDFT was associated with a reduction in ICU length of stay and costs and a decrease in postoperative

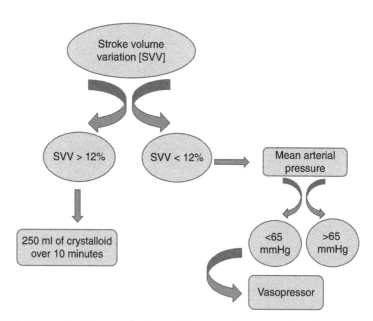

Figure 17.1 Goal-directed fluid therapy algorithm. A black and white version of this figure will appear in some formats. For the color version, please refer to the plate section.

morbidity.[32] In patients with aneurysmal SAH, it has been observed that TEE-guided GDFT maintained intraoperative MAP with significantly lower fluid volumes in comparison with fluid management guided by CVP monitoring, with no adverse impact on postoperative complications.[33] In patients with supratentorial brain tumors scheduled for mass excision, the PPV-guided GDFT group has been observed to have more intraoperative fluid, more urine output and low serum lactate level in comparison with the control group who received standard care. PPV-guided GDFT improved peripheral perfusion without increasing brain swelling in these patients.[34] In an another study in patients with supratentorial brain tumors, authors did not find any benefit of GDFT over standard fluid therapy in terms of incidence of postoperative complications, hospital and ICU stay and Glasgow outcome scores at-discharge. However, the use of GDFT led to the better perioperative fluid management and brain relaxation scores.[35] Prone position for spine surgery often leads to airway edema, and using static parameters for fluid assessment can worsen the upper airway edema since standard fluid therapy has been associated with volume overload. GDFT using a cardiac output monitor is becoming popular for fluid management during complex spine surgical procedures. GDFT significantly reduces airway edema in patients undergoing complex spine surgeries in prone position. As compared with standard therapy, GDFT also reduces postoperative incidence of sore throat, hoarseness of voice and duration of ICU stay.[36] It has been observed that GDFT based on SVV in patients undergoing major spine surgeries is also associated with reduced blood losses and transfusions, better postoperative respiratory performance as well as faster return of bowel function.[37] In middle-aged and elderly patients undergoing spine surgery, PPV-guided GDFT has been found to reduce the incidence of postoperative delirium (POD), possibly by stabilizing perioperative hemostat and improving the supply and demand of oxygen. Intraoperative MAP, cardiac index (CI) and regional cerebral oxygenation (rSO$_2$) values were higher in the GDT group than in the restricted fluid (RF) group ($P < 0.05$).[38] In patients undergoing complex spine surgeries in prone position, PPV-guided GDFT did not show any significant advantage over standard therapy with respect to intraoperative hypotension, blood transfusion or postoperative complications ($P > 0.5$).[39] Literature is limited for studies assessing hemodynamic monitoring to guide fluid therapy in TBI patients.

Conclusion

A strategic approach in fluid management is essential for all neurosurgical procedures and perioperative management of neurological patients. Optimum fluid administration is essential for maintenance of perfusion pressures through the brain and the spinal cord. It appears logical to use isotonic crystalloids and avoid colloids as far as possible. Data are limited in recommending the use of balanced solutions, although the results with their use are encouraging. Hyperglycemia or hypoglycemia has to be avoided under all circumstances. Hemodynamic monitoring to guide fluid therapy in neurosurgical patients has a positive impact on patient outcome. While dynamic parameters are more reliable in assessing fluid responsiveness, static parameters are considered less effective. Large randomized trials with sufficiently powered methodology are required to detect the effect of GDFT on clinical outcome in neurosurgical patients.

References

1. Shenkin HA, Bezier HS, Bouzarth WF. Restricted fluid intake. Rational management of the neurosurgical patient. *J Neurosurg.* 1976;**45**:432–6,

2. Perel P, Roberts I, Ker K. Colloids versus crystalloids for fluid resuscitation in critically ill patients. *Cochrane Database Syst Rev.* 2013;**2**:CD000567.

3. Tommasino C. Fluids in the neurosurgical patient. *Anesthesiology Clin N Am.* 2002;**20**:329–46.

4. Perel A, Pizov R, Cotev S. Respiratory variations in the arterial pressure during mechanical ventilation reflect volume status and fluid responsiveness. *Intensive Care Med.* 2014;**40**:798–807.

5. Zimmermann M, Feibicke T, Keyl C, et al. Accuracy of stroke volume variation compared with Pleth variability index to predict fluid responsiveness in mechanically ventilated patients undergoing major surgery. *Eur J Anaesthesiol.* 2010;**27**:555–61.

6. Prabhakar H, Singh GP, Anand V, et al. Mannitol versus hypertonic saline for brain relaxation in patients undergoing craniotomy. *Cochrane Database Syst Rev.* 2014;**7**:CD010026.

7. Xia J, He Z, Cao X, et al. The brain relaxation and cerebral metabolism in stroke-volume variation-directed fluid therapy during supratentorial tumor resection: crystalloid solution versus colloid solution. *J Neurosurg Anesthesiol.* 2014;**26**:320–7.

8. Ibrahim GM, Macdonald RL. The effects of fluid balance and colloid administration on outcomes in patients with aneurismal subarachnoid hemorrhage: a propensity score-matched analysis. *Neurocrit Care.* 2013;**19**:140–9.

9. Dankbaar JW, Slooter AJ, Rinkel GJ, et al. Effect of different components of triple-H therapy on cerebral perfusion in patients with aneurysmal subarachnoid haemorrhage: a systematic review. *Crit Care.* 2010;**14**:R23.

10. Roquilly A, Loutrel O, Cinotti R, et al. Balanced versus chloride-rich solutions for fluid resuscitation in brain-injured patients: a randomised double-blind pilot study. *Crit Care.* 2013;**17**:R77.

11. Lehmann L, Bendel S, Uehlinger DE, et al. Randomized, double-blind trial of the effect of fluid composition on electrolyte, acid-base, and fluid homeostasis in patients early after subarachnoid hemorrhage. *Neurocrit Care.* 2013;**18**:5–12.

12. Verbalis JG. Management of disorders of water metabolism in patients with pituitary tumors. *Pituitary.* 2002;**5**:119–32,

13. SAFE Study Investigators. Saline or albumin for fluid resuscitation in patients with traumatic brain injury. *N Engl J Med.* 2007;**357**:874–84.

14. Simma B, Burger R, Falk M, et al. A prospective, randomized, and controlled study of fluid management in children with severe head injury: lactated Ringer's solution versus hypertonic saline. *Crit Care Med.* 1998;**26**:1265–70.

15. Van Aken HK, Kampmeier TG, Ertmer C, et al. Fluid resuscitation in patients with traumatic brain injury: what is a SAFE approach? *Curr Opin Anaesthesiol.* 2012;**25**:563–5.

16. Tan PG, Cincotta M, Clavisi O, et al. Prehospital fluid management in traumatic brain injury. *Emerg Med Australas.* 2011;**23**:665–76.

17. Zheng F, Cammisa FP, Sandhu HS, et al. Factors predicting hospital stay, operative time, blood loss and transfusion in patients undergoing revision posterior lumbar spine decompression, fusion, and segmental instrumentation. *Spine.* 2002;**15**:818–24.

18. Siemionow K, Cywinski J, Kusza K, et al. Intraoperative fluid therapy and pulmonary complications. *Orthopedics.* 2012;**35**:e184–91.

19. Geerts BF, Maas JJ, de Wilde RBP, et al. Hemodynamic assessment in the Dutch intensive care unit. *Neth J Crit Care.* 2009;**13**:178–84.

20. Marik PE, Monnet X, Teboul JL. Hemodynamic parameters to guide fluid therapy. *Ann Intensive Care.* 2011;**1**:1.

21. Marik PE, Baram M, Vahid B. Does central venous pressure predict fluid responsiveness? A systematic review of the literature and the tale of seven mares. *Chest.* 2008;**134**:172.

22. Magder S. Fluid status and fluid responsiveness. *Curr Opin Crit Care.* 2010;**16**:289–96.

23. Lopes MR, Oliveira MA, Pereira VO, et al. Goal-directed fluid management based on pulse pressure variation monitoring during high-risk surgery: a pilot randomized controlled trial. *Crit Care.* 2007;**11**:R100.

24. Sakka SG, Becher L, Kozieras J, et al. Effects of changes in blood pressure and airway pressures on parameters of fluid responsiveness. *Eur J Anaesthesiol.* 2009;**26**:322–7.

25. Jhanji S, Vivian-Smith A, Lucena-Amaro S, et al. Haemodynamic optimisation improves tissue microvascular flow and oxygenation after major surgery: a randomised controlled trial. *Crit Care.* 2010;**14**:R151.

26. Sangkum L, Liu GL, Yu L, et al. Minimally invasive or noninvasive cardiac output measurement: an update. *J Anesth.* 2016;**30**:461.

27. Marx G, Cope T, McCrossan L, et al. Assessing fluid responsiveness by stroke volume variation in mechanically ventilated patients with severe sepsis. *Eur J Anaesthesiol.* 2004;**21**:132–8.

28. Michard F. Changes in arterial pressure during mechanical ventilation. *Anesthesiology.* 2005;**103**:419–28.

29. Perner A, Faber T. Stroke volume variation does not predict fluid responsiveness in patients with septic shock on pressure support ventilation. *Acta Anaesthesiol Scand.* 2006;**50**:1068–73.

30. De Backer D, Heenen S, Piagnerelli M, et al. Pulse pressure variations to predict fluid responsiveness: influence of tidal volume. *Intensive Care Med.* 2005;**31**:517–23.

31. Wrzosek A, Jakowicka-Wordliczek J, Zajaczkowska R, et al. Perioperative restrictive versus goal-directed fluid therapy for adults undergoing major non-cardiac surgery. *Cochrane Database Syst Rev.* 2019;**12**:CD012767.

32. Luo J, Xue J, Liu J, et al. Goal-directed fluid restriction during brain surgery: a prospective randomized controlled trial. *Ann Intensive Care.* 2017;**7**:16.

33. Bloria SD, Panda NB, Jangra K, et al. Goal-directed fluid therapy versus conventional fluid therapy during craniotomy and clipping of cerebral aneurysm: a prospective randomized controlled trial. *J Neurosurg Anesthesiol.* 2022;**34**:407–14.

34. Hasanin A, Zanata T, Osman S, et al. Pulse pressure variation-guided fluid therapy during supratentorial brain tumour excision: a randomized controlled trial. Open *Access Maced J Med Sci.* 2019;**7**:2474–9.

35. Mishra N, Rath GP, Bithal PK, et al. Effect of goal-directed intraoperative fluid therapy on duration of hospital stay and postoperative complications in patients undergoing excision of large supratentorial tumors. *Neurol India.* 2022;**70**:108–14.

36. Prasad C, Radhakrishna N, Pandia MP, et al. The effect of goal-directed fluid therapy versus standard fluid therapy on the cuff leak gradient in patients undergoing complex spine surgery in prone position. *J Neurosci Rural Pract.* 2021;**12**:745–50.

37. Bacchin MR, Ceria CM, Giannone S, et al. Goal-directed fluid therapy based on stroke volume variation in patients undergoing major spine surgery in the prone position: a cohort study. *Spine (Phila Pa 1976).* 2016;**41**:E1131–E1137.

38. Wang DD, Li Y, Hu XW, et al. Comparison of restrictive fluid therapy with goal-directed fluid therapy for postoperative delirium in patients undergoing spine surgery: a randomized controlled trial. *Perioper Med (Lond).* 2021;**10**:48.

39. Wongtangman K, Wilartratsami S, Hemtanon N, et al. Goal directed fluid therapy based on pulse pressure variation compared with standard fluid therapy in patients undergoing complex spine surgery: a randomized controlled trial. *Asian Spine J.* 2022;**16**:352–60.

Fluid and Hemodynamic Monitoring in Trauma

Marie Werner, Sean Coeckelenbergh and Anatole Harrois

Introduction

Hemorrhagic shock and traumatic brain injury (TBI) account for the two leading causes of death in trauma patients. Fluid resuscitation is a fundamental cornerstone to trauma management as it restores circulatory volume during hemorrhage and can prevent hypotension in TBI patients. A substantial amount of fluid is administered at the initial phase of trauma care to achieve these goals (Table 18.1). This commonly causes a positive fluid balance whose severity is associated with worse outcome. Consequently, patients should benefit from a targeted approach to fluid therapy that aims to administer only therapeutic amounts of fluids. Fluids are varied and display different properties related to their nature (i.e., colloid vs. crystalloid), their osmolarity, and their composition (balanced or non-balanced). As every patient has specific comorbidities and injuries, no fluid exists that can be universally administered to every trauma patient. For these reasons, clinicians must carefully determine what fluid best fits the patient's injuries and how to safely administer it.

Table 18.1 Fluid volume given in traumatic brain injury or post-traumatic hemorrhagic shock in representative studies

Reference	n	Population	Study period	Fluid volume, mL
Holcomb et al. 2015 [61]	680	Trauma and severe bleeding	24 hr of admission	6 500
Wiegers et al. 2021 [15]	2 125	Traumatic brain injury	Daily	2 910 (2 150–3 600)
Young et al. 2014 [29]	46	Trauma and severe bleeding	24 hr of admission	10 300 ± 6 500
Sperry et al. 2018 [62]	501	Trauma and SBP < 70 mmHg or SBP < 90 mmHg and HR >108 bpm	24 hr of admission	4 500 (3 000–6 800)

bpm, beats per minute; HR, heart rate; SBP, systolic blood pressure. Figures are given in mean±standard deviation or median (interquartile range).

Fluid Resuscitation Strategy in Trauma

Early Resuscitation

Severe trauma can decrease venous return through multiple mechanisms. Hemorrhage decreases cardiac preload through hypovolemia, while the early release of inflammatory mediators and damage associated molecular patterns cause vasodilation.[1,2] Several compensatory mechanisms initially maintain venous return, such as sympathetic activation and transcapillary refill, but ongoing hemorrhage results in a drop in arterial oxygen transport and blood pressure that ultimately leads to tissue hypoperfusion. At a given point, the oxygen debt may become irreversible in spite of resuscitation and transfusion and cause refractory multiorgan failure.[1] Fluid resuscitation aims to restore circulating volume to prevent cardiovascular collapse and tissue hypoperfusion during the initial critical and surgical stabilization. On the other hand, administration of fluid can worsen coagulopathy, through hemodilution, and bleeding, if blood pressure increases excessively. In a randomized-controlled trial (RCT) conducted in 598 patients with penetrating torso trauma, Bickel et al. reported that delayed fluid resuscitation started in the prehospital setting improved survival when compared with an immediate fluid resuscitation strategy.[3] In this study, immediate fluid resuscitation led to a significantly greater systolic blood pressure (SBP) than in the no fluid group (79 ± 46 mmHg vs. 72 ± 43 mmHg) by administrating a greater volume of fluid (870 ± 667 mL vs. 92 ± 309 mL). However, this resulted in more blood transfusions and a lower survival rate (62% vs. 70%, $p = 0.04$).[3] Of note, transportation time to the trauma center was 13 minutes, a short time explained by the urban enrollment of injured patients in the study. Opposite results were reported by Hampton et al. in a multicenter, prospective, observational study where prehospital fluid resuscitation was associated with improved survival as compared with no fluid resuscitation (<150 mL) in 1 200 severe trauma patients (64% blunt and 36% penetrating trauma).[4] In this study, prehospital fluid administration did not result in a higher blood pressure on arrival to the emergency department in comparison with patients receiving no fluid. Furthermore, 500 mL or more of fluid resuscitation in the prehospital setting is associated with an improvement in blood pressure and shock index in severe trauma patients, but the greater the fluid volume, the greater the risk of transfusion.[5] Systematic administration of a high volume of fluid (2 000 mL) was associated with worse survival when compared with a tailored strategy aiming to reverse shock signs by successive boluses of 250 mL of crystalloids.[6] Clearly, fluid therapy improves heart rate and blood pressure, and consequently shock index, but a reproducible pattern of morbidity caused by fluid excess also exists. This observation led clinicians to introduce specific strategies to improve trauma patient outcome during fluid resuscitation, such as hypotensive resuscitation.

Hypotensive resuscitation aims to target a subnormal blood pressure level that remains compatible with survivable organ perfusion through a more moderated administration of fluid. A hypotensive fluid strategy has now become part of the damage-control resuscitation with early blood products administration and has been shown to improve outcome following trauma laparotomy.[7] Thresholds of 70–90 mmHg of SBP or 50–65 mmHg of mean BP have been proposed as targets for hypotensive resuscitation.[8] It seems however that a low mean BP of 50 mmHg is hard to maintain and does not provide additional benefit in comparison with a hypotensive target of 60–65 mmHg.[9] The European guidelines now recommend an SBP of 80 to 90 mmHg or a mean BP of 60 mmHg in trauma patients suffering from hemorrhagic shock that do not have TBI.[10] If severe TBI occurs, a higher mean BP of 80 mmHg (SBP of 110 mmHg) is recommended. It is important to underline that a dogmatic approach that is based on the belief that only one treatment (i.e., a fixed fluid volume) can fit all trauma patients is flawed. Instead, fluid resuscitation should focus on an individualized approach that achieves hemodynamic targets which take into account the specific characteristics of each patient (e.g., time to trauma center, hemorrhage severity, associated TBI).

Post-Acute Resuscitation

Following the initial phase of trauma care, fluid resuscitation continues to be essential in hemodynamic optimization. Strict management of fluid resuscitation is necessary since a positive fluid balance is associated with the occurrence of abdominal compartment syndrome,[11] acute kidney injury (AKI),[12] and poor outcome.[13–15] Losses from ongoing hemorrhage, surgeries, and capillary leakage from exacerbated inflammation lead to an increase in fluid requirements, which rarely allow for a neutral fluid balance during initial management. Goal-directed fluid therapy using advanced hemodynamic monitoring may help to adjust fluid resuscitation and optimize stroke volume. Cardiac output monitoring was indeed associated with a decreased intensive care unit (ICU) length of stay in trauma-related acute respiratory distress syndrome (ARDS) or multiple trauma patients in two RCTs.[16,17] Implementing hemodynamic monitoring as soon as possible is valuable, but this is often only achievable after initial management, during surgery, or at ICU admission.

What Fluid in Trauma?

Colloids

Colloids are natural (e.g., albumin) or synthetic (e.g., gelatins, starches, dextrans) and display better volume expansion properties than crystalloids.[18] Theoretically, crystalloids require three times more volume than colloids for the same volume effect. This is a consequence of the increased oncotic pressure provided by colloids that prevents interstitial leakage and leads to a similar intravascular effect at a lesser volume. From a historical perspective, trauma protocols have often used colloids as the fluid of choice for restoring circulating volume during uncontrolled bleeding.

However, over the past decades, clinical data have decreased the popularity of colloids. The ratio of 3 to 1 has only exceptionally been reported, and studies that randomized crystalloids versus colloids as the fluid for resuscitation in surgical and critically ill patients showed a mean ratio closer to 1.50 [confidence interval (CI) 95% 1.36–1.65] and even a lower ratio of 1.33 (CI 95% 1.17–1.50) in the past decade.[19] In a recent multicenter study conducted in 775 high-risk patients undergoing major abdominal surgery, where fluid administration was guided by hemodynamic monitoring to optimize stroke volume, those assigned to receive colloids were given the same amount of fluid than those assigned to crystalloids [33.4 ± 3.4 mL/kg in the hydroxyethyl starch (HES) group versus 34.6 ± 5.8 mL/kg in the 0.9% NaCl group, $p = 0.15$]. Moreover, AKI was more common in the HES group than in the 0.9% NaCl group.[20] In trauma patients, discrepancies exist with regards to fluids according to the kind of trauma. For example, significantly less HES than 0.9% NaCl was used to achieve fluid resuscitation in penetrating trauma, while the amount required in blunt trauma was comparable.[21] Nevertheless, HES has detrimental effects on coagulation properties in major elective surgery with a decrease in clot strength measured by thromboelastographic devices as compared with crystalloids, which led to more surgical bleeding with HES.[22] This analysis translates clinically in trauma patients. James et al. reported in their RCT that there was a significantly greater amount of blood product administration when using HES, in comparison with crystalloids, for fluid resuscitation in blunt trauma.[21]

The effect of fluids on renal function has also been studied. When trauma and surgical patients were studied from previous randomized trials, HES did not increase the risk of AKI. [23,24] However, in the CHEST study that enrolled 7 000 ICU patients, the use of HES, when compared with 0.9% NaCl, was associated with a greater risk for renal replacement therapy. Due to its interaction with hemostasis, its possible nephrotoxic effect, and the lack of benefit when compared with crystalloids, the European Medicines Agency recommended to suspend HES solution from the market in 2022. Gelatins provide an alternative to HES but data regarding their use in fluid resuscitation in trauma patients are scarce. In cardiac surgery, gelatin administration increased biomarkers of renal tubular injury in comparison with crystalloids [25] and was associated with an increased risk for AKI.[26] Moreover, their use was shown to increase bleeding in this population.[27]

In conclusion, due to their interaction with coagulation and the associated increased risk for AKI, current evidence does not support the use of colloids for fluid resuscitation in trauma patients.

Crystalloids

Sodium 0.9% has been the standard trauma resuscitation fluid for years. However, due to its high chloride concentration, there is no strong ion difference (SID = 0 mmol/L, Table 18.2), and hyperchloremic acidosis is a risk if administered in excess. There are also concerns regarding the impact of 0.9% NaCl on renal function. When compared

Table 18.2 Composition of main balanced and non-balanced solutions in comparison with human plasma

Variables	Plasma	NaCl 0.9%	Lactated Ringer's	Plasma-Lyte	Isofundin
Na	140	154	130	140	145
Cl	100	154	109	98	127
K	5	0	5.4	5	4
Mg	1	0	0	1.5	1
Ca	2.2	0	2.7	0	2.5
Acetate/lactate	0	0	0/29	27/0	24/0
Gluconate/malate	0	0	0	23/0	0/5
SID	40	0	26	50	20
Osmolarity	280 −296	308	273	295	309

Figures are given in mmol/L. SID, strong ion difference.

with balanced fluids that attempt to have physiological concentrations of chloride and a SID close to 40 mmol/L (Table 18.2), 0.9% NaCl increases the risk for hyperchloremia. Hyperchloremia can reduce renal perfusion through vasoconstriction of glomerular afferent arterioles.[28] Balanced crystalloids prevent hyperchloremic acidosis in trauma patients.[29] In addition, while 0.9% NaCl makes urinary pH acidotic, balanced crystalloids preserve a neutral urinary pH. This decreases the risk for myoglobin precipitation in rhabdomyolysis, a frequent condition following trauma.[30] In a large single-center, open, randomized trial including 15 802 patients admitted to ICU of whom 3 328 were trauma patients, balanced crystalloids (i.e., Ringer's lactate or Plasma-Lyte) were compared with 0.9% NaCl. These balanced fluids reduced the occurrence of the composite outcome of death, renal replacement therapy, or persistent doubling of creatinine at day 30.[31] This result was not confirmed, however, in two recent RCTs that enrolled 11 052 (BASICS study) and 5 037 (PLUS study) critically ill patients to receive Plasma-Lyte or 0.9% NaCl.[31,32] No difference in mortality or AKI was found in both studies. In the BASICS study, 60% of patients were included once admitted to ICU following surgery. Patients had thus received a substantial volume of intraoperative fluid before randomization to Plasma-Lyte or 0.9% NaCl.[32] This may have attenuated any difference between fluids. A secondary analysis of the BaSICS study reported the positive effects on survival of balanced crystalloids when started at the initial phase of resuscitation in critically ill patients. [33] In the PLUS study, patients received a median fluid volume of 3 900 mL over their ICU stay, and only a median of 1 500 mL their first day of ICU admission. Trauma patients suffering from hemorrhagic shock usually require a much greater volume of fluid during initial care (see Table 18.1). This may explain the lack of difference, as a retrospective study indicated that the beneficial impact of balanced crystalloids over 0.9% NaCl increases with large fluid volumes, particularly those exceeding 7 000 mL. [34] A recent meta-analysis of RCTs concluded that the use of balanced crystalloids, when compared with 0.9% NaCl, is associated with a maximum mortality decrease of 9% in the ICU.[35] However, in the subgroup of trauma patients (3 863 trauma patients without TBI), no significant benefit was reported. Of note, trauma patients were included in those RCTs only upon ICU admission. They thus had potentially received fluids before hospital admission, in the emergency department, and in the ICU before randomization. This clearly implies that patients received various fluids before randomization, which could have hidden any potential difference between the crystalloids.

The current evidence indicates that balanced crystalloids are superior to 0.9% NaCl in the care of trauma patients, especially when administered in large volumes. There still remains a considerable gap in knowledge, however, in determining the ideal fluid for trauma, as contemporary literature consists of studies that include heterogeneous patients of various levels of severity who may have received considerable amounts of fluids before randomization. It is important to underline that in some cases, patients may benefit from one type of fluid over the others. Future studies should investigate an individualized approach to fluid therapy that not only aims to target ideal blood pressure and stroke volume for the given injuries, but also to administer the ideal electrolyte combination for a given imbalance. In the absence of studies that touch upon these specific questions in trauma care, international guidelines recommend the use of balanced crystalloid during the initial phase of trauma resuscitation.[10]

Hypertonic Solutes

Hypertonic solutions display interesting properties for fluid resuscitation when compared to isotonic fluids since they can achieve similar hemodynamic effects with less volume.[36] They cause less organ edema than isotonic fluids [36] and decrease cerebral edema in patients experiencing severe TBI. In clinical trials, however, the use of hypertonic saline (HTS) failed to prevent organ failure or improve survival. Of note, these trials commonly used hypertonic saline combined with dextran, a colloid, which can skew the interpretation of HTS effects given that colloids do interact with coagulation and promote AKI (cf. colloids section). The administration of 7.5% NaCl–dextran, when compared with Ringer's lactate, failed to decrease the rate of ARDS in hypotensive patients with blunt trauma.[37] In patients with clinical criteria of hemorrhagic shock [SBP < 70 mmHg or SBP 71–90 mmHg with a heart rate greater than 108 beats per minute (bpm)], 7.5% NaCl-dextran had no effect on mortality.[38] In a study derived from the same cohort, HTS (with or without dextran) worsened hypocoagulability and hyperfibrinolysis.[39] A meta-analysis including 2932 patients of 12 randomized studies showed no difference in mortality between HTS (or HTS with dextran) and isotonic solutions, and no difference in fluid volume was reported. [40] For these reasons, hypertonic saline is not recommended for initial fluid resuscitation in trauma patients.[10,41] High osmotic load, however, has interesting properties for treating patients suffering from severe TBI with pupil abnormalities and hemorrhagic shock.

Traumatic Brain Injury: A Specific Setting

Isotonic Crystalloids

Fluid resuscitation is largely used (see Table 18.1) to optimize hemodynamics and prevent hypotension, which is independently associated with increased mortality in TBI patients.[42] The osmotic profile of solutions used for fluid resuscitation for TBI patients is of utmost importance. The use of isotonic solution (280 to 310 mosmol/L), as opposed to hypotonic solution (<280 mosmol/L), is recommended to avoid causing cerebral edema. The prehospital use of Ringer's lactate (osmolarity = 273 mosmol/L) was indeed reported to be associated with a worse outcome in TBI patients as compared to 0.9% NaCl.[43] Few studies have compared the effects of isotonic balanced crystalloids with 0.9% NaCl in TBI, however. Roquilly et al. found no difference between isofundin (osmolarity 309 mosmol/L, see Table 18.2) and 0.9% NaCl on intracranial pressure (ICP) in 40 severe TBI patients.[44] More recently, 11052 ICU patients were randomized in Brazil to receive Plasma-Lyte (290 mosmol/L) or 0.9% NaCl during their ICU stay. In the subgroup of TBI patients (n = 486), those assigned to Plasma-Lyte had a significantly increased risk of death.[32] A similar result was reported in a meta-analysis that enrolled patients in three RCTs that compared 0.9% NaCl with balanced crystalloids [45] but one of them allowed the use of Ringer's lactate, a hypotonic solution, in the balanced crystalloid group.[46] These studies have led to the conclusion that 0.9% NaCl appears thus to be the safest option for fluid resuscitation in TBI patients.

Hypertonic Fluids

Continuous hyperosmolar infusion therapy has been proposed to prevent or treat intracranial hypertension in TBI patients. In an RCT that enrolled 370 patients to receive either a continuous prophylactic hyperosmolar therapy of 20% NaCl (with the goal of maintaining a blood sodium level of up to 155 mmol/L to prevent/treat intracranial hypertension) to 0.9% NaCl, there was no difference in the development of intracranial hypertension (33.7% vs. 36.4%), 6-month mortality or 6-month GOS-E (Glasgow Outcome Scale–Extended) score [odds ratio (OR) 1.02 CI 95%: 0.71–1.47].[47] A recent meta-analysis including six trials assessing continuous hyperosmolar infusion therapy in TBI patients ($n = 1\,521$) reported an improvement in neurological outcome at day 90, but most studies were observational.[48] Further studies are necessary to explore the beneficial effect of continuous hyperosmolar therapy in TBI patients.

When ICP rises above 22 mmHg, however, hyperosmolar therapy is clearly indicated for lowering ICP by decreasing intracellular volume through increased serum osmolality. Mannitol and hypertonic saline are both used for this purpose. Given in equimolar dose, they achieve the same effect on ICP for the same length of time in TBI patients experiencing intracranial hypertension.[49] However, both display potential harmful effects on kidney function. Mannitol may indeed cause osmotic nephrosis, [50] especially when given repeatedly, while hypertonic saline causes hyperchloremia, which is associated with decreased renal perfusion.[28] Observational studies reported mannitol use to be associated with worse outcome [51] in TBI patients. In a multicenter study derived from the EPO-TBI study, the use of mannitol was associated with an increased risk for AKI.[52] Of note, mannitol was administered in patients having more severe symptoms [pupil abnormalities, lower Glasgow Coma Scale (GCS) score] in both studies, and since more severe patients received mannitol, it may be a confounding factor in these studies. While waiting for prospective randomized studies to compare mannitol and hypertonic saline, mannitol should not be used repeatedly to treat intracranial hypertension.

Another potential fluid, hypertonic sodium lactate, was presented as an alternative to HTS with effective hyperosmolar effects and a decreased risk for hyperchloremia. When compared with an equimolar load of mannitol, hyperosmolar sodium lactate led to a more pronounced decrease in ICP in TBI patients.[53,54] Moreover, it offers a favorable cerebral metabolic profile.[55] This promising hypertonic fluid requires more investigations and may become a treatment of choice in patients suffering from TBI. Until then, its availability will continue to be limited in most countries.

Few data are available regarding the use of synthetic colloids in TBI patients. In an observational study of 2 213 trauma patients, 497 received HES, which was independently associated with AKI and death, especially in the subgroup of patients with severe TBI.[56] The SAFE study showed that 4% albumin administration, when compared with 0.9% NaCl, had no adverse effect on renal function and blood coagulation in ICU patients but was associated with a worse outcome in TBI patients.[57,58] This effect was possibly due to the hypotonic content of the 4% albumin administered in the study [Albumex® (CSL, Melbourne)], which only had a tonicity of 260 mosmol/L. This may have contributed to a more elevated ICP.[59] Consequently, the current evidence pleads against the use of colloids, including albumin, when caring for TBI patients.[60]

Conclusion

Fluid resuscitation strategies in severe trauma patients relies on goal-directed resuscitation to achieve a systolic BP of 80 to 90 mmHg during the initial phase of bleeding control. This systolic BP goal has to be raised to 110 mmHg (mean BP of 80 mmHg) in patients with TBI while waiting for an ICP monitor to be inserted. In addition to BP monitoring, cardiac output monitoring is an appropriate option to optimize volume status. Its use should be considered as soon as possible, including during initial trauma management. Regarding the nature of fluid in trauma, colloids have shown no benefit over crystalloids for fluid resuscitation and have been reported to interact with coagulation and renal function. Balanced crystalloids have less adverse effects on acid–base balance than 0.9% NaCl and may thus be favored for initial trauma management in the absence of TBI. Sodium 0.9% remains a safe option, however, for TBI patients. Future studies will determine which crystalloid is best for this specific population.

References

1. Rixen D, Siegel JH. Bench-to-bedside review: oxygen debt and its metabolic correlates as quantifiers of the severity of hemorrhagic and post-traumatic shock. *Crit Care*. 2005;**9**:441–53.

2. Timmermans K, Kox M, Vaneker M, et al. Plasma levels of danger-associated molecular patterns are associated with immune suppression in trauma patients. *Intensive Care Med*. 2016;**42**:551–61.

3. Bickell WH, Wall MJ, Pepe PE, et al. Immediate versus delayed fluid resuscitation for hypotensive patients with penetrating torso injuries. *N Engl J Med*. 1994;**331**:1105–9.

4. Hampton DA, Fabricant LJ, Differding J, et al. Prehospital intravenous fluid is associated with increased survival in trauma patients. *J Trauma Acute Care Surg*. 2013;**75**:S9–15.

5. Geeraedts LMG, Pothof LAH, Caldwell E, de Lange-de Klerk ESM, D'Amours SK. Prehospital fluid resuscitation in hypotensive trauma patients: do we need a tailored approach? *Injury*. 2015;**46**:4–9.

6. Schreiber MA, Meier EN, Tisherman SA, et al. A controlled resuscitation strategy is feasible and safe in hypotensive trauma patients: results of a prospective randomized pilot trial. *J Trauma Acute Care Surg*. 2015;**78**:687–97.

7. Joseph B, Azim A, Zangbar B, et al. Improving mortality in trauma laparotomy through the evolution of damage control resuscitation: analysis of 1,030 consecutive trauma laparotomies. *J Trauma Acute Care Surg*. 2017;**82**:328–33.

8. Owattanapanich N, Chittawatanarat K, Benyakorn T, Sirikun J. Risks and benefits of hypotensive resuscitation in patients with traumatic hemorrhagic shock: a meta-analysis. *Scand J Trauma Resusc Emerg Med*. 2018;**26**:107.

9. Carrick MM, Morrison CA, Tapia NM, et al. Intraoperative hypotensive resuscitation for patients undergoing laparotomy or thoracotomy for trauma: early termination of a randomized prospective clinical trial. *J Trauma Acute Care Surg*. 2016;**80**:886–96.

10. Spahn DR, Bouillon B, Cerny V, et al. The European guideline on management of major bleeding and coagulopathy following trauma: fifth edition. *Crit Care*. 2019;**23**:98.

11. Strang SG, Van Lieshout EM, Van Waes OJ, Verhofstad MH. Prevalence and mortality of abdominal compartment syndrome in severely injured patients: a systematic review. *J Trauma Acute Care Surg*. 2016;**81**:585–92.

12. Hatton GE, Du RE, Wei S, et al. Positive fluid balance and association with

post-traumatic acute kidney injury. *J Am Coll Surg.* 2020;**230**:190-199e1.

13. Kasotakis G, Sideris A, Yang Y, et al. Aggressive early crystalloid resuscitation adversely affects outcomes in adult blunt trauma patients: an analysis of the Glue Grant database. *J Trauma Acute Care Surg.* 2013;**74**:1215–22.

14. Mezidi M, Ould-Chikh M, Deras P, et al. Influence of late fluid management on the outcomes of severe trauma patients: a retrospective analysis of 294 severely-injured patients. *Injury.* 2017;**48**:1964–71.

15. Wiegers EJA, Lingsma HF, Huijben JA, et al. Fluid balance and outcome in critically ill patients with traumatic brain injury (CENTER-TBI and OzENTER-TBI): a prospective, multicentre, comparative effectiveness study. *Lancet Neurol.* 2021;**20**:627–38.

16. Yuanbo Z, Jin W, Fei S, et al. ICU management based on PiCCO parameters reduces duration of mechanical ventilation and ICU length of stay in patients with severe thoracic trauma and acute respiratory distress syndrome. *Ann Intensive Care.* 2016;**6**:113.

17. Chytra I, Pradl R, Bosman R, et al. Esophageal Doppler-guided fluid management decreases blood lactate levels in multiple-trauma patients: a randomized controlled trial. *Crit Care.* 2007;**11**:R24.

18. Bradley CR, Bragg DD, Cox EF, El-Sharkawy AM, Buchanan CE, Chowdhury AH, et al. A randomized, controlled, double-blind crossover study on the effects of isoeffective and isovolumetric intravenous crystalloid and gelatin on blood volume, and renal and cardiac hemodynamics. *Clinl Nutr.* 2020;**39**:2070–9.

19. Orbegozo Cortes D, Gamarano Barros T, Njimi H, Vincent JL. Crystalloids versus colloids: exploring differences in fluid requirements by systematic review and meta-regression. *Anesth Analg.* 2015;**120**:389–402.

20. Futier E, Garot M, Godet T, et al. Effect of hydroxyethyl starch vs saline for volume replacement therapy on death or postoperative complications among high-risk patients undergoing major abdominal surgery: the FLASH randomized clinical trial. *JAMA.* 2020;**323**:225.

21. James MF, Michell WL, Joubert IA, et al. Resuscitation with hydroxyethyl starch improves renal function and lactate clearance in penetrating trauma in a randomized controlled study: the FIRST trial (Fluids in Resuscitation of Severe Trauma). *Br J Anaesth.* 2011;**107**:693–702.

22. Rasmussen KC, Secher NH, Pedersen T. Effect of perioperative crystalloid or colloid fluid therapy on hemorrhage, coagulation competence, and outcome: a systematic review and stratified meta-analysis. *Medicine.* 2016;**95**:e4498.

23. Chappell D, van der Linden P, Ripollés-Melchor J, James MFM. Safety and efficacy of tetrastarches in surgery and trauma: a systematic review and meta-analysis of randomised controlled trials. *Br J Anaesth.* 2021;**127**:556–68.

24. Tseng C-H, Chen T-T, Wu M-Y, et al. Resuscitation fluid types in sepsis, surgical, and trauma patients: a systematic review and sequential network meta-analyses. *Crit Care.* 2020;**24**:698

25. Smart L, Boyd C, Litton E, et al. A randomised controlled trial of succinylated gelatin (4%) fluid on urinary acute kidney injury biomarkers in cardiac surgical patients. *Intensive Care Med Exp.* 2021;**9**:48.

26. Heringlake M, Berggreen AE, Reemts E, et al. Fluid therapy with gelatin may have deleterious effects on kidney function: an observational trial. *J Cardiothorac Vasc Anesth.* 2020;**34**:2674–81.

27. Koponen T, Musialowicz T, Lahtinen P. Gelatin and the risk of bleeding after cardiac surgery. *Acta Anaesthesiol Scand.* 2020;**64**:1438–45.

28. Chowdhury AH, Cox EF, Francis ST, Lobo DN. A randomized, controlled, double-blind crossover study on the effects of 2-L infusions of 0.9% saline and Plasma-Lyte(R) 148 on renal blood flow

velocity and renal cortical tissue perfusion in healthy volunteers. *Ann Surg.* 2012;**256**:18–24.

29. Young JB, Utter GH, Schermer CR, et al. Saline versus Plasma-Lyte A in initial resuscitation of trauma patients: a randomized trial. *Ann Surg.* 2014;**259**:255–62.

30. Cho YS, Lim H, Kim SH. Comparison of lactated Ringer's solution and 0.9% saline in the treatment of rhabdomyolysis induced by doxylamine intoxication. *Emerg Med J.* 2007;**24**:276–80.

31. Finfer S, Micallef S, Hammond N, et al. Balanced multielectrolyte solution versus saline in critically ill adults. *N Engl J Med.* 2022;**386**:815–26.

32. Zampieri FG, Machado FR, Biondi RS, et al. Effect of intravenous fluid treatment with a balanced solution vs 0.9% saline solution on mortality in critically ill patients: the BaSICS randomized clinical trial. *JAMA.* 2021;**326**:818.

33. Zampieri FG, Machado FR, Biondi RS, et al. Association between type of fluid received prior to enrollment, type of admission, and effect of balanced crystalloid in critically ill adults: a secondary exploratory analysis of the BaSICS clinical trial. *Am J Respir Crit Care Med.* 2022;**205**:1419–28.

34. Zampieri FG, Ranzani OT, Azevedo LC, et al. Lactated Ringer is associated with reduced mortality and less acute kidney injury in critically ill patients: a retrospective cohort analysis. *Crit Care Med.* 2016;**44**:2163–70.

35. Hammond NE, Zampieri FG, Di Tanna GL, et al. Balanced crystalloids versus saline in critically ill adults – a systematic review with meta-analysis. *NEJM Evid.* 2022 1.

36. Prunet B, Cordier P-Y, Prat N, et al. Short-term effects of low-volume resuscitation with hypertonic saline and hydroxyethylstarch in an experimental model of lung contusion and haemorrhagic shock. *Anaesth Crit Care Pain Med.* 2018;**37**:135–40.

37. Bulger EM, Jurkovich GJ, Nathens AB, et al. Hypertonic resuscitation of hypovolemic shock after blunt trauma: a randomized controlled trial. *Arch Surg.* 2008;**143**:139–48; discussion 149.

38. Bulger EM, May S, Kerby JD, et al. Out-of-hospital hypertonic resuscitation after traumatic hypovolemic shock: a randomized, placebo controlled trial. *Ann Surg.* 2011;**253**:431–41.

39. Delano MJ, Rizoli SB, Rhind SG, et al. Prehospital resuscitation of traumatic hemorrhagic shock with hypertonic solutions worsens hypocoagulation and hyperfibrinolysis. *Shock.* 2015;**44**:25–31.

40. Wu H, Larsen CP, Hernandez-Arroyo CF, et al. AKI and collapsing glomerulopathy associated with COVID-19 and *APOL 1* high-risk genotype. *J Am Soc Nephrol.* 2020;**31**:1688–95.

41. Joannes-Boyau O, Le Conte P, Bonnet M-P, et al. Guidelines for the choice of intravenous fluids for vascular filling in critically ill patients, 2021. *Anaesth Crit Care Pain Med.* 2022;**41**:101058.

42. Spaite DW, Hu C, Bobrow BJ, et al. Mortality and prehospital blood pressure in patients with major traumatic brain injury: implications for the hypotension threshold. *JAMA Surg.* 2017;**152**:360.

43. Rowell SE, Fair KA, Barbosa RR, et al. The impact of pre-hospital administration of lactated Ringer's solution versus normal saline in patients with traumatic brain injury. *J Neurotrauma.* 2016;**33**:1054–9.

44. Roquilly A, Loutrel O, Cinotti R, et al. Balanced versus chloride-rich solutions for fluid resuscitation in brain-injured patients: a randomised double-blind pilot study. *Crit Care.* 2013;**17**:R77.

45. Dong W-H, Yan W-Q, Song X, Zhou W-Q, Chen Z. Fluid resuscitation with balanced crystalloids versus normal saline in critically ill patients: a systematic review and meta-analysis. *Scand J Trauma Resusc Emerg Med.* 2022;**30**:28.

46. Semler MW, Self WH, Wanderer JP, et al. Balanced crystalloids versus saline in critically ill adults. *N Engl J Med.* 2018;**378**:829–39.

47. Roquilly A, Moyer JD, Huet O, et al. Effect of continuous infusion of hypertonic saline vs standard care on 6-month neurological outcomes in patients with traumatic brain injury: the COBI randomized clinical trial. *JAMA.* 2021;**325**:2056.

48. Hourmant Y, Huard D, Demeure Dit Latte D, et al. Effect of continuous infusion of hypertonic saline solution on survival of patients with brain injury: a systematic review and meta-analysis. *Anaesth Crit Care Pain Med.* 2023;**42**:101177.

49. Francony G, Fauvage B, Falcon D, et al. Equimolar doses of mannitol and hypertonic saline in the treatment of increased intracranial pressure. *Crit Care Med.* 2008;**36**:795–800.

50. Nomani AZ, Nabi Z, Rashid H, et al. Osmotic nephrosis with mannitol: review article. *Ren Fail.* 2014;**36**:1169–76.

51. Anstey J, Taccone F, Udy A, et al. Early osmotherapy in severe traumatic brain injury: an international multicentre study. *J Neurotrauma.* 2020;**37**:178–84.

52. Skrifvars MB, Bailey M, Moore E, et al. A post hoc analysis of osmotherapy use in the erythropoietin in traumatic brain injury study – associations with acute kidney injury and mortality. *Crit Care Med.* 2021;**49**:e394–403.

53. Ichai C, Armando G, Orban J-C, et al. Sodium lactate versus mannitol in the treatment of intracranial hypertensive episodes in severe traumatic brain-injured patients. *Intensive Care Med.* 2009;**35**:471–9.

54. Ichai C, Payen J-F, Orban J-C, et al. Half-molar sodium lactate infusion to prevent intracranial hypertensive episodes in severe traumatic brain injured patients: a randomized controlled trial. *Intensive Care Med.* 2013;**39**:1413–22.

55. Quintard H, Patet C, Zerlauth J-B, et al. Improvement of neuroenergetics by hypertonic lactate therapy in patients with traumatic brain injury is dependent on baseline cerebral lactate/pyruvate ratio. *J Neurotrauma.* 2016;**33**:681–7.

56. Lissauer ME, Chi A, Kramer ME, Scalea TM, Johnson SB. Association of 6% hetastarch resuscitation with adverse outcomes in critically ill trauma patients. *Am J Surg.* 2011;**202**:53–8.

57. Finfer S, Bellomo R, Boyce N, et al. A comparison of albumin and saline for fluid resuscitation in the intensive care unit. *N Engl J Med.* 2004;**350**:2247–56.

58. SAFE Study Investigators; Australian and New Zealand Intensive Care Society Clinical Trials Group; Australian Red Cross Blood Service; et al. Saline or albumin for fluid resuscitation in patients with traumatic brain injury. *N Engl J Med.* 2007;**357**:874–84.

59. Cooper DJ, Myburgh J, Heritier S, et al. Albumin resuscitation for traumatic brain injury: is intracranial hypertension the cause of increased mortality? *J Neurotrauma.* 2013;**30**:512–18.

60. Oddo M, Poole D, Helbok R, et al. Fluid therapy in neurointensive care patients: ESICM consensus and clinical practice recommendations. *Intensive Care Med.* 2018;**44**:449–63.

61. Holcomb JB, Tilley BC, Baraniuk S, et al. Transfusion of plasma, platelets, and red blood cells in a 1:1:1 vs a 1:1:2 ratio and mortality in patients with severe trauma: the PROPPR randomized clinical trial. *JAMA.* 2015;**313**:471–82.

62. Sperry JL, Guyette FX, Brown JB, et al. Prehospital plasma during air medical transport in trauma patients at risk for hemorrhagic shock. *N Engl J Med.* 2018;**379**:315–26.

Chapter 19

Fluid and Hemodynamic Monitoring in Pediatrics

Robert Sümpelmann and Nils W. Dennhardt

Introduction

An adequate fluid therapy is essential for the perioperative stabilization of the homeostasis of children, whereas dosing errors or an inappropriate use of unphysiologically composed solutions may lead to life-threatening complications. As a consequence, it is important first to understand and respect the physiology of children, second to use suitable composed infusion solutions, and third to monitor the patient carefully for close guidance of the fluid therapy. In the following, well-established strategies, based on physiology, scientific studies, and clinical experience in large pediatric centers, are presented with safety and efficacy as first priorities.[1,2]

Physiology

The total body water (TBW), consisting of intracellular fluid (ICF) and extracellular fluid (ECF), represents up to 90% of the body weight in neonates, and reaches adult levels of about 60% after 1 year of age. The ECF represents the main part of TBW and decreases in parallel from 40% in term neonates to adult levels of 20–25% after 1 year of age.[3] The composition of ECF or plasma is similar in neonates, children, and adults, but dehydration occurs more rapidly in the younger age groups because of the higher fluid need.

At birth, the kidneys are still undeveloped and the reabsorptive areas of the tubular cells are small. As a consequence, neonates cannot concentrate urine effectively or excrete large salt loads. After a month, the kidneys reach about 60% of maturation, but the reabsorptive areas of the tubular cells are still small and the capacity, that is, for glucose reabsorption or potassium excretion, is lower than in adults. In the first two years the maturity and function of the kidneys increase greatly and reach adult levels.[4]

The newborn heart has a lower density of contractile elements and therefore it has less reserve and does not respond to stress as well as the adult heart. A higher percentage of noncontractile elements result in decreased ventricular compliance and less responsiveness to changes in vascular tone and preload. The cardiac output is tightly coupled with oxygen consumption, which is several times higher in neonates and infants than in adults. The stroke volume of the small hearts is limited, and therefore the high cardiac output depends strongly on a high heart rate. Normally, the heart pumps all of the venous return (VR) it receives, and under most conditions the VR is the main determinant of the cardiac output in all age groups. VR depends strongly on the intravascular volume. Underestimation of hypovolemia and bleeding are the most common causes of perioperative cardiac arrest in children.[5] Therefore, maintaining normovolemia is of paramount importance in the young age groups to maintain circulatory function and to stabilize the high tissue perfusion needed.[6]

Perioperative Fasting

The main aim of preoperative fasting is to minimize the volume of gastric contents to lessen the risk of pulmonary aspiration during induction of anesthesia. Many hospitalized children are suffering from prolonged fasting periods, leading to dehydration, hypotension, keto-acidosis, and uncooperative behavior.[7] When the fasting times are optimized, infants have a more stable acid–base balance with lower ketone body concentrations and less hypotension after induction of anesthesia.[8] An oral fluid uptake is generally preferable to an intravenous fluid therapy whenever possible. A previous clinical study showed no increased incidence in pulmonary aspiration in children with clear fluid fasting times shortened from 2 hours to 1 hour.[9] In accordance, the updated European guideline recommends shortened fasting times of 4 hours for formula milk, 3 hours for breast milk, and 1 hour for clear fluids in children.[10] With child-friendly shortened preoperative fasting periods, perioperative fluid therapy is often not really necessary for very short surgical procedures (duration < 1 hour). Postoperatively, a liberal fluid and food intake as wanted by the children should be favored, which leads to a better mental state without increasing the frequency of nausea and vomiting.[11]

Maintenance Infusion

Maintenance fluid therapy in children should meet the normal needs of water, electrolytes, and glucose. For half a century, this has been based on Holliday and Segar's recommendations, suggesting first the use of hypotonic fluids with 5% glucose added and second the 4–2–1 rule for infusion rate.[12] In recent years, many studies and case reports have shown that the routine use of such fluids may lead to serious hyponatremia and hyperglycemia, and may occasionally result in permanent neurological damage or death.[13] The two main factors for the development of perioperative hyponataemia are first a stress-induced secretion of antidiuretic hormone leading to an impaired ability to excrete free water and second the administration of hypotonic solutions as a source of free water.[14] Hyponatremia leads to an influx of water into the brain, primarily through glial cell swelling, initially largely preserving neuronal cell volume. This process will ultimately lead to cerebral oedema, brain stem herniation, and death. Prepubescent children are a high-risk group for a poor outcome associated with hyponatremic encephalopathy because of the presence of a high brain size to cranial vault ratio and reduced Na^+-K^+-ATPase activity compared with the adult brain.[15]

Infants are also at increased risk of perioperative lipolysis and hypoglycemia owing to a higher metabolic rate compared with adults. If hypoglycemia does occur, this will induce a stress response as well as alter cerebral blood flow and metabolism.[16] Permanent neurodevelopmental impairment can result if hypoglycemia goes unrecognized and untreated. However, intraoperative administration of 5% glucose solutions for prevention of hypoglycemia will often result in hyperglycemia due to stress-induced insulin resistance. [17] Hyperglycemia may also be detrimental to the brain due to an accumulation of lactate, a decrease in intracellular pH, and subsequently compromised cellular function in the context of global or focal cerebral ischemia.[18] Lastly, the administration of glucose free solutions increases the risk of lipolysis with the release of ketone bodies and free fatty acids.[19]

Against the above-mentioned background, the intraoperative maintenance infusion of isotonic balanced fluids with lower glucose concentrations (i.e., 1% to 2.5%) represents a well-accepted compromise to avoid hyponatremia, hypoglycemia, lipolysis, and hyperglycemia in children in many European countries (Table 19.1).[2,20,21] A higher infusion rate than calculated by the 4–2–1 rule can be used intraoperatively to compensate possible pre- and postoperative deficits in routine surgeries (i.e., 10 ml/kg/hr).[22] Infusion pumps are recommendable to prevent accidental fluid overload, especially in neonates and small infants. In prolonged surgeries, the maintenance infusion should be adapted, that is, after 1 hour in accordance to the patient's needs.

In nonsurgical or postoperative children, the current trend is also to use isotonic balanced electrolyte solutions instead of hypotonic solutions, both with 5% glucose, for maintenance infusion, as recent clinical studies and reviews have shown a lower incidence of hyponatremia and no change in hypernatremia.[23,24]

Fluid Replacement Therapy

Fluid replacement using crystalloid solutions aims to compensate an extracellular fluid deficit as a result of cutaneous, enteral, or renal fluid loss. Intraoperative bleeding is leading to a shift of interstitial fluid into the intravascular space (autotransfusion), and the resulting extracellular fluid deficit should be corrected by the infusion of crystalloid solutions as a first step. Theoretically, the intravascular volume effect of crystalloids depends on the ratio between the intravascular and the extracellular fluid volume (ECFV). The ECFV of neonates and infants is larger than in adults,[3] and the intravascular volume effect of crystalloids is therefore in theory lower in the younger age groups.

The composition of ECF is independent of age, and therefore similar crystalloid solutions can be used for fluid replacement in both pediatric and adult anesthesia. Ideally, the composition of crystalloid solutions should mimic the composition of extracellular fluid as close as possible, and each deviation could have unwanted effects on the homeostasis of the patients. Generally, infusion solutions for fluid replacement should be isotonic with a theoretical osmolarity (without glucose) comparable to saline 0.9% (308 mosmol·L^{-1}) or a real osmolality comparable to plasma (288 mosmol·kg H$_2$O^{-1}). The disparity is due to some of the infused electrolytes not being osmotically effective.[25] Saline 0.9% contains no bicarbonate precursor and unphysiological high chloride concentrations. It therefore may cause unwanted bicarbonate dilution and hyperchloremic acidosis with renal vasoconstriction and impaired renal function. Ringer's lactate contains lactate as bicarbonate precursor but is hypotonic (theoretical osmolarity 276 instead of 308 mosmol/l) and therefore may increase the intracranial pressure and may worsen cerebral edema when infused in high volumes. This can all be avoided by the use of balanced electrolyte solutions (BEL) containing a more physiological osmolarity and electrolyte composition and metabolic anions (i.e., acetate, lactate, or malate) as bicarbonate precursors for acid–base stabilization (Table 19.1).[25–27]

Most cases with minor or moderate surgical procedures can be managed with maintenance infusion plus extra volumes of 10–20 ml/kg BEL as needed to replace ECF or blood loss. In major cases with significant blood loss and restrictive transfusion, the infusion of very high volumes of crystalloids may lead to unwanted intravascular hypovolemia and interstitial fluid overload, which may worsen recovery and outcome.[28]

Volume Replacement Therapy

Volume replacement using colloid solutions aims to replace blood loss, and to maintain or restore hemodynamics and tissue perfusion, especially when the use of crystalloids alone is not effective and blood products are not indicated.[2] In the past, human albumin (HA) was

Table 19.1 Composition of extracellular fluid (ECF) and various intravenous fluids for children (in mmol/l)

Fluid	Cations				Anions					Theoretical osmolarity[5]	Real osmolality[6]
	Na$^+$	K$^+$	Ca^{2+}	Mg^{2+}	Cl$^-$	HCO$_3^-$	Acetate	Lactate	Glucose		
ECF	142	4.5	2.5	1.25	103	24	-	1.5	2.78–5	291	288
BEL[1] + 1% glucose	140	4	2	2	118	-	30	-	55.5	296	275
BEL[1]	145	4	2.5	1	127	-	24 (Malat 5)	-	-	309	287
Saline 0.9%	154	-	-	-	154	-	-	-	-	308	286
RL[2]	130	5	1	1	112	-	-	27	-	276	256
bal- GEL[3]	151	4	1	1	103	-	24	-	-	284	264
bal- HES[4]	140	4	2.5	1	118	-	24 (Malat 5)	-	-	296	275

[1]balanced electrolyte solution, [2]Ringer's lactate, [3]balanced gelatin, [4]balanced hydroxyethyl starch,
[5]Σ (cations+anions) in mosmol/l, [6]osmolality · osmotic coefficient 0.926/water content 0.997 in mosmol/kg H$_2$O.

used frequently in children but currently artificial colloids are a well-established alternative because of a comparable risk–benefit ratio and lower costs.[29]

In clinical studies, hydroxyethyl starch (HES, molecular weight 130 kDa) was shown to be safe and effective in children undergoing major pediatric surgery,[30,31] and a meta-analysis found no impairment of renal function, blood loss and transfusion volume in children with perioperative HES infusion.[32] Nevertheless, in 2018, the European Medicines Agency considered removing HES from the market because it possibly results in a renal function impairment in adult intensive care patients.[33] As a consequence, HES has been used more restrictively, including in pediatric anesthesia, which has resulted in increased interest in gelatin (GEL) as a possible alternative.

Studies from neonatology found a high level of safety of GEL even when used in preterms,[34] and a recent observational study showed a very low incidence of adverse effects in children with GEL infusion undergoing major pediatric surgery.[35] Possible adverse drug reactions of both GEL and HES include anaphylactoid reactions, coagulation disorders, and renal function impairment. In adults, anaphylactoid reactions occurred more frequently after GEL than after HES, but generally the risk of severe anaphylactoid reactions is lower in the younger age groups. Animal experiments and clinical studies in pediatric patients showed stable coagulation parameters after moderate doses (10–20 ml/kg) of GEL or HES but significant impairment of clot formation after profound hemodilution of more than 50% of the estimated blood volume.[36,37] GEL- or HES-induced renal insufficiency could not be detected perioperatively in animals or children with normal renal function. [30,35,38] The acid–base balance was more stable when using GEL or HES in a balanced electrolyte solution instead of saline.[30,35]

Monitoring

Conscious children, especially neonates and small infants, manage to maintain blood pressure for long periods of time through vasoconstriction in the presence of larger fluid deficits even if a shock situation has already occurred. In deeply anesthetized children, however, some or all of the regulation mechanisms are suppressed so that hypotension is more likely to occur in the presence of reduced blood volume. Shallow anesthesia, on the other hand, may mask hypovolemia. As a consequence, a low normal blood pressure and a normal oxygen saturation are no guarantees for a sufficient tissue perfusion. The leg-raise test for evaluation of fluid responsiveness is not effective in small children because of their limited body height. Therefore, apart from the standard parameters of heart rate and arterial blood pressure, other parameters need to be used to estimate a child's volume status and tissue perfusion.[39] A short manual pressure on the liver can be used to shift blood volume from intraabdominal to intrathoracic and to analyze the consequences of the change in venous return on blood flow or expiratory carbon dioxide tension (Fig. 19.1). Alternatively, recurrent small fluid boluses in a short time interval while tracking hemodynamic changes may help to confirm fluid responsiveness.[40] Other possible parameters to evaluate fluid responsiveness are respiratory-synchronous changes in the invasive blood pressure curve or perfusion or Pleth Variability Index calculated by recent pulse oximeter algorithms. Stable base excess values and lactate concentrations are reflecting stable tissue perfusion perioperatively. Major surgical procedures should there-fore be accompanied by regular blood gas analyses at induction of anesthesia and in hourly intervals thereafter for early detection of negative trends. When a central venous

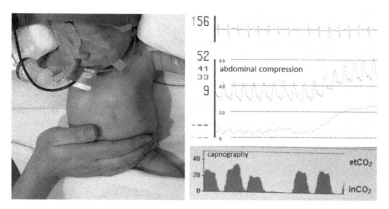

Figure 19.1 Abdominal pressure maneuver as test for fluid responsiveness in small children. A black and white version of this figure will appear in some formats. For the color version, please refer to the plate section.

catheter is inserted, measurement of central venous oxygen saturation is very valuable to evaluate the ratio between oxygen consumption and oxygen delivery.[39] Other useful parameters for estimating volume status and tissue perfusion include recapillarization time and measurement of regional oxygen saturation by near infrared spectroscopy or cardiac output by echocardiography or transpulmonary thermodilution.[40,41] In patients with hemodynamic instability, echocardiography is valuable to evaluate the contractility and filling of the heart and to target specific interventions.[40] Generally, individual parameters on which the infusion therapy is based should not be assessed in isolation, but rather as trend monitoring under consideration of the overall clinical constellation and the other monitoring parameters.[2]

Clinical Recommendations

The main aims of perioperative fluid therapy are to maintain a normal blood volume, a normal tissue perfusion, and a normal water–acid–base–metabolite–electrolyte balance. In line with current recommendations, children should be allowed to drink clear fluids until 1 hour before induction of anesthesia unless other considerations mandate otherwise. For preterm infants, neonates, and toddlers, it is always advisable to compensate at least the deficit from preoperative fasting and the intraoperative maintenance requirements using BEL with 1–2% glucose for example. If such solutions are not available commercially, they can be prepared extemporaneously in the hospital pharmacy or by users themselves (e.g., by adding 6–12 ml of glucose 40% to 250 ml of IV fluid).[22,42] To compensate preoperative deficits (e.g., from fasting), the overall infusion rate in the first hour may be 10 ml/kg/hr. As blood glucose concentrations increase, glucose-containing IV fluids should be reduced or stopped, infusing correspondingly more glucose-free BEL. Older toddlers and school-age children may also be given glucose-free BEL within the recommended fasting periods. In case of hemodynamic instability or bleeding, repetitive doses of BEL (single-bolus dose 10–20 ml/kg) first and GEL or HES (single-bolus dose 5–10 ml/kg) thereafter may additionally be administered as required. Postoperatively, children should be allowed to take oral fluids again as wanted unless other considerations mandate otherwise (Table 19.2).

Table 19.2 Suggested perioperative intravenous fluid therapy for neonates, infants, and toddlers

Before surgery	Minimize fasting periods (formula milk up to 4 hr, breast milk up to 3 hr, clear fluids up to 1 hr preop)
Minor procedures	Intraop maintenance infusion of 10 ml/kg/hr of a balanced electrolyte solution with 1–2% glucose (add 6–12 ml of glucose 40% to 250 ml of balanced electrolyte solution); older toddlers and school-age children may also be given glucose-free balanced electrolyte solutions
Larger procedures	Adapt maintenance infusion to patient's need after 1 hr, use additional balanced electrolyte solution for fluid replacement; consider artificial colloids in case of persistent hypovolemia – the objective is to achieve normal blood volume, normal tissue perfusion, normoglycemia, and normal water–acid–base–electrolyte balance
Major procedures	Same as larger procedures; administer blood products in case of critical hemodilution
After surgery	Permit oral fluid soon after surgery as wanted by the children

References

1. Sümpelmann R, Becke K, Zander R, Witt L. Perioperative fluid management in children: can we sum it all up now? *Curr Opin Anaesthesiol.* 2019;**32**:384–91.

2. Sümpelmann R, Becke K, Brenner S, et al. Perioperative intravenous fluid therapy in children: guidelines from the Association of the Scientific Medical Societies in Germany. *Paediatr Anaesth,* 2017;**27**:10–18.

3. Friis-Hansen B. Body water compartments in children: changes during growth and related changes in body composition. *Pediatrics.* 1961;**28**:169–81.

4. Bissonnette B. *Pediatric Anesthesia.* Shelton: People's Medical Publishing House; 2011.

5. Bhananker SM, Ramamoorthy C, Geiduschek JM, et al. Anesthesia-related cardiac arrest in children: update from the Pediatric Perioperative Cardiac Arrest Registry. *Anesth Analg.* 2007;**105**:344–50.

6. Nichols D, Ungerleider R, Spevak PEA. *Critical Heart Disease in Infants and Children.* Philadelphia: Mosby Elsevier; 2006.

7. Frykholm P, Schindler E, Sümpelmann R, Walker R, Weiss M. Preoperative fasting in children: review of existing guidelines and recent developments. *Br J Anaesth.* 2018;**120**:469–74.

8. Dennhardt N, Beck C, Huber D, et al. Optimized preoperative fasting times decrease ketone body concentration and stabilize mean arterial blood pressure during induction of anesthesia in children younger than 36 months: a prospective observational cohort study. *Paediatr Anaesth,* 2016;**26**:838–43.

9. Beck CE, Rudolph D, Mahn C, et al. Impact of clear fluid fasting on pulmonary aspiration in children undergoing general anesthesia: results of the German prospective multicenter observational (NiKs) study. *Paediatr Anaesth.* 2020;**30**:892–9.

10. Frykholm P, Disma N, Andersson H, et al. Preoperative fasting in children: guideline from the European Society of Anaesthesiology and Intensive Care. *Eur J Anaesthesiol.* 2022;**39**:4–25.

11. Radke OC, Biedler A, Kolodzie K, et al. The effect of postoperative fasting on vomiting

in children and their assessment of pain. *Paediatr Anaesth*. 2009;**19**:494–9.

12. Holliday MA, Segar WE. The maintenance need for water in parenteral fluid therapy. *Pediatrics*. 1957;**19**:823–32.

13. Moritz ML, Ayus JC. Hospital-acquired hyponatremia: why are there still deaths? *Pediatrics*. 2004;**113**:1395–6.

14. Arieff AI. Postoperative hyponatraemic encephalopathy following elective surgery in children. *Paediatr Anaesth*. 1998;**8**:1–4.

15. Ayus JC, Achinger SG, Arieff A. Brain cell volume regulation in hyponatremia: role of sex, age, vasopressin, and hypoxia. *Am J Physiol Renal Physiol*. 2008;**295**:F619–24.

16. Sieber FE, Traystman RJ. Special issues: glucose and the brain. *Crit Care Med*. 1992;**20**:104–14.

17. Welborn LG, McGill WA, Hannallah RS, et al. Perioperative blood glucose concentrations in pediatric outpatients. *Anesthesiology*. 1986;**65**:543–7.

18. Bailey AG, McNaull PP, Jooste E, Tuchman JB. Perioperative crystalloid and colloid fluid management in children: where are we and how did we get here? *Anesth Analg*. 2010;**110**:375–90.

19. Nishina K, Mikawa K, Maekawa N, Asano M, Obara H. Effects of exogenous intravenous glucose on plasma glucose and lipid homeostasis in anesthetized infants. *Anesthesiology*. 1995;**83**:258–63.

20. Berleur MP, Dahan A, Murat I, Hazebroucq G. Perioperative infusions in paediatric patients: rationale for using Ringer-lactate solution with low dextrose concentration. *J Clin Pharm Ther*. 2003;**28**:31–40.

21. Sümpelmann R, Becke K, Crean P, et al. European Consensus Statement for Intraoperative Fluid Therapy in Children. *Eur J Anaesthesiol*. 2011;**28**:637–9.

22. Sümpelmann R, Mader T, Eich C, Witt L, Osthaus WA. A novel isotonic-balanced electrolyte solution with 1% glucose for intraoperative fluid therapy in children: results of a prospective multicentre observational Post-Authorization Safety

Study (PASS). *Paediatr Anaesth*. 2010;**20**:977–81.

23. McNab S, Duke T, South M, et al. 140 mmol/L of sodium versus 77 mmol/L of sodium in maintenance intravenous fluid therapy for children in hospital (PIMS): a randomised controlled double-blind trial. *Lancet*. 2014;**385**:1190–7.

24. McNab S, Ware RS, Neville KA, et al. Isotonic versus hypotonic solutions for maintenance intravenous fluid administration in children. *Cochrane Database Syst Rev*. 2014:CD009457.

25. Zander R. *Fluid Management*. Melsungen: Bibliomed; 2009.

26. Witt L, Osthaus WA, Bunte C, et al. A novel isotonic-balanced electrolyte solution with 1% glucose for perioperative fluid management in children – an animal experimental preauthorization study. *Paediatr Anaesth*. 2010;**20**:734–40.

27. Disma N, Mameli L, Pistorio A, et al. A novel balanced isotonic sodium solution vs normal saline during major surgery in children up to 36 months: a multicenter RCT. *Paediatr Anaesth*. 2014;**24**:980–6.

28. Arikan AA, Zappitelli M, Goldstein SL, et al. Fluid overload is associated with impaired oxygenation and morbidity in critically ill children. *Pediatr Crit Care. Med* 2011;**13**:253–8.

29. Saudan S. Is the use of colloids for fluid replacement harmless in children? *Curr Opin Anaesthesiol*. 2010;**23**:363–7.

30. Sümpelmann R, Kretz FJ, Luntzer R, et al. Hydroxyethyl starch 130/0.42/6:1 for perioperative plasma volume replacement in 1130 children: results of an European prospective multicenter observational Postauthorization Safety Study (PASS). *Paediatr Anaesth*. 2012;**22**:371–8.

31. Van der Linden P, Dumoulin M, Van Lerberghe C, et al. Efficacy and safety of 6% hydroxyethyl starch 130/0.4 (Voluven) for perioperative volume replacement in children undergoing cardiac surgery: a propensity-matched analysis. *Crit Care*. 2015;**19**:87.

32. Thy M, Montmayeur J, Julien-Marsollier F, et al. Safety and efficacy of peri-operative administration of hydroxyethyl starch in children undergoing surgery: a systematic review and meta-analysis. *Eur J Anaesthesiol.* 2018;**35**:484–95.

33. European Medicines Agency. Hydroxymethyl starch (HES) containing medicinal products. Accessed 5.4.2022 at: www.ema.europa.eu/en/medicines/huma n/referrals/hydroxyethyl-starch-hes-con taining-medicinal-products.

34. Northern Neonatal Nursing Initiative Trial Group. Randomised trial of prophylactic early fresh-frozen plasma or gelatin or glucose in preterm babies: outcome at 2 years. *Lancet.* 1996;**348**:229–32.

35. Sümpelmann R, Camporesi A, Gálvez I, et al. Modified fluid gelatin 4% for perioperative volume replacement in pediatric patients (GPS): results of a European prospective non-interventional multicenter study. *Paediatr Anaesth.* 2022;**32**:825–33.

36. Osthaus WA, Witt L, Johanning K, et al. Equal effects of gelatin and hydroxyethyl starch (6% HES 130/0.42) on modified thrombelastography in children. *Acta Anaesthesiol Scand.* 2009;**53**:305–10.

37. Witt L, Osthaus WA, Jahn W, et al. Isovolaemic hemodilution with gelatin and hydroxyethylstarch 130/0.42: effects on

hemostasis in piglets. *Paediatr Anaesth.* 2012;**22**:379–85.

38. Witt L, Glage S, Lichtinghagen R, et al. Impact of high doses of 6% hydroxyethyl starch 130/0.42 and 4% gelatin on renal function in a pediatric animal model. *Paediatr Anaesth.* 2016;**26**:259–65.

39. Osthaus WA, Huber D, Beck C, et al. Correlation of oxygen delivery with central venous oxygen saturation, mean arterial pressure and heart rate in piglets. *Paediatr Anaesth.* 2006;**16**:944–7.

40. Singh Y, Villaescusa JU, da Cruz EM, et al. Recommendations for hemodynamic monitoring for critically ill children-expert consensus statement issued by the cardiovascular dynamics section of the European Society of Paediatric and Neonatal Intensive Care (ESPNIC). *Crit Care.* 2020;**24**:620.

41. Weber F, Scoones GP. A practical approach to cerebral near-infrared spectroscopy (NIRS) directed hemodynamic management in noncardiac pediatric anesthesia. *Paediatr Anaesth.* 2019;**29**:993–1001.

42. Sümpelmann R, Mader T, Dennhardt N, et al. A novel isotonic balanced electrolyte solution with 1% glucose for intraoperative fluid therapy in neonates: results of a prospective multicentre observational Postauthorisation Safety Study (PASS). *Paediatr Anaesth.* 2011;**21**:1114–18.

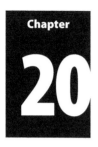

Fluid Therapy for Liver and Renal Transplantation

Laurence Weinberg

Introduction

With improvements in surgical skills, anesthetic techniques, graft preservation and perioperative management, liver and renal transplantations have become established treatments for patients with acute and chronic liver failure and irreversible chronic kidney disease. In these contexts, transplantation is a therapeutic intervention that improves survival and quality of life, and controls and/or reverses many of the comorbidities associated with organ failure.

The scientific literature provides little evidence-based guidance in amount (quantitative fluid intervention) or type (qualitative fluid intervention) of fluid to optimize outcomes during liver and renal transplantation. Fluid intervention and vasoactive pharmacological support for transplantation depend on clinician preference, institutional resources and practice culture. This chapter provides a contemporary overview of the fundamental principles underpinning fluid intervention for adult liver and renal transplantations.

Fluid Intervention for Liver Transplantation

A contemporary systematic review [1] that included expert panel recommendations for the perioperative fluid management and outcomes for adults undergoing liver transplantation (LT) recommended:

1. A moderately restrictive or replacement-only fluid regime, especially during the dissection phase of the LT (Quality of Evidence: Moderate; Grade of Recommendation: Weak)
2. The avoidance of sustained hypervolemia, based on absence of fluid responsiveness, elevated filling pressures and/or echocardiographic findings (Quality of Evidence: Moderate; Grade of Recommendation: Strong)
3. Defending a mean arterial blood pressure greater than 60–65 mmHg (Quality of Evidence: Low; Grade of Recommendation: Strong)
4. Avoidance of 130/0.4 hydroxyethyl starch (HES) given the high incidence of acute kidney injury (AKI) in high-risk surgical patients (Quality of Evidence: Low; Grade of Recommendation: Strong)
5. The evidence supporting the preferential use of any other specific colloid or any crystalloid for routine volume replacement is weak.

Patients undergoing LT should be managed on an individualized basis. No single approach will be effective. Overarching principles in the setting of LT are to normalize the microcirculation by maintaining intravascular volume, tissue perfusion and tissue oxygenation, thereby protecting the new graft and other organs. Fluid intervention and use of vasoactive medications during LT are critically dependent on a comprehensive understanding of the three stages of LT, as summarized in Table 20.1.

Factors Influencing Volume and Type of Fluid for Liver Transplantation

As LT imposes a major pathophysiological insult on the patient, the volume and type of fluid intervention utilized depend on the presence and severity of the following perioperative sequelae.

Hemodynamic Changes

Patients with end-stage liver disease have a hyperdynamic resting circulation with high cardiac output states and low systemic vascular resistance and tachycardia. Intraoperatively, this state is amplified. The potential for massive bleeding is common and can result in sudden and catastrophic hypovolemia. This can be compounded by obstruction or clamping of the inferior vena cava, or surgical manipulation of the liver that decreases venous return and cardiac output. In addition, profound vasoplegia is common, particularly at reperfusion. Patients with end-stage liver disease suffer from glycocalyx alterations, and ischemia reperfusion injury during transplantation further exacerbates endothelial damage. [2] The endothelial glycocalyx participates in the maintenance of vascular integrity, and its perturbations cause capillary leakage, loss of vascular responsiveness and enhanced adhesion of leukocytes and platelets. Reperfusion syndrome can result in profound hemodynamic embarrassment and cardiac arrest.[3,4]

Biochemical Derangements

Severe biochemical derangements are common and include citrate toxicity, metabolic acidosis, hypocalcemia, osmolality changes and rapid potassium influx. Massive blood transfusion results in large volumes of citrated blood being administered and the development of a metabolic acidosis. There is limited hepatic function to metabolize citrate; therefore, citrate intoxication can occur and resultant hypocalcemia is frequent. Ionized calcium levels must be frequently monitored, and calcium chloride should be administered when appropriate. Mild to moderate acidosis can be safely tolerated during transplantation; however, in the author's institution a base deficit of greater than −15 or a pH less than 7.1 means that a titration of 8.4% sodium bicarbonate is administered to reduce the risk of reperfusion arrhythmias and impaired myocardial contractility. Sodium bicarbonate must be used cautiously as aggressive correction of preexisting hyponatremia can impose a risk of serious neurological complications from pontine and extra pontine myelinolysis. Intravenous sterile water is frequently administered to control hypernatremia.

Coagulopathy

Fluid intervention for the management of coagulopathy is beyond the scope of this review; however, there are multiple causes of coagulopathy during LT.[5–7] These include preexisting coagulopathy due to chronic liver insufficiency and reduced synthesis of clotting factors, preexisting enhanced fibrinolytic activity, thrombocytopenia,

Table 20.1 Stages of liver transplantation and associated hemodynamic challenges

Surgical phase	Surgical technique	Challenges	Hemodynamic and fluid goals
Stage 1: Pre-anhepatic or dissection phase	Commences with surgical incision and extends until the portal vessels are clamped. Mobilization and dissection of native liver.	Hemodynamic instability can be pronounced due to: – Decompression of ascites – Bleeding from extensive collateral circulation due to portal hypertension – Bleeding from adhesions due to previous surgery – Effects of liver retraction of the inferior venae cava (IVC) with compromised venous return to the right atrium Most cirrhotic patients have increased blood volumes and cardiac output; therefore, they will tolerate 15–20% blood loss with little volume.	Maintenance of baseline vascular filling pressures with a combination of vasoactive pharmacotherapy (e.g., noradrenalin) and fluids. Some centers advocate restrictive fluid therapy, with low central venous pressure (CVP) to minimize Stage 1 blood loss. Most cirrhotic patients have increased blood volumes and cardiac output; therefore, they will tolerate 15–20% blood loss with little volume intervention or vasoactive support needed. Volume reduction of this magnitude can be tolerated if mean arterial pressure is greater than 65 mmHg and cardiac index is above 2.0 L/min/m². **Advantages of Stage 1 restrictive fluid intervention:** – Less bleeding may lower venous pressure and intravascular volume of abdominal collateral vessels. – In cases of caval injury, less brisk bleeding can facilitate faster control and repair. **Disadvantages of Stage 1 restrictive fluid intervention:** – Increased risk of air embolism. – May result in impaired organ perfusion rather than decreased venous pressures. – Increase risk of postoperative acute renal failure.

Stage		

Stage 2: Anhepatic phase	• Begins with transection of the portal vessels and ends with reperfusion.	• Portal vein clamping can induce portal hypertension and splanchnic congestion making dissection more difficult.
		• Splanchnic congestion can cause renal congestion and subsequent renal dysfunction.
		• Surgeons frequently apply side clamps to IVC to facilitate surgery.
		• Depending on extent, type and duration of surgical clamping of the IVC, venous return will be compromised.
		• Temporary portal caval shunts associated with preservation of the IVC have been used safely without the need for venous-venous bypass and associated with better hemodynamic stability.
		• If hemodynamically unstable, veno-venous bypass can be considered.
			• IVC clamp reduces venous return by 50%.
			• Consider judicious volume loading prior to IVC clamp.
			• Once IVC clamp is applied, avoid aggressive volume loading unless replacing ongoing blood losses.
			• Aggressive volume loading can precipitate volume overload and right heart failure on reperfusion.
			• Aggressive volume loading can result in high CVP during Stage 3, increasing venous congestion in the new graft.
			• As the portal vein anastomosis is nearing completion ensure:
			  – Calcium > 1.1 mmol/L
			  – Potassium < 5.0 mmol/L

Stage 3: Reperfusion & neohepatic phase	• Begins with removal of caval clamps and passive washout from hepatic veins. • Surgical testing of the caval hepatic anastomoses is then performed with	• Reperfusion results in release of CO_2, tumor necrosis factor and other active mediators and cytokines. • Reperfusion syndrome: diagnosed by sustained reduction in mean arterial pressure by 30% for greater than 1 minute.	• Significant hemodynamic changes occur in ~30–50% of patients including arrhythmias and hypotension. • Reperfusion mediators are negative inotropes and can result in acute right cardiac dysfunction, elevated pulmonary artery pressures and increased right ventricular afterload.

Table 20.1 (cont.)

Surgical phase	Surgical technique	Challenges	Hemodynamic and fluid goals

	back-pressure before portal venous flow is restored.
	• After reperfusion of the liver with portal venous blood, the hepatic arterial anastomosis is completed.
	• Biliary anastomosis is finally completed (either a duct-to-duct anastomosis connection or a Roux-en-Y choledochojejunostomy).
	• After the vascular and biliary anastomosis, perfect surgical hemostasis must be achieved prior to closure.
		• Reperfusion syndrome occurs in 8–30% of transplants and is caused by acidemia, metabolic derangements, emboli of air and microthrombus and release of vasoactive substances from the ischemic liver.
		• Throughout the neohepatic phase, signs of improving graft function include:
		  – Improvements in coagulation
		  – Falling potassium
		  – Improving acid–base physiology
		  – Falling lactate
		  – Improved urine output
		  – Improvement hemodynamics
		  – Production of bile from new graft
			• Right ventricular distension limits left ventricular filling and can cause profound hemodynamic embarrassment.
			• Reperfusion can result in life threatening hyperkalemia.
			• Drugs used to treat reperfusion syndrome and hyperkalemia include adrenalin, noradrenalin calcium, atropine, insulin/dextrose and bicarbonate.
			• Vasopressin and methylene blue can be used for refractory vasoplegia.
			• If right cardiac dysfunction is present, large volume fluid intervention/resuscitation may increase CVP, precipitate right cardiac failure and cardiac arrest. Use of transesophageal echocardiography is useful to guide fluid intervention and assess the hemodynamic state in this scenario.

variable disseminated intravascular coagulopathy and coagulopathy from hemodilution and massive blood transfusion. Patients with primary biliary cirrhosis, primary sclerosing cholangitis or underlying hepatoma and pediatric patients may have a hypercoagulable state; in contrast, patients with advanced cirrhosis often present with preexisting enhanced fibrinolytic activity. During Stages 2 and 3 of the surgery, there is lack of hepatic clearance of tissue plasminogen activator and progressive thrombocytopenia reaching a nadir post-reperfusion. In addition, if University of Wisconsin solution is used for graft preservation, platelet aggregation due to the adenosine can occur post-reperfusion. Heparin activity can also occur post-reperfusion due to release of exogenous heparin from the graft and the release of endogenous heparinoids from damaged endothelium. Hypothermia slows enzymatic reactions, prolongs factor reaction time and reduces platelet aggregation.

Renal Dysfunction

Acute kidney injury (AKI) is a common after LT associated with inferior patient and graft outcomes.[8–11] Whilst the etiology is multifactorial, common causes include preexisting ischemic acute tubular necrosis, cyclosporine toxicity and sepsis. Patients with acute renal failure from hepato-renal syndrome will recovery in most cases, although recovery may be delayed up to 6 months. The risk of chronic kidney disease is approximately 18% at 5 years and increases to approximately 25% by 10 years after transplantation. Although preoperative, intraoperative and post-transplant factors may contribute to the development of post-transplantation chronic renal failure, pre-transplant chronic renal failure appears to be one of the most important risk factors.[12]

Physiochemical Considerations for Choice of Fluids

The liver has a vital function in acid–base regulation, and severe metabolic derangements during transplantation are common and frequently profound. Choice of fluid for LT should consider the important role that the liver plays in the maintenance of acid–base homeostasis. Clinicians should have a fundamental understanding of the physiochemical properties of the available intravenous solutions to individualize therapy to the patient's underlying pathophysiological condition. The physiochemical composition of the commonly available crystalloid solutions used in LT are summarized in Table 20.2.

Metabolic Acidosis

Accumulating data and expert opinion suggest that large volumes of saline 0.9% result in the hyperchloremic metabolic acidosis.[13–15] Severe acidemia can result in impaired cardiac contractility, arrhythmias, pulmonary hypertension, renal and splanchnic vasoconstriction and impaired coagulation,[16] all of which are common during LT. Correction of acidemia during LT is contentious, as the physiological benefits of acidemia include improved oxygen delivery via the Bohr effects and protection against hypoxic stress.[16] Experimental evidence has shown that the optimal strong ion difference for an intravenous fluid not to influence blood pH should be approximately 24 mEq/L.[17,18] Saline (0.9%), with its equal concentrations of sodium and chloride, has a strong ion different of zero. Use of 0.9% saline during transplantation will significantly reduce the strong ion difference of plasma and exacerbate the severity of any metabolic acidosis. Use of buffered solutions with a high

Table 20.2 Characteristics of common crystalloid solutions compared with human plasma

	Human plasma	0.9% saline (unbuffered solution)	Compound sodium lactate (lactate-buffered solution)	Ringer's lactate (lactate-buffered solution)	Ionosteril® (acetate-buffered solution)	Sterofundin ISO® (acetate- & malate-buffered solution)	Plasma-Lyte 148® (acetate- & gluconate-buffered solution)
Sodium (mmol/L)	136–145	154	129	130	137	145	140
Potassium (mmol/L)	3.5–5.0		5	4	4	4	5
Magnesium (mmol/L)	0.8–1.0				1.25	1	1.5
Calcium (mmol/L)	2.2–2.6		2.5	3	1.65	2.5	
Chloride (mmol/L)	98–106	154	109	109	110	127	98
Acetate (mmol/L)					36.8	24	27
Gluconate (mmol/L)							23
Lactate (mmol/L)			29	28			
Malate (mmol/L)						5	
eSID (mEq/L)	42		27	28	36.8	25.5	50

Theoretical osmolarity (mosmol/L)	291	308	278	273	291	309	295
Actual or measured* osmolality (mosmol/kg H$_2$O)	287	286	256	256	270	Not stated	271
pH	7.35–7.45	4.5–7	5–7	5.0–7	6.9–7.9	5.1–5.9	4–8

* Freezing point depression

eSID, effective strong ion difference.

Plasma-Lyte 148 manufactured by Baxter Healthcare, Toongabie, NSW, Australia

Ringer's lactate manufactured by Baxter Healthcare, Deerfield, IL, USA

Hartmann's solution manufactured by Baxter Healthcare, Toongabie, NSW, Australia

Ionosteril manufactured by Fresenius Medical Care, Schweinfurt, Germany

Sterofundin ISO manufactured by B. Braun Melsungen AG, Melsungen, Germany effective strong ion difference composition can minimize the severity of metabolic acid–base disturbances in this setting, whilst restoring intravascular volume deficit.

Inorganic Anions

The liver plays a vital role in its capacity to metabolize various organic anions, which results in consumption of hydrogen ions and regeneration of the extracellular bicarbonate buffer. Anions may be exogenous (e.g., citrate in blood transfusion, or acetate gluconate, acetate and lactate from buffered crystalloid solutions), or endogenous such as lactate from active glycolysis or anaerobic metabolism. During LT hepatic metabolism is severely or completely compromised; therefore, organic anions present in delivered buffered fluid solutions may not be able to be adequately metabolized to generate bicarbonate.

Theoretically, the use of acetate-buffered solutions confers several advantages over the lactate-buffered solutions in the setting of LT.[19] Use of lactate-based crystalloid solutions can result in hyperlactatemia, as lactate anions are ineffectively metabolized. Lactate levels may therefore be an unreliable index of the severity of graft function. Hyperlactatemia has also been shown to be an important prognostic marker after liver resection,[20] shock states and critical illness,[21,22] correlating strongly with increased risks of complications and death. Unlike lactate, acetate is metabolized widely throughout the body and not reliant entirely on hepatic metabolism. A canine study showed that acetate metabolism is well preserved in profound shock while lactate metabolism was significantly impaired.[23] Acetate is metabolized more rapidly than lactate with an increase in bicarbonate levels evident after 15 minutes after the start of an administered acetate infusion.[24,25] Acetate is also more alkalinizing than lactate, with may be advantageous for patients undergoing LT.

More recently, in a larger clinical trial of 78 critically ill trauma patients resuscitated with sodium acetate as an alternative to 0.9% saline or lactated Ringer's solution, patients receiving acetate had stable hemodynamic profiles without evidence of hemodynamic instability. Normalization of hyperchloremia and metabolic acidosis occurred faster in the patients who received acetate.[26] Acetate turnover shows no age-related differences,[27] and acetate may protect against malnutrition by replacing fat as an oxidative fuel without affecting glucose oxidation or causing hyperglycemia.[28,29] Finally, acetate metabolism does not result in changes in glucose or insulin concentrations,[30] whereas exogenously administered lactate can be converted to glucose via gluconeogenesis resulting in significant hyperglycemia.[31] In diabetic patients, intraoperative glucose levels have been shown to double following administration of exogenous lactate solutions.[30] Compared with bicarbonate, lactate or acetate, the alkalizing effect of gluconate is almost zero;[32,33] therefore, its clinical effects in vivo as a metabolizable anion appear to be limited.

Historically, adverse effects of acetate have been observed with high doses and high rates of acetate infusions, particularly in the setting of hemodialysis. The generalizability of these findings to LT is unknown. Small quantities of acetate present in various dialysis fluids (usually 35 mmol/L) have resulted in plasma acetate concentration of 10 to 40 times physiological levels.[34–36] Moreover, sodium acetate produced a direct dose-related decrease in myocardial contractility and blood pressure in a dog model, whereas a slow infusion of sodium acetate did not result in adverse hemodynamic effects.[33,37] Hypoxia and hypotension have been reported in patients with end-stage renal disease dialysed against solutions containing acetate.[38–40] In a crossover study involving 12 patients undergoing hemodiafiltration randomized to either acetate or bicarbonate (acetate-free) dialysate, exposure to acetate-free dialysate was associated with less deterioration in systemic hemodynamics and less suppression of myocardial contractility.[41] Similarly, exposure of myocardial tissue to acetate concentrations as low as 5 mmol/L selectively impaired fatty acid metabolism in cardiac tissue issue, decreased ATP production and tissue ATP concentrations, which in turn resulted in impaired contractile function.[42] In contrast, the effects of acetate on left ventricular contractility and function were evaluated before and after a 20-minute sodium acetate infusion during dialysis.[43] Angiographically determined left ventricular volumes and pressures were used to calculate the ventricular function indices. A plasma acetate concentration of 3.13 mmol/L increased ejection fraction and cardiac index.

Avoidance of Hyperchloremia

Use of fluid solutions with physiological concentrations of chloride during LT may be beneficial. A review of 22 851 surgical patients undergoing non-cardiac surgery with normal preoperative serum chloride concentration and renal function reported that postoperative hyperchloremia was associated with postoperative renal dysfunction and 30-day mortality. [44] Accordingly, the implementation of a chloride-restrictive strategy may reduce the incidence of acute kidney injury and use of renal replacement therapy.[45] A systematic review and meta-analysis that assessed the relationship between the chloride content of intravenous resuscitation fluids and patient outcomes in the perioperative and intensive care settings reported a weak but significant association between higher chloride content fluids and unfavorable outcomes were found, although mortality was unaffected.[46] Mechanisms of hyperchloremic-induced renal injury include inability of the proximal tubule capacity to reabsorb chloride, resulting in greater chloride delivery to the thick ascending limb of the distal tubule from inactivation of tubuloglomerular feedback by the macula densa and a reduction in glomerular filtration,[47–49] hyperchloremic-induced thromboxane release with associated vasoconstriction [50] and an alteration in the expression of inflammatory cytokines.[51]

Plasma Osmolality

An understanding of intravenous solutions' osmolality is important during LT. Hartmann's solution or Ringer's lactate are hypotonic solutions with a calculated in vivo osmolality (tonicity) of approximately 254 mosmol/kg H_2O (see Table 20.2). Hypotonic fluids must be used cautiously, if at all, in patients undergoing LT with fulminant liver failure. The most common cause of death in fulminant liver failure is intractable intracranial hypertension from cerebral edema, present in approximately 50–80% of patients with fulminant liver failure. Permissive hypernatremia and use of hypertonic saline solutions are frequently used in this specific setting. Saline (0.9%) is considered a relatively hypertonic solution because the sum of its osmotically active components gives a theoretical in vitro osmolality of 308 mosmol/kg H_2O (154 mmol/L sodium plus 154 mmol/L chloride). However, 0.9% saline is an isotonic solution as its constituents – sodium and chloride – are only partially active with an osmotic coefficient of 0.926.[52] The calculated in vivo osmolality (tonicity) of saline is 285 mosmol/kg H_2O, which is the same as plasma osmolality (tonicity). Saline may therefore be a more appropriate fluid in the setting of transplantation for fulminant liver failure. Finally, administration of hypotonic fluids can represent a significant free water load that may not be easily excreted in the presence of the high antidiuretic hormone concentrations commonly associated with physiological stress.[53] Failure to excrete water in a timely fashion may result in postoperative transplantation positive fluid balance, edema and weight gain.

Colloids and Liver Transplantation

In a survey evaluating the use of fluids during LT,[54] albumin was reported to be the most common used colloid (85%), followed by HES. There are no large-scale prospective studies guiding the efficacy and safety of any colloids in the setting of LT. In a small single-center study, 40 patients undergoing living donor LT were prospectively randomized to receive albumin or HES. The use of HES as an alternative to human albumin resulted in equivalent renal outcomes.[55] In a larger single-center observational study that evaluated the influence of HES on renal function in 394 patients undergoing orthotopic LT, the perioperative use of HES had no significant effect on renal function in the first postoperative week.[56] In contrast, a retrospective cross-sectional analysis of 147 adult patients who underwent orthotopic LT reported that patients receiving HES had an increased odds of acute kidney injury compared with patients receiving 5% albumin.[57]

Significant concerns regarding HES and the risk of AKIs in critically unwell patients have resulted in cautious perioperative use in the context of LT.[58–61] Four landmark trials – CHEST,[62] 6S,[63] VISEP,[64] and CRYSTMAS [65] – have reported that HES might increase the risk of AKIs, need for renal replacement therapy or mortalities. These findings were supported by a meta-analysis examining HES solutions for resuscitating patients with sepsis [66] and critically ill patients requiring volume resuscitation.[58] A recent reanalysis of a Cochrane collaboration analysis of trials examining colloids versus crystalloids for fluid resuscitation in critically ill patients concluded that HES solutions are associated with an increased risk of AKIs. Therefore, the research suggests that HES should not be used to treat critically ill patients.[67] These findings would be generalizable to patients undergoing LT.

These findings are further supported by robust evidence evaluating the effects of HES on postoperative kidney function in 44 176 patients undergoing non-cardiac surgeries.[68] After controlling for confounding variables, the odds of developing more serious AKIs with Hextend was found to be 21% (6–38%) greater than with crystalloids only. More recently, the fluid loading in abdominal surgery (FLASH) trial evaluated the effects of HES 130/0.4 compared with 0.9% saline for intravascular volume expansion on mortality and postoperative complications after major abdominal surgery.[69] The authors concluded that HES should not be used for volume replacement therapy in such patients.

There is a greater paucity of data regarding the use of gelatin-based solutions in LT. The associations of gelatins and adverse effects on hemostasis and coagulation have been the main detractions for its use in LT given that coagulopathy during transplantation is common, pronounced and often refractory.[69–71] Both gelatin and HES solutions have been associated with adverse effects on blood coagulation.[70,72] There are fewer effects on blood coagulation using crystalloids compared with colloids, and it is possible that adverse coagulation effects of both gelatin and HES solutions may be similar. There appears to be no differences in adverse coagulation effects between balanced HES 130/0.42 and non-balanced HES 130/0.4.[72] Use of gelatin has been recently shown to cause more impairment in renal function in elective living-donor LT compared with HES solutions.[73] Despite years of clinical use, there is insufficient quality of clinical trials to confirm both the safety and efficacy of gelatin in the setting of LT.[74] Finally, in the Victorian Consultative Council on Anaesthetic Morbidity and Mortality report for the Triennium 2003–2005, 27 cases of anaesthesia related anaphylactic reactions to HES solutions and gelatin were reported, 5 of which were fatal.[75] This again has specific relevance to patients undergoing LT given the severe hemodynamic challenges faced with each case.

Albumin is the most common colloid used in LT. Specific to LT, advantages include maintenance of colloid osmotic pressure, preservation of kidney function, pleiotropic physiological benefits on endothelial integrity, improving the endothelial integrity by substantially protecting the glycocalyx of endothelial cells,[76,77] facilitation of negative fluid balance in hypoproteinemia states that are common in transplant patients and maintenance of glomerular filtration via hemodynamic and oncotic mechanisms.[78–80] Biological plausibility, freedom from nephrotoxicity (safety) and reduction of renal morbidity in liver cirrhosis (effectiveness) support the use of albumin in LT.[81] In contrast to other colloids, fluid resuscitation with human albumin is not considered nephrotoxic.

Albumin has been extensively reappraised a resuscitation fluid by Finfer.[82] Available as iso-oncotic and iso-osmolar 4–5% solutions and hyperoncotic 20–25% solutions, albumin is both suspended in sodium chloride and contains octanoate as the anion stabilizer. It remains an attractive colloid for LT with 4–5% albumen providing plasma volume expansion by an amount approximately equal to the volume infused, whilst concentrated albumen expands the plasma volume by approximately 4–5 times the volume infused.[82] Relevant to LT, albumin might be harmful in patients with traumatic brain injury;[82,83] therefore, large volumes of albumin should be used cautiously in fulminant LT recipients with raised intracranial pressure.

The pooled analysis of mortality data from large studies of volume therapy with human albumin in sepsis, namely, the SAFE and ALBIOS studies,[62,84] confirm that administration of albumen could significantly reduce mortality in patients with severe sepsis or septic shock.[60,83] In the ALBIOS study,[84] patients in the albumin group not only achieved more frequently hemodynamic stabilization but also had prognostically favorable negative fluid balance.[83] A meta-analysis by Patel et al. confirmed that albumen appears to be safe in the settings of critical illness.[85]

Crystalloids and Liver Transplantation

There is no consensus community regarding the optimal type of crystalloid for LT. In the survey by Schumann et al. evaluating the use of fluids during LT,[86] in the same representative sample of 61 US academic institutions with a comprehensive liver transplant program, 0.9% saline was the most frequent crystalloid used (81%), followed by a pH-adjusted buffered/balanced crystalloid solution, Plasma-Lyte 148 (74%). Least favored were glucose-containing normal saline solutions (43%). Such practice variation is related to the paucity of prospective evidence regarding the comparative safety and efficacy of available crystalloid solutions for both fluid resuscitation and maintenance therapy in the perioperative setting.

Observational studies have associated saline with an increased risk of AKI in surgical patients.[44–46,87–89] However, such observational studies may be affected by selection bias and do not account for confounders, making causal inferences problematic.

The 0.9% saline versus Plasma-Lyte 148 for intensive care unit therapy (SPLIT) trial [90] and the saline against lactated Ringer's or Plasma-Lyte (SALT) trial [91] were prospective fluid intervention pilot studies conducted in intensive care units (ICU). Both studies evaluated the effects of buffered crystalloid solutions versus saline and reported no differences between the rates of major AKIs. The patients in the SALT trial [91] were admitted to the ICU mainly for sepsis or respiratory failure, whereas those in the SPLIT trial were predominantly surgical patients.[90] Both studies had low fluid administration volumes, with median crystalloid volumes of less than 2000 mL received in both arms, which is clearly not generalizable to patients undergoing LT, who require much larger volume infusions. Notably, the SALT trial found a significant difference between treatment arms in the rate of major AKIs within 30 days experienced by patients who received larger fluid volumes.

More recently, two large multiple crossover trials involving 13 347 non-critically ill [92] and 7942 critically ill [93] adult patients found lower rates of renal injuries using balanced crystalloids (Ringer's solution or Plasma-Lyte) compared with saline. These studies did not discriminate against major surgery patients and were not double-blind in design. Despite some recent positive findings, pooled meta-analyses of studies performed in the critical care setting have found no differences in the hospital mortality, AKI or renal replacement therapy rates between patients receiving balanced crystalloids and those receiving saline.[94]

A large pragmatic single-center study evaluating the effects of restricting the perioperative use of IV chloride on AKI after cardiac surgery showed that a perioperative fluid strategy to restrict IV chloride administration was not associated with an altered incidence of AKIs or other metrics of renal injuries.[95] More recently, the saline or lactated Ringer's trial (SOLAR trial) studied the risk of a combination of in-hospital mortalities and major postoperative complications among 8616 patients undergoing elective orthopedic and colorectal surgery.[96] The trial included renal, respiratory, infectious and hemorrhagic complications, and AKIs were reported as a secondary outcome. No clinically meaningful difference was found between those patients who received unblinded saline and those who received lactated Ringer's solution. Further, for postoperative AKIs, the Acute Kidney Injury Network's Stages I–III versus zero occurred in 6.6% of patients who received lactated Ringer's solution versus 6.2% of those who received saline. This was a lower incidence than is observed in this study, with an estimated relative risk of 1.18. The absolute differences between the treatment groups for AKIs and all other outcomes were less than 0.5% and are, therefore, not clinically meaningful. The generalizability of these findings to patients undergoing LT is unknown.

Fluid Intervention for Renal Transplantation

Crystalloids and Renal Transplantation

While fluid therapy remains the first therapeutic approach to maintaining or restoring circulatory function in every patient undergoing kidney transplantation, a coherent evidence-based perioperative strategy for fluid management in this setting has also been elusive with a dearth of – and a desperate need for – large-scale, well-designed fluid interventional and hemodynamic trials. The ideal intravenous fluid for renal transplantation has also not been defined.[97] Traditionally, crystalloids are the mainstay and first choice of perioperative fluid intervention in renal transplantation.

The consensus statement of the Committee on Transplant Anesthesia of the American Society of Anesthesiologists (ASA) guidelines underscores the importance of perioperative fluid intervention – with respect to achieving favorable patient outcomes – in the context of kidney transplantation.[98] Four strong recommendations were made: –

1. Do not routinely use of albumin over crystalloids. (Quality of Evidence: moderate; Grade of Recommendation: weak)
2. Balanced crystalloid solutions are at least equal, if not better, than 0.9% saline (Quality of Evidence: moderate; Grade of Recommendation: Strong)
3. Kidney donor HES exposure is associated with increased risk of delayed graft function (Quality of Evidence: poor; Grade of Recommendation: Strong)
4. Do not use central venous pressure as an endpoint for fluid administration. (Quality of Evidence: weak; Grade of Recommendation: weak)

Conventionally, 0.9% saline is widely advocated due to concerns about hyperkalemia from the balanced/buffered solutions, which all contain potassium. A 2016 Cochrane review [99] that examined six studies [100–105] investigated the effects of lower-chloride solutions versus normal saline on delayed graft function, hyperkalemia and acid–base status in kidney transplant recipients. The review concluded that balanced electrolyte solutions are associated with less hyperchloremic metabolic acidosis compared with normal saline; however, it remains uncertain whether lower chloride solutions lead to improved graft outcomes compared with normal saline. These findings were confirmed with more recent randomized-controlled trials that reported that for patients undergoing renal transplantation, participants receiving normal saline had a greater incidence of hyperkalemia and hyperchloremia and were more acidemic compared with those receiving a balanced crystalloid solution.[106,107] These biochemical differences were not associated with adverse clinical outcomes.

To address the question of which fluid type to use, the Better Evidence for Selecting Transplant Fluids (BEST-Fluids) trial was a large multicenter, double-blind randomized-controlled trial that compared the effect of a balanced, low-chloride solution (Plasma-Lyte 148) versus 0.9% saline on the incidence of delayed graft function in deceased-donor kidney transplant recipients.[108] Results from this study showed that the low-chloride solution was followed by a lower incidence of delayed graft function (DGF, 30% vs. 40%), which should guide clinical decision making regarding the choice of crystalloid fluid in kidney transplant recipients.

Colloids and Renal Transplantation

Many of the adverse effects of colloid solutions outlined in the section "Colloids and Liver Transplantation" are relevant to patients undergoing kidney transplantation. Specific to renal transplantation, there have been historical concerns regarding the use of HES solutions and impaired renal function.[109] An early prospective randomized trial in 1993 comparing HES and gelatin for plasma-volume expansion in brain-dead organ donors found that HES was associated with impaired immediate renal function in kidney transplant recipients.[110] Renal biopsies demonstrated osmotic, nephrosis-like lesions in the HES treated group.[111] Similar findings have been reported by other investigators.[112] In the absence of direct chemical toxicity, the most likely attributed mechanism for HES-induced renal dysfunction is swelling and vacuolization of tubular cells and tubular obstruction due to the production of hyperviscous urine. Renal dysfunction from high plasma colloid osmotic pressure is thought to increases with repeated doses of concentrated HES of high molecular weight and high degree of substitution.[113] Findings from these older studies have been recently confirmed by Patel et al., who evaluated the impact of HES in organ donors after neurological determination of death on recipient renal graft outcomes. In that study, 986 kidneys were transplanted from 529 donors. Forty-two percent received HES and 35% developed delayed graft function. Hydroxyethyl starch use during donor management was independently associated with a 41% increase in the risk of delayed graft function.[114]

Albumin's theoretical advantages result in continued advocacy for use in renal transplant recipients, including increased plasma oncotic pressure, antioxidant properties, enhanced protein transport, anti-inflammatory properties and buffering capacity.[98] Potential risks associated with albumin include increased cost, availability and immunogenicity.[98] Recent available evidence suggests that there is no advantage of albumin over crystalloid alone in kidney transplantation and use should be selective rather than per protocol.

Conclusions

Fluid prescription for liver and renal transplantation is complex. Whilst there is physiologically rational and biologically plausible data to suggest certain fluids may confer metabolic, organ and outcome benefits, there is no unequivocal data to support the use any single fluid. Clinicians should have a fundamental understanding of the physiochemical properties of the available crystalloid and colloid solutions to individualize therapy to the patient's underlying pathophysiological condition. It is imperative to continue to conduct further large-scale clinical trials to determine both the optimal type and dose of fluid for patients undergoing both liver and renal transplantation.

References

1. Morkane CM, Sapisochin G, Mukhtar AM, et al.; ERAS4OLT.org Working Group. Perioperative fluid management and outcomes in adult deceased donor liver transplantation – a systematic review of the literature and expert panel recommendations. *Clin Transplant.* 2022;**36**:e14651.

2. Schiefer J, Lebherz-Eichinger D, Erdoes G, et al. Alterations of endothelial glycocalyx during orthotopic liver transplantation in patients with end-stage liver disease. *Transplantation.* 2015;**99**:2118–23.

3. Bukowicka B, Akar RA, Olszewska A, et al. The occurrence of postreperfusion syndrome in orthotopic liver transplantation and its significance in terms of complications and short-term survival. *Ann Transplant.* 2011;**16** 26–30.

4. Paugam-Burtz C, Kavafyan J, Merckx P, et al. Postreperfusion syndrome during liver transplantation for cirrhosis: outcome and predictors. *Liver Transpl.* 2009;**15**:522–9.

5. Sabate A, Dalmau A, Koo M, et al. Coagulopathy management in liver transplantation. *Transplant Proc.* 2012;**44**:1523–5.

6. Porte RJ. Coagulation and fibrinolysis in orthotopic liver transplantation: current views and insights. *Semin Thromb Hemost.* 1993;**19**:191–6.

7. Massicotte L, Lenis S, Thibeault L, et al. Effect of low central venous pressure and phlebotomy on blood product transfusion requirements during liver transplantations. *Liver Transpl.* 2006;**12**:117–23.

8. de Haan JE, Hoorn EJ, de Geus HRH. Acute kidney injury after liver transplantation: Recent insights and future perspectives. *Best Pract Res Clin Gastroenterol.* 2017;**31**:161–9.

9. Dong V, Nadim MK, Karvellas CJ. Post-liver transplant acute kidney injury. *Liver Transpl.* 2021;**27**:1653–64.

10. Sirivatanauksorn Y, Parakonthun T, Premasathian N, et al. Renal dysfunction after orthotopic liver transplantation. *Transplant Proc.* 2014;**46**:818–21.

11. Yalavarthy R, Edelstein CL, Teitelbaum I. Acute renal failure and chronic kidney disease following liver transplantation. *Hemodial Int.* 2007;11(Suppl 3):S7–12.

12. Tinti F, Umbro I, Giannelli V, et al. Acute renal failure in liver transplant recipients: role of pretransplantation renal function and 1-year follow-up. *Transplant Proc.* 2011;**43**:1136–8.

13. Scheingraber S, Rehm M, Sehmisch C, Finsterer U. Rapid saline infusion produces hyperchloremic acidosis in patients undergoing gynecologic surgery. *Anesthesiology.* 1999;**90**:1265–70.

14. Waters JH, Miller LR, Clack S, Kim JV. Cause of metabolic acidosis in prolonged surgery. *Crit Care Med.* 1999;**27**:2142–6.

15. Prough DS, Bidani A. Hyperchloremic metabolic acidosis is a predictable consequence of intraoperative infusion of 0.9% saline. *Anesthesiology.* 1999;**90**:1247–9.

16. Morgan TJ. The ideal crystalloid – what is "balanced"? *Curr Opin Crit Care.* 2013;**4**:299–307.

17. Morgan TJ, Venkatesh B. Designing "balanced" crystalloids. *Crit Care Resusc.* 2003;**5**:284–91.

18. Omron EM. Omron RM. A physicochemical model of crystalloid infusion on acid-base status. *J Intensive Care Med.* 2010;**25**:271–80.

19. Zander R. *Fluid Management.* Melsungen: Bibliomed; 2009. Accessed 14/4/2015 at: www.bbraun.com/documents/Knowledge/Fluid_Management_0110.pdf

20. Watanabe I, Mayumi T, Arishima T, et al. Hyperlactaemia can predict the prognosis after liver resection. *Shock.* 2007;**28**:35–8.

21. Jansen TC, van Bommel J, Bakker J. Blood lactate monitoring in critically ill patients: a systematic health technology assessment. *Crit Care Med.* 2009;**37**:2827–39.

22. Kveim M, Nesbakken R. Bakker J, et al. Serial blood lactate levels can predict the development of multiple organ failure following septic shock. *Am J Surg.* 1996;**171**:221–6.

23. Nakatani T. Utilization of exogenous acetate during canine haemorrhagic shock. *Scand J Clin Lab Invest.* 1979;**39**:653–8.

24. Mudge GH, Manning JA, Gilman A. Sodium acetate as a source of fixed base. *Proc Soc Exp Biol Med.* 1949;**71**:136–8.

25. Hamada T, Yamamoto M, Nakamura K, et al. The pharmacokinetics of D-lactate, L-lactate and acetate in humans. *Masui.* 1997;**46**:229–36.

26. McCague A, Dermendjieva M, Hutchinson R, Wong DT, Dao N. Sodium acetate infusion in critically ill trauma patients for hyperchloremic acidosis. *Scand J Trauma Resusc Emerg Med.* 2011;**19**:24.

27. Skutches CL, Holroyde CP, Myers RN, et al. Plasma acetate turnover and oxidation. *J Clin Invest.* 1979;**64**:708–13.

28. Akanji AO, Bruce MA, Frayn KN: Effect of acetate infusion on energy expenditure and substrate oxidation rates in non-diabetic and diabetic subjects. *Eur J Clin Nutr.* 1989;**43**:107–15.

29. Akanji AO, Hockaday TDR. Acetate tolerance and the kinetics of acetate utilization in diabetic and nondiabetic subjects. *Am J Clin Nutr.* 1990;**51**:112–8.

30. Thomas DJ, Alberti KG. Hyperglycaemic effects of Hartmann's solution during surgery in patients with maturity onset diabetes. *Br J Anaesth.* 1978;**50**:185–8.

31. Arai K, Mukaida K, Fujioka Y, et al. A comparative study of acetated Ringer's solution and lactated Ringer's solution as intraoperative fluids. *Hiroshima J Anesth.* 1989;**25**:357–63.

32. Naylor JM, Forsyth GW. The alkalinizing effects of metabolizable bases in the healthy calf. *Can J Vet Res*. 1986;**50**:509–16.

33. Kirkendol PL, Starrs J, Gonzalez FM. The effect of acetate, lactate, succinate and gluconate on plasma pH and electrolytes in dogs. *Trans Am Soc Artif Intern Organs*. 1980;**26**:323–7.

34. Coll E, Perez-Garcia R, Rodriguez-Benitez P, et al. Clinical and analytical changes in hemodialysis without acetate. *Nefrologia*. 2007;**27**:742–8.

35. Bottger I, Deuticke U, Evertz-Prusse E, Ross BD, Wieland O. On the behavior of the free acetate in the miniature pig. Acetate metabolism in the miniature pig. *Z Gesamte Exp Med*. 1968;**145**:346–52.

36. Fournier G, Potier J, Thebaud HE, et al. Substitution of acetic acid for hydrochloric acid in the bicarbonate buffered dialysate. *Artif Organs*. 1998;**22**:608–13.

37. Kirkendol NW, Gonzalez FM, Devia CJ. Cardiac and vascular effects of infused sodium acetate in dogs. *Trans Am Soc Artif Intern Organs*. 1978;**24**:714–18.

38. Thaha M, Yogiantoro M, Soewanto, Pranawa. Correlation between intradialytic hypotension in patients undergoing routine hemodialysis and use of acetate compared in bicarbonate dialysate. *Acta Med Indones*. 2005;**37**:145–8.

39. Veech RL, Gitomer WL. The medical and metabolic consequences of administration of sodium acetate. *Adv Enzyme Regul*. 1988;**27**:313–43.

40. Quebbeman EJ, Maierhofer WJ, Piering WF. Mechanisms producing hypoxemia during hemodialysis. *Crit Care Med*. 1984;**12**:359–63.

41. Selby NM, Fluck RJ, Taal MW, McIntyre CW. Effects of acetate-free double-chamber hemodiafiltration and standard dialysis on systemic hemodynamics and troponin T levels. *ASAIO J*. 2006;**52**:62–9.

42. Jacob AD, Elkins N, Reiss OK, Chan L, Shapiro JI. Effects of acetate on energy metabolism and function in the isolated perfused rat heart. *Kidney Int*. 1997;**52**:755–60.

43. Nitenberg A, Huyghebaert MF, Blanchet F, Amiel C. Analysis of increased myocardial contractility during sodium acetate infusion in humans. *Kidney Int*. 1984;**26**:744–51.

44. McCluskey SA, Karkouti K, Wijeysundera D, et al. Hyperchloremia after noncardiac surgery is independently associated with increased morbidity and mortality: a propensity-matched cohort study. *Anesth Analg*. 2013;**117**:412–21.

45. Yunos NM, Bellomo R, Hegarty C, et al. Association between a chloride-liberal vs chloride-restrictive intravenous fluid administration strategy and kidney injury in critically ill adults. *JAMA*. 2012;**308**:1566–72.

46. Krajewski ML, Raghunathan K, Paluszkiewicz SM, Schermer CR, Shaw AD. Meta-analysis of high- versus low-chloride content in perioperative and critical care fluid resuscitation. *Br J Surg*. 2015;**102**:24–36.

47. Wilcox CS. Regulation of renal blood flow by plasma chloride. *J Clin Invest*. 1983;**71**:726–35.

48. Salomonsson M, Gonzalez E, Kornfeld M, Persson AE. The cytosolic chloride concentration in macula densa and cortical thick ascending limb cells. *Acta Physiol Scand*. 1993;**147**:305–13.

49. Hashimoto S, Kawata T, Schnermann J, Koike T. Chloride channel blockade attenuates the effect of angiotensin II on tubuloglomerular feedback in WKY but not spontaneously hypertensive rats. *Kidney Blood Press Res*. 2004;**27**:35–42.

50. Bullivant EM, Wilcox CS, Welch WJ. Intrarenal vasoconstriction during hyperchloremia: role of thromboxane. *Am J Physiol*. 1989;**256**:F152–F157.

51. Zhou F, Peng ZY, Bishop JV, et al. Effects of fluid resuscitation with 0.9% saline versus a balanced electrolyte solution on acute kidney injury in a rat model of sepsis. *Crit Care Med*. 2014;**42**:e270–8.

52. Guidet B, Soni N, Della Rocca G, et al. A balanced view of balanced solutions. *Crit Care*. 2010;**14**:25.

53. McLoughlin PD, Bell DA. Hartmann's solution – osmolality and lactate. *Anaesth Intensive Care*. 2010;**38**:1135–6.

54. Schumann R, Mandell S, Michaels MD, Klinck J, Walia A. Intraoperative fluid and pharmacologic management and the anesthesiologist's supervisory role for nontraditional technologies during liver transplantation: a survey of US academic centers. *Transplant Proc*. 2013;**45**:2258–62.

55. Mukhtar A, Aboulfetouh F, Obayah G, et al. The safety of modern hydroxyethyl starch in living donor liver transplantation: a comparison with human albumin. *Anesth Analg*. 2009;**109**:924–30.

56. Zhou ZB, Shao XX, Yang XY et al. Influence of hydroxyethyl starch on renal function after orthotopic liver transplantation. *Transplant Proc*. 2015;**47**:1616–19.

57. Hand WR, Whiteley JR, Epperson TI, et al. Hydroxyethyl starch and acute kidney injury in orthotopic liver transplantation: a single-center retrospective review. *Anesth Analg*. 2015;**120**:619–26.

58. Zarychanski R, Abou-Setta AM, Turgeon AF, et al. Association of hydroxyethyl starch administration with mortality and acute kidney injury in critically ill patients requiring volume resuscitation: a systematic review and meta-analysis. *JAMA*. 2013;**309**:678–88.

59. Lewis SR, Pritchard MW, Evans DJ, et al. Colloids versus crystalloids for fluid resuscitation in critically ill people. *Cochrane Database Syst Rev*. 2018;**8**:CD000567.

60. Bagshaw SM, Chawla LS. Hydroxyethyl starch for fluid resuscitation in critically ill patients. *Can J Anaesth*. 2013;**60**:709–13.

61. Haase N, Perner A. Hydroxyethyl starch for resuscitation. *Curr Opin Crit Care*. 2013;**19**:321–5.

62. Myburgh JA, Finfer S, Bellomo R, et al. Hydroxyethyl starch or saline for fluid resuscitation in intensive care. *N Engl J Med*. 2012;**367**:1901–11.

63. Perner A, Haase N, Guttormsen AB, et al. Hydroxyethyl starch 130/0.42 versus Ringer's acetate in severe sepsis. *N Engl J Med*. 2012;**367**:124–34.

64. Brunkhorst FM, Engel C, Bloos F et al. Intensive insulin therapy and pentastarch resuscitation in severe sepsis. *N Engl J Med*. 2008;**358**:125–39.

65. Guidet B, Martinet O, Boulain T, et al. Assessment of hemodynamic efficacy and safety of 6% hydroxyethylstarch 130/0.4 vs. 0.9% NaCl fluid replacement in patients with severe sepsis: the CRYSTMAS study. *Crit Care Lond Engl*. 2012;**16**:R94.

66. Haase N, Perner A, Hennings LI, et al. Hydroxyethyl starch 130/0.38–0.45 versus crystalloid or albumin in patients with sepsis: systematic review with meta-analysis and trial sequential analysis. *BMJ*. 2013;**346**:f839.

67. Perel P, Roberts I, Ker K. Colloids versus crystalloids for fluid resuscitation in critically ill patients. *Cochrane Database Syst Rev*. 2013;**28**:CD000567.

68. Kashy BK, Podolyak A, Makarova N, et al. Effect of hydroxyethyl starch on postoperative kidney function in patients having noncardiac surgery. *Anesthesiology*. 2014 Oct;**121**(4):730–9.

69. Niemi TT, Suojaranta-Ylinen RT, Kukkonen SI, Kuitunen AH. Gelatin and hydroxyethyl starch, but not albumin, impair hemostasis after cardiac surgery. *Anesth Analg*. 2006;**102**:998–1006.

70. Konrad C, Markl T, Schuepfer G, Gerber H, Tschopp M. The effects of in vitro hemodilution with gelatin, hydroxyethyl starch, and lactated Ringer's solution on markers of coagulation: an analysis using SONOCLOT. *Anesth Analg*. 1999;**88**:483–8.

71. Hartog CS, Reuter D, Loesche W, Hofmann M, Reinhart K. HES 130/0.4 influence of hydroxyethyl starch (HES) 130/0.4 on hemostasis as measured by viscoelastic device analysis: a systematic review. *Intensive Care Med*. 2011;**37**:1725–37.

72. Casutt M, Kristoffy A, Schuepfer G, Spahn DR, Konrad C. Effects on coagulation of balanced (130/0.42) and non-balanced (130/0.4) hydroxyethyl starch or gelatin compared with balanced Ringer's solution: an in vitro study using two different viscoelastic coagulation tests ROTEMTM and SONOCLOTTM. *Br J Anaesth*. 2010;**105**:273–81.

73. Demir A, Aydınlı B, Toprak HI, et al, Impact of 6% starch 130/0.4 and 4% gelatin infusion on kidney function in living-donor liver transplantation. *Transplant Proc*. 2015;**47**:1883–9.

74. Thomas-Rueddel DO, Vlasakov V, Reinhart K, et al. Safety of gelatin for volume resuscitation–a systematic review and meta-analysis. *Intensive Care Med*. 2012;**38**:1134–42.

75. Victorian Consultative Council on Anaesthetic Mortality and Morbidity. *Tenth Report of the Victorian Consultative Council on Anaesthetic Mortality and Morbidity*. Department of Health, Melbourne, Victoria, May 2011. Accessed 21/6/2022 at: www.health.vic.gov.au/publications/tenth-report-of-the-victorian-consultative-council-on-anaesthetic-mortality-and

76. Jacob M, Paul O, Mehringer L, et al. Albumin augmentation improves condition of guinea pig hearts after 4 hr of cold ischemia. *Transplantation*. 2009;**87**:956–65.

77. Kozar RA, Peng Z, Zhang R, et al. Plasma restoration of endothelial glycocalyx in a rodent model of hemorrhagic shock. *Anesth Analg*. 2011;**112**:1289–95.

78. Dawidson IJ, Sandor ZF, Coorpender J, et al. Intraoperative albumin administration affects the outcome of cadaver renal transplantation. *Transplantation*. 1992;**53**:774–82.

79. Pockaj BA, Yang JC, Lotze MT, et al. A prospective randomized trial evaluating colloid versus crystalloid resuscitation in the treatment of the vascular leak syndrome associated with interleukin-2 therapy. *J Immunother Tumor Immunol*. 1994;**15**:22–8.

80. Stevens AP, Hlady V, Dull RO. Fluorescence correlation spectroscopy can probe albumin dynamics inside lung endothelial glycocalyx. *Am J Physiol Lung Cell Mol Physiol*. 2007;**293**:L328–35.

81. Wiedermann CJ, Joannidis M. Nephroprotective potential of human albumin infusion: a narrative review. *Gastroenterol Res Pract*. 2015;**2015**:912839.

82. Finfer S. Reappraising the role of albumin for resuscitation. Curr Opin Crit Care. 2013;**19**:315–20.

83. The SAFE Study Investigators. Saline or albumin for fluid resuscitation in patients with traumatic brain injury. *N Engl J Med*. 2007;**357**:874–84.

84. Caironi P, Tognoni G, Masson S, et al., Albumin replacement in patients with severe sepsis or septic shock. *N Engl J Med*. 2014;**370**:1412–21.

85. Patel A, Laffan MA, Waheed U, Brett SJ. Randomised trials of human albumin for adults with sepsis: systematic review and meta-analysis with trial sequential analysis of all-cause mortality. *BMJ*. 2014;**349**: g4561.

86. Schumann R, Mandell S, Michaels MD, Klinck J, Walia A. Intraoperative fluid and pharmacologic management and the anesthesiologist's supervisory role for nontraditional technologies during liver transplantation: a survey of US academic centers. *Transplant Proc*. 2013;**45**:2258–62.

87. Raghunathan K, Shaw A, Nathanson B, et al. Association between the choice of IV crystalloid and in-hospital mortality among critically ill adults with sepsis. *Crit Care Med*. 2014;**42**:1585–91.

88. Shaw AD, Perner SM, Goldstein SL, et al. Major complications, mortality, and resource utilization after open abdominal surgery: 0.9% saline compared to Plasma-Lyte. *Ann Surg*. 2012;**255**:821–9.

89. Weinberg L, Li M, Churilov L, et al. Associations of fluid amount, type, and balance and acute kidney injury in patients undergoing major surgery. *Anaesth Intensive Care*. 2018;**46**:79–87.

90. Young P, Bailey M, Beasley R, et al. Effect of a buffered crystalloid solution vs saline on acute kidney injury among patients in the intensive care unit: the SPLIT randomized clinical trial. *JAMA*. 2015;**314**:1701–10.

91. Semler MW, Wanderer JP, Ehrenfeld JM, et al.; SALT Investigators and the Pragmatic Critical Care Research Group; SALT Investigators. Balanced crystalloids versus saline in the intensive care unit. The SALT Randomized Trial. *Am J Respir Crit Care Med*. 2017;**195**:1362–72.

92. Self WH, Semler MW, Wanderer JP, et al. Balanced crystalloids versus saline in noncritically ill adults. *New Eng J Med*. 2018;**378**:819–28.

93. Semler MW, Self WH, Wanderer JP, et al. Balanced crystalloids versus saline in critically ill adults. *New Eng J Med*. 2018;**378**:829–39.

94. Zayed YZM, Aburahma AMY, Barbarawi MO, et al. Balanced crystalloids versus isotonic saline in critically ill patients: systematic review and meta-analysis. *J Intensive Care*. 2018;**6**:51.

95. McIlroy D, Murphy D, Kasza J, et al. Effects of restricting perioperative use of intravenous chloride on kidney injury in patients undergoing cardiac surgery: the LICRA pragmatic controlled clinical trial. *Intensive Care Med*. 2017;**43**:795–806.

96. Maheshwari K, Turan A, Makarova N, et al. Saline versus lactated Ringer's solution. The saline or lactated Ringer's (SOLAR) trial. *Anesthesiology*. 2020;**132**:614–24.

97. Weinberg L, Collins MG, Peyton P. Urine the right direction: the consensus statement from the Committee on Transplant Anesthesia of the American Society of Anesthesiologists on fluid management during kidney transplantation. *Transplantation*. 2021 **105**:1655–7.

98. Wagener G, Bezinover D, Wang C, et al. Fluid management during kidney transplantation: a consensus statement of the Committee on Transplant Anesthesia of the American Society of Anesthesiologists. *Transplantation*. 2021;**105**:1677–84.

99. Wan S, Roberts MA, Mount P. Normal saline versus lower-chloride solutions for kidney transplantation. *Cochrane Database Syst Rev*. 2016;**8**:CD010741.

100. O'Malley CM, Frumento RJ, Hardy MA, et al. A randomized, double-blind comparison of lactated Ringer's solution and 0.9% NaCl during renal transplantation. *Anesth Analg*. 2005;**100**:1518–24.

101. Hadimioglu N, Saadawy I, Saglam T, et al. The effect of different crystalloid solutions on acid-base balance and early kidney function after kidney transplantation. *Anesth Analg*. 2008;**107**:264–9.

102. Khajavi MR, Etezadi F, Moharari RS, et al. Effects of normal saline vs. lactated ringer's during renal transplantation. *Ren Fail*. 2008;**30**:535–9.

103. Kim SY, Huh KH, Lee JR, et al. Comparison of the effects of normal saline versus Plasmalyte on acid-base balance during living donor kidney transplantation using the Stewart and base excess methods. *Transplant Proc*. 2013;**45**:2191–6.

104. Potura E, Lindner G, Biesenbach P, et al. An acetate-buffered balanced crystalloid versus 0.9% saline in patients with end-stage renal disease undergoing cadaveric renal transplantation: a prospective randomized controlled trial. *Anesth Analg*. 2015;**120**:123–9.

105. Modi MP, Vora KS, Parikh GP, et al. A comparative study of impact of infusion of Ringer's Lactate solution versus normal saline on acid-base balance and serum electrolytes during live related renal transplantation. *Saudi J Kidney Dis Transpl*. 2012;**23**:135–7.

106. Weinberg L, Harris L, Bellomo R, et al. Effects of intraoperative and early postoperative normal saline or Plasma-Lyte 148® on hyperkalaemia in deceased donor renal transplantation: a double-blind randomized trial. *Br J Anaesth*. 2017;**119**:606–15.

107. Arslantas R, Dogu Z, Cevik BE. Normal saline versus balanced crystalloid solutions for kidney transplantation. *Transplant Proc.* 2019;**51**:2262–4.

108. Collins MG, Fahim MA, Pascoe EM, et al.; BEST-Fluids Investigators and the Australasian Kidney Trials Network. Balanced crystalloid solution versus saline in increased donor kidney transplantation (BEST-Fluids): a pragmatic double-blind, randomised, controlled trial. *Lancet.* 2023;**402**:105–17.

109. Schnuelle P, Johannes van der Woude F. Perioperative fluid management in renal transplantation: a narrative review of the literature. *Transpl Int.* 2006;**19**:947–59.

110. Legendre C, Thervet E, Page B, et al. Hydroxyethylstarch and osmotic-nephrosis-like lesions in kidney transplantation. *Lancet.* 1993;**342**:248–9.

111. Cittanova ML, Leblanc I, Legendre C, et al. Effect of hydroxyethylstarch in brain-dead kidney donors on renal function in kidney-transplant recipients. *Lancet.* 1996;**348**:1620.

112. Bernard C, Alain M, Simone C, et al. Hydroxyethylstarch and osmotic nephrosis-like lesions in kidney transplants. *Lancet.* 1996;**348**:1595.

113. Baron JF. Adverse effects of colloids on renal function. In JL Vincent (ed.), *Yearbook of Intensive Care and Emergency Medicine.* Berlin: Springer; 2000: 486–93.

114. Patel MS, Niemann CU, Sally MB, et al. The impact of hydroxyethyl starch use in deceased organ donors on the development of delayed graft function in kidney transplant recipients: a propensity-adjusted analysis. *Am J Transplant.* 2015;**15**:2152–8.

Fluid and Hemodynamic Monitoring in Burns

Emmanuel Dudoignon, François Depret, Benjamin Deniau and Matthieu Legrand

Severe burn injury induces an early and profound hypovolemia, followed rapidly by systemic inflammatory response syndrome (SIRS), resulting in a distributive shock.[1] Hemodynamic management is the cornerstone of early resuscitation for severely burned patients, since both under- or over-resuscitation may worsen a patient's outcome.[2] Therefore, the aim of this chapter is to provide a pathophysiological approach to the hemodynamic consequences of severe burn injuries and to use the available evidence-based strategies for initial hemodynamic management.

Cardiovascular Consequences of Severe Burn Injury

Burn Edema

To understand the pathogenesis of burn-related edema, one must remember the two main factors involved: (1) the conventional Starling law and (2) the glycocalyx. The SIRS induced by the burned tissues and the burn increase vascular permeability, allowing albumin to diffuse from the intravascular to the extravascular compartment, leading to a decrease in intravascular oncotic pressure. The endothelial glycocalyx, one of the main factors involved in vascular integrity,[3] is a 0.2 μm to 2 μm thick layer composed of proteoglycans (the backbone of glycocalyx) and sulfated glycosaminoglycans. Under normal conditions, glycocalyx is permeable to small molecules and restricts larger molecules like albumin. Therefore, the oncotic gradient pressure is set between glycocalyx and the plasma and not between the plasma and the extravascular space as historically proposed by the Starling equation. In many pathological situations (e.g., burn injury, sepsis, trauma, hemorrhagic shock), glycocalyx is impaired, leading to fluid and albumin leakage into the interstitial compartment.[3] Glycocalyx shedding can be assessed by dosing plasmatic syndecan-1. In a small cohort including 39 severely burned patients, Osuka et al. observed that syndecan-1 was associated with increased fluid requirement ($P = 0.04$) even after adjustment.[4] Whether strategies aiming at protecting glycocalyx during burn resuscitation would improve patient outcome remains to be explored.

Burn Shock

Severe burn injuries initially lead to a characteristic hypovolemic shock state with a profound hypovolemia secondary to increased vascular permeability and a systemic and pulmonary vasoconstriction (related to hemolysis and endogenous catecholamine release). All of this results in a low cardiac output (CO) and low oxygen transportation.[1] Therefore, within 24 to 48 hours, the patient will develop a hyperdynamic and vasoplegic shock state

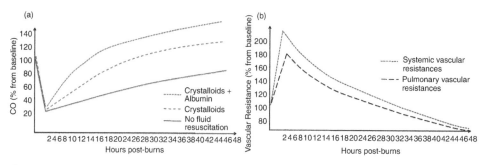

Figure 21.1 Trends of (a) cardiac output and (b) systemic vascular resistance after burn injury without and with fluid resuscitation, from [17].

characterized by a high CO, an increase in oxygen transportation and decreased systemic and pulmonary vascular resistances [5] (Fig. 21.1). This pattern appears earlier and with a higher CO with fluid resuscitation.[1]

Burn-Associated Cardiac Injury

A cardiac dysfunction can be observed after severe burn injury, including systolic left ventricular dysfunction and decreased diastolic performances (i.e., slowed isovolemic relaxation and decreased diastolic compliance).[6,7] Furthermore, acute respiratory syndrome secondary to burn injury and/or smoke inhalation can be responsible for an increased arterial pulmonary pressure leading to a right ventricular failure.[8] Therefore, we suggest assessing the cardiac function of a severely burned patient using echocardiography and to reassess this function during the course of management in patients with hemodynamic instability.

Burn and Microcirculation

Microcirculatory disorders in severely burned patients have been described both in injured and non-injured tissue. In one observational study, these disorders have been found to be associated with organ failure and poor outcome in severely burned patients.[9] Pathophysiology of microcirculatory disorders implies tissue edema, intravascular disseminated coagulation and altered erythrocyte deformability.[10] To date, microcirculation monitoring in burn patients remains in the field of research.

Risks Associated with Under- and Over-Resuscitation in Severely Burned Patients

The goal of fluid resuscitation in the early management of severely burned patients is to prevent under-resuscitation that would lead to organ hypoperfusion and damage [e.g., acute kidney injury (AKI), mesenteric ischemia], avoiding over-resuscitation, which is associated with the risk of acute respiratory distress syndrome (ARDS), acute abdominal compartment syndrome (ACS) and AKI. Larger volumes of fluid have been associated with respiratory failure in both pediatric and adults burn patients.[11,12] Hypervolemia promotes fluid leakage into the interstitial space due to alteration of glycocalyx, increasing vascular permeability and increasing distance of diffusion of oxygen from erythrocytes to organ cells.[13] Hypervolemia can also lead to increased venous pressures, leading to organ venous congestion and altered perfusion.

Hemodynamic Targets in Early Resuscitation of Critically Ill Burn Patients

Formulas have been commonly used to predict the required crystalloid volumes. The most familiar is the Parkland formula, which has long been considered the most accurate. However, if it can be used as a rough estimate the Parkland formula has been shown to be poorly accurate to guide fluid resuscitation for several reasons. First, this formula has been developed in the general population and does not take into account interindividual variability related to different host responses to burn injury, age and comorbidities. Second, many factors associated with the burn can influence the volume of fluid required, such has the depth of the burn injury, the presence of smoke inhalation, early escharotomy or fasciotomy and burn mechanism. Finally, in the early stage of management, it can be challenging to estimate the total body burn surface area or the weight of the patient, leading to errors in the volume of crystalloid required.

The Parkland formula can be used to estimate the initial crystalloid flow rate; it should be secondarily adjusted according to therapeutic targets and responses to treatment. In a retrospective study including 40 critically ill burn patients, low stroke volume and cardiac index at admission were independently associated with 90 days' mortality.[14] Of note, mean arterial pressure and/or urine output (UO) values can be misleading to guide fluid resuscitation.[15] Mean arterial pressure can remain normal despite severe hypovolemia given intense increased systemic vascular resistances (Fig. 21.1). Urine output can be influenced by intrarenal causes of AKI such as hemolysis, rhabdomyolysis and oxaluria (in case of hydroxocobalamin administration). Furthermore, in cases of over-resuscitation compartment abdominal syndrome, venous congestion can be observed leading to oliguria. Taken altogether, persistent oliguria despite fluid resuscitation should always lead to further investigation to assess systemic hemodynamics (e.g., echocardiography, venous Doppler). Systematically increasingly crystalloids in cases of persistent oliguria would lead to fluid overload and its deleterious effects (e.g., ACS, ARDS, AKI).[16]

Goal-Directed Resuscitation Therapy

Goal-directed fluid therapy based on advanced hemodynamic targets can be used to tailor resuscitation in burn patients.[10,17] Many biomarkers have been found to be associated with poor outcome in severely burned patients (e.g., serum lactate, base deficit, stroke volume or oxygen delivery). However, only a few randomized-controlled trials (RCTs) have assessed the utility of a goal-directed fluid therapy compared with a fluid resuscitation. In a prospective study including 30 severely burned patients, Aboelatta and Abdelsalam compared a resuscitation strategy guided by transpulmonary thermodilution technique (TTT) with a resuscitation following the Parkland formula [18] and observed high volume of fluids using TTT. Similarly, Holm et al. observed that a resuscitation guided by TTT using static targets [i.e., intrathoracic blood volume index above 800 ml/m^2 and cardiac index (CI) above 3.5 l/min/m^2] was associated with an increased volume of crystalloid compared with the Parkland formula [19] with a higher UO and lower serum creatinine. Due to the small sample size, the investigators did not observe differences between groups concerning stronger outcomes

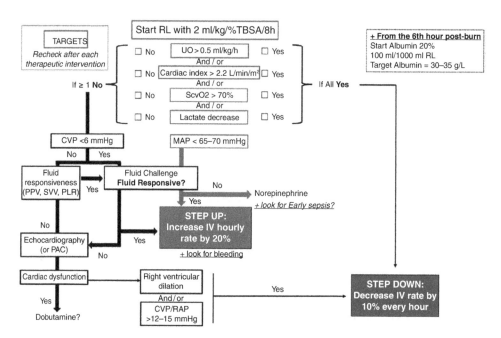

Figure 21.2 Proposed Saint Louis Hospital algorithm for hemodynamic management in severely burn patients, from [17]. CVP, central venous pressure; MAP, mean arterial pressure; PAC, pulmonary artery catheter; PLR, passive leg raising; PPV, pulse pressure variation; RAP, right arterial pressure; RL, Ringer's lactate; ScvO$_2$, central venous oximetry; SVV, stroke volume variation; TBSA, total body surface area; UO, urinary output.

[e.g., mortality, intensive care unit (ICU) length of stay]. In a monocenter prospective study, Csontos et al. compared a resuscitation strategy guided by TTT with UO-guided resuscitation. Multiple organ dysfunction score was significantly higher in the UO-guided group at 48 and 72 hours.[20] When using dynamic parameters such as pulse pressure variation (PPV), Tokarik et al. observed a decreased volume of fluid administered.[21] In our center, we combine static and dynamic biomarkers to adjust fluid volumes administration (Fig. 21.2).

Types of Fluids

Crystalloid Solutions

Balanced crystalloids are the most commonly used fluid in severely burned patients. Pathophysiological and clinical evidence suggests that a large amount of saline would lead to hyperchloremic metabolic acidosis and AKI (i.e., through vasoconstriction of the afferent glomerular artery). Meta-analyses in non-burned critically ill patients show better survival with balanced crystalloids compared with saline in terms of outcome.[22,23] Due to the large amount of crystalloid in the first 24–48 hours of hemodynamic resuscitation in severely burned patients, balanced crystalloids are the preferred resuscitation solution. In a single-center randomized trial, fluid resuscitation with severely ill burned patients using Ringer's lactate or Plasma-Lyte did not lead to significant differences in acid–base status, but Plasma–Lyte was associated with more hypocalcemia, likely due to the chelation of ionized calcium with gluconate.[24]

Colloid Solutions

The use of albumin in severely burned patients is controversial. The increase of capillary permeability leads to a passage of large molecules in the interstitial compartment. Endothelial dysfunction assessed by using the albumin/creatinine ratio was highest 2 hours after the burn injury.[25] There is no available RCT addressing the question of the impact of albumin resuscitation on outcomes in burn patients. However, in a meta-analysis published in 2017, after exclusion of studies at high risk of bias, albumin use was associated with a reduced mortality and a decrease in the occurrence of ACS.[26] In an observational study performed in North America,[27] authors prospectively assessed the use of albumin in severely burned adult patients [i.e., age above 18 years and total body surface area (TBSA) burned above 20%]. In this study, two-thirds of patients received albumin. Total fluid volume was higher in patients receiving albumin when compared with patients receiving crystalloid (5.2 ± 2.3 vs. 3.7 ± 1.7 mL/kg/% TBSA burn/24 hr). Of note, patients in the albumin group were older, had larger burns, higher admission Sequential Organ Failure Assessment (SOFA) scores and more inhalation injury. This study suggests wide variabilities in terms of albumin administration between centers. In our algorithm we propose the use of albumin from 6 hours after the burn injury with a target of albumin plasmatic level between 30 and 35 g/L. Whether albumin perfusion improves a severely burned patient's outcome should be assessed in a well-conducted, international RCT.

Catecholamine Use in Early Burn Shock

Data concerning the choice of catecholamine in severely burned patients are limited. Norepinephrine is often required during the "distributive phase" (i.e., after 12 to 36 hr post-injury). However, a rapid increase in norepinephrine doses in a severely burned patient should prompt a search for a cause such as an early sepsis, a bleeding or a cardiac dysfunction.

Adjunctive Therapies

As in septic shock, in a small RCT, use of low-dose hydrocortisone has been found to be associated with a reduced duration of norepinephrine without making a difference in strong outcome (i.e., mortality). Therefore, this possible benefit has to be counterbalanced with the potential immunosuppressive effect and the increased risk of infection.[28]

Due to its antioxidant properties, ascorbic acid administered in high doses (66 mg/kg/h) during the first 24 hours post-burn has been proposed and associated with a significant reduction of fluid volume requirements (5.5 vs. 3.0 ml/kg/% TBSA, $P < 0.01$).[29] However, this work was a monocentric and unblinded study. In 2019, Nakajima ct al. performed a retrospective study using a propensity score to evaluate the effect of ascorbic acid in severely burned patients.[30] This study suggests that when administered above 10 g within 2 days of patient admission, vitamin C is associated with a reduced in-hospital mortality (risk ratio, 0.79; 95% confidence interval, 0.66–0.95; $p = 0.006$); however, when higher dosage was used (>24 g threshold), this benefit was not observed (risk ratio, 0.83; 95% confidence interval, 0.68–1.02; $p = 0.068$). Therefore, this retrospective study suggests administering between 10 and 24 g of vitamin C within 2 days of admission. These data require confirmation in a dedicated RCT.

Conclusions

Fluid resuscitation using balanced crystalloids and albumin remains the cornerstone of hemodynamic resuscitation of severely ill burn patients. This initial resuscitation is challenging with the risk of under- and over-resuscitation justifying an invasive hemodynamic monitoring. However, many knowledge gaps remain to be filled regarding the role of albumin, hemodynamic targets, adjuvant therapy (i.e., ascorbic acid), type of vasopressor and their impact on outcome.

References

1. Asch MJ, Feldman RJ, Walker HL, et al. Systemic and pulmonary hemodynamic changes accompanying thermal injury. Ann Surg. 1973;**178**:218. https://doi.org/10.1097/00000658-197308000-00020

2. Mason SA, Nathens AB, Finnerty CC, et al. Hold the pendulum: rates of acute kidney injury are increased in patients who receive resuscitation volumes less than predicted by the Parkland equation. Ann Surg. 2016;**264**:1142–7. https://doi.org/10.1097/SLA.0000000000001615

3. Kottke MA, Walters TJ. Where's the leak in vascular barriers? A review. Shock. 2016;**46**:20–36. https://doi.org/10.1097/SHK.0000000000000666

4. Osuka A, Kusuki H, Yoneda K, et al. Glycocalyx shedding is enhanced by age and correlates with increased fluid requirement in patients with major burns. Shock. 2018;**50**:60–5. https://doi.org/10.1097/SHK.0000000000001028

5. Holm C, Melcer B, Hörbrand F, et al. Haemodynamic and oxygen transport responses in survivors and non-survivors following thermal injury. Burns. 2000;**26**:25–33. https://doi.org/10.1016/S0305-4179(99)00095-9

6. Abu-Sittah GS, Sarhane KA, Dibo SA, Ibrahim A. Cardiovascular dysfunction in burns: review of the literature. Ann Burns Fire Disasters. 2012;**25**:26–37

7. Tapking C, Popp D, Herndon DN, et al. Cardiac dysfunction in severely burned patients: current understanding of etiology, pathophysiology, and treatment. Shock. 2020;**53**:669–78. https://doi.org/10.1097/SHK.0000000000001465

8. Maybauer MO, Asmussen S, Platts DG, et al. Transesophageal echocardiography in the management of burn patients. Burns. 2014;**40**:630–5. https://doi.org/10.1016/j.burns.2013.08.032

9. Lorente JA, Ezpeleta A, Esteban A, et al. Systemic hemodynamics, gastric intramucosal PCO2 changes, and outcome in critically ill burn patients. Crit Care Med. 2000;**28**:1728–35

10. Soussi S, Legrand M. Hemodynamic coherence in patients with burns. Best Pract Res Clin Anaesthesiol. 2016;**30**:437–43. https://doi.org/10.1016/j.bpa.2016.10.004

11. Blot S, Hoste E, Colardyn F. Acute respiratory failure that complicates the resuscitation of pediatric patients with scald injuries. J Burn Care Rehabil. 2000;**21**:289–90

12. Klein MB, Hayden D, Elson C, et al. The association between fluid administration and outcome following major burn: a multicenter study. Ann. Surg. 2007;**245**:622–8. https://doi.org/10.1097/01.sla.0000252572.50684.49

13. Jedlicka J, Becker BF, Chappell D. Endothelial glycocalyx. Crit Care Clin, 2020;**36**:217–32. https://doi.org/10.1016/j.ccc.2019.12.007

14. Soussi S, Deniau B, Ferry A, et al. Low cardiac index and stroke volume on admission are associated with poor outcome in critically ill burn patients: a retrospective cohort study. Ann Intensive Care. 2016;**6**:87. https://doi.org/10.1186/s13613-016-0192-y

15. Dries DJ, Waxman K. Adequate resuscitation of burn patients may not be

measured by urine output and vital signs. *Crit Care Med.* 1991;**19**:327–9. https://doi.org/10.1097/00003246-199103000-00007

16. Derkenne C, Prunet B. Letter to the Editor re: Greeenhaigh, "Management of Burns." *N Engl J Med.* 2019;**381**:1188–9. https://doi.org/10.1056/NEJMc1909342

17. Soussi S, Dépret F, Benyamina M, Legrand M. Early hemodynamic management of critically ill burn patients, *Anesthesiology.* 2018;**129**:583–9. https://doi.org/10.1097/ALN.0000000000002314

18. Aboelatta Y, Abdelsalam A. volume overload of fluid resuscitation in acutely burned patients using transpulmonary thermodilution technique. *J Burn Care Res.* 2013;**34**:349–54. https://doi.org/10.1097/BCR.0b013e3182642b32

19. Holm C, Mayr M, Tegeler J, et al. A clinical randomized study on the effects of invasive monitoring on burn shock resuscitation. *Burns.* 2004;**30**:798–807. https://doi.org/10.1016/j.burns.2004.06.016

20. Csontos C, Foldi V, Fischer T, Bogar L. Arterial thermodilution in burn patients suggests a more rapid fluid administration during early resuscitation: fluid resuscitation after burn injury. *Acta Anaesthesiol Scand.* 2008;**52**:742–9. https://doi.org/10.1111/j.1399-6576.2008.01658.x

21. Tokarik M, Sjöberg F, Balik M, et al. Fluid therapy LiDCO controlled trial – optimization of volume resuscitation of extensively burned patients through noninvasive continuous real-time hemodynamic monitoring LiDCO. *J Burn Care Res.* 2013;**34**:537–42. https://doi.org/10.1097/BCR.0b013e318278197e

22. Hammond NE, Zampieri FG, Tanna GLD, et al. Balanced crystalloids versus saline in critically ill adults: a systematic review with meta-analysis. *NEJM Evid.* 2022;**1**. https://doi.org/10.1056/EVIDoa2100010

23. Zwager CL, Tuinman PR, de Grooth H-J, et al. Why physiology will continue to guide the choice between balanced crystalloids and normal saline: a systematic review and meta-analysis. *Crit Care,* 2019;**23**:366. https://doi.org/10.1186/s13054-019-2658-4

24. Chaussard M, Dépret F, Saint-Aubin O, et al. Physiological response to fluid resuscitation with Ringer lactate versus Plasmalyte in critically ill burn patients. *J Appl Physiol.1985).* 2020;**128**:709–14. https://doi.org/10.1152/japplphysiol.00859.2019

25. Vlachou E, Gosling P, Moiemen NS. Microalbuminuria: a marker of endothelial dysfunction in thermal injury. *Burns.* 2006;**32**:1009–16. https://doi.org/10.1016/j.burns.2006.02.019

26. Eljaiek R, Heylbroeck C, Dubois M-J. Albumin administration for fluid resuscitation in burn patients: a systematic review and meta-analysis. *Burns.* 2017;**43**:17–24. https://doi.org/10.1016/j.burns.2016.08.001

27. Greenhalgh DG, Cartotto R, Taylor SL, et al. Burn resuscitation practices in North America: results of the Acute Burn ResUscitation Multicenter Prospective Trial (ABRUPT). *Ann Surg.* 2023;**277**:512–19. https://doi.org/10.1097/SLA.0000000000005166

28. Venet F, Plassais J, Textoris J, et al. Low-dose hydrocortisone reduces norepinephrine duration in severe burn patients: a randomized clinical trial. *Crit Care.* 2015;**19**:21. https://doi.org/10.1186/s13054-015-0740-0

29. Tanaka H. Reduction of resuscitation fluid volumes in severely burned patients using ascorbic acid administration: a randomized, prospective study. *Arch Surg.* 2000;**135**:326. https://doi.org/10.1001/archsurg.135.3.326

30. Nakajima M, Kojiro M, Aso S, et al. Effect of high-dose vitamin C therapy on severe burn patients: a nationwide cohort study. *Crit Care.* 2019;**23**:407. https://doi.org/10.1186/s13054-019-2693-1

Chapter

22

Optimizing Hemodynamic Therapy by Monitoring Microcirculation: One Step Forward in Matching Tissue Oxygen Delivery to Consumption

Sean Coeckelenbergh, Hiromi Kato, Salima Naili and Jacques Duranteau

Goal-Directed Hemodynamic Therapy and Microcirculation

Hemodynamic resuscitation ultimately aims to optimize organ microcirculation and tissue oxygenation. The microcirculation regulates blood flow and oxygen transport, in close synergy with the macrocirculation, by matching oxygen delivery to demand. Arteriolar tone, blood viscosity, microvascular endothelium, red blood cells, and the glycocalyx are central regulatory factors. Goal-directed hemodynamic therapy is used throughout the world during moderate- to high-risk surgery. This approach focuses mainly on macrovascular parameters (e.g., blood pressure, stroke volume, arterial oxygen transport, dynamic preload-dependent parameters). During normal physiological conditions, changes in macrocirculation usually lead to concomitant changes in microcirculation. During surgery, however, alterations in macrocirculation to microcirculation coupling can occur. Inflammation from surgical stress, the occurrence of hemorrhagic shock, and hemodynamic therapies (e.g., fluids, transfusion, and vasopressors) all affect microvascular flow and arterial oxygen transport to tissues.

Due to this potential uncoupling during surgery in the absence of microvascular monitoring, it is difficult to determine whether optimized macrocirculation corresponds to optimal tissue perfusion. With the exception of a few surrogate markers of oxygen delivery to consumption mismatching, such as arterial lactate, which increases after the start of anaerobic metabolism, contemporary goal-directed therapy protocols continue to focus almost exclusively on macrocirculatory criteria. Current strategies thus largely ignore early alterations in microcirculation that may cause tissue hypoperfusion and organ damage during the postoperative period. An important gap in hemodynamic optimization still exists, and future studies need to elucidate the potential of different approaches to assess tissue perfusion. Several novel surrogate markers are available today, but direct visualization of capillaries is also possible. Hand-held vital microscopes offer a window to microcirculation monitoring, most notably by analyzing the mucosa under the tongue. This perspective provides information on the flow of erythrocytes in capillaries, the density of capillaries, and the heterogeneity of microvascular perfusion. In addition, these techniques can be used to observe the behavior of leukocytes and indirectly assess the integrity of the glycocalyx.

The aim of this chapter is to offer a brief overview of important and novel ways to measure tissue oxygen delivery, the potential matching of this delivery with tissue oxygen consumption, and how to integrate these tools into care packages for treating patients undergoing surgery.

Monitoring of Microcirculation during Surgery

The clinical implications of coupling microvascular and macrovascular physiology remains a challenge in contemporary medicine. Many studies have investigated the potential of maximizing oxygen delivery to consumption ratio with the hopes of improving patient outcome.[1–3] However, when applying a goal-directed strategy, it is indispensable to have those goals made clear. Macrovascular goals, such as a specific value for blood pressure, stroke volume, or a dynamic indicator of fluid responsiveness (e.g., stroke volume variation), are simple to measure and assess continuously. Microvascular goals, on the other hand, are more difficult due to the complexity of truly measuring the microcirculation's capacity to deliver oxygen for the tissues' needs despite several surrogate measures being easily available during surgery. Some, such as arterial lactate, have become part of standard care protocols, while others, such as the veno-arterial difference in the partial pressure of carbon dioxide ($Pv\text{-}aCO_2$ gap), show potential but have yet to be implemented into goal-directed hemodynamic protocols at a large scale. Studying microvascular flow allows immediate assessment of capillary perfusion (e.g., sublingual microcirculation monitoring) and may become a powerful new tool for hemodynamic optimization.

Lactate

Measuring arterial lactate in patients suffering from hemodynamic instability and shock, including surgery, is today considered standard care.[4] Increases in lactate concentration often correlate to tissue hypoxia, but other causes exist. For example, liver failure and metformin toxicity can both lead to increased lactate through non-hypoxic causes.[5] In addition to lactate's limited specificity, decreases in lactate are relatively slow (i.e., several hours), which also restricts its use when evaluating acute events (e.g., immediate effects of fluid challenges or transfusions). Nonetheless, lactate concentration and assessing its evolution over hours are extremely useful.[6]

A lactate value above 1.5 meq L^{-1} is considered abnormal and may even indicate the start of shock.[4] However, since hyperlactatemia is not specific to tissue hypoxia, other tools, such as direct analysis of sublingual microcirculation, may help rule out non-ischemic causes. Furthermore, hyperlactatemia as a consequence of poor tissue oxygenation only appears after anaerobic metabolism has occurred. In other words, it is not an early, but rather a delayed indicator of poor oxygen delivery to consumption matching.

Respiratory Exchange Ratio

The respiratory exchange ratio (RER) has recently been shown to be of considerable interest during abdominal surgery. The RER provides a continuous measure of anaerobic metabolism in mechanically ventilated patients using values derived from the standard anesthesia machine gas analyzer. By applying a simple formula $-RER = (FeCO_2 - FiCO_2) / (FiO_2 - FeO_2)$ – one can easily measure this surrogate of oxygen distribution to consumption matching. Values above 0.9 should be a warning of potential mismatching and values above 1 are considered pathological. These variables can thus be easily measured in any patient receiving mechanical ventilation. In both laparoscopic and open abdominal surgery, the RER has been shown to predict postoperative complications.[7] Elevated values have also been shown to correlate with increased lactate at the end of surgery.[8] In patients undergoing liver transplantation, the RER predicted postoperative complications with higher sensitivity and specificity than other surrogates of tissue perfusion, such as SvO_2, Pv-aCO_2 gap, and lactate.[9] This marker, which has been only recently introduced into clinical practice, is thus a potentially useful tool to determine whether hyperlactatemia is present in the absence of an arterial line. Furthermore, if hyperlactatemia is present, it may help to determine whether the cause is due to hypoxia or another cause of increased lactate.

Veno-Arterial Difference in the Partial Pressure of Carbon Dioxide

The Pv-aCO_2 gap, which is measured by subtracting the venous partial pressure of CO_2 by the arterial partial pressure of CO_2, is another potential surrogate marker of tissue perfusion and oxygenation.[10] A growing amount of evidence has shown its interest when shock is suspected as it increases exponentially with decreasing cardiac output. It is thus extremely useful in tracking low cardiac output states. Furthermore, increased Pv-aCO_2 gap at the end of surgery in high-risk patients has been shown to correlate with increased complications. [11] This indicates a potential for this measurement to be part of a goal-directed hemo-dynamic therapy package. Future studies will determine whether its implementation can improve patient outcome.

Sublingual Microcirculation

Hand-held vital microscope studies have largely focused on the sublingual surface because it is an easily accessible zone for visualizing mucosal microcirculation. These orthogonal polarization spectral imaging and sidestream dark field imaging microscopes can visualize mucosal capillaries in real time.[12,13] The live videos directly visualize the density of perfused capillaries, which corresponds to diffusive transport of oxygen (also referred to as functional capillary density) and the flow of red blood cells through the capillaries, which represents the convective transport of oxygen. The emitted light, corresponding to the wavelength of hemoglobin absorption, displays each erythrocyte in black on a light back-ground. The greatest care has to be taken to avoid pressure artifacts, however, as pressure can distort flow.[13] Several scores arc used today to offer a systematic way of measuring microcirculation. The most common are:

1. The microvascular flow index: a qualitative evaluation of the microvascular flow where the image is divided into four quadrants, and the predominant type of flow in very small vessels (i.e., diameter less than 20 μm) is assessed in each quadrant using a scale from 0 to 3 score (0 = no flow, 1 = intermittent flow, 2 = sluggish flow, 3 = normal flow). The overall score is the sum of each quadrant score divided by the number of quadrants.
2. The percentage of perfused vessels: equals 100 × (total number of vessels – [no flow + intermittent flow])/total number of vessels.
3. The perfused vessel density (also known as functional capillary density): equals the area of perfused vessels divided by the total area of interest.
4. The heterogeneity index: equals the highest site microvascular flow index – lowest site microvascular flow index divided by the mean of the microvascular flow index of all sublingual sites.

Current Evidence for Perioperative Sublingual Microcirculation Monitoring

Several studies have analyzed how sublingual microcirculation evolves during and after surgery. Since sublingual mucosa is easily accessible, it offers an ideal location for a hand-held vital microscope to measure qualitative microvascular flow and quantitative microcirculatory functional parameters, including functional capillary density and red blood cell velocity. During abdominal surgery, Bouattour et al. [14] found that preload dependence identified by variation in pulse pressure was associated with decreased convective and diffusive microcirculatory capacity. These parameters were restored by a fluid bolus. This study suggests that microcirculatory parameters derived from hand-held vital microscopy (HVM) could be additional non-invasive indices of preload dependence that could serve as strong adjuncts to the classical indices of preload dependence. This tool is thus of particular interest when administering fluids, especially when no invasive monitoring is available or if hemodynamic monitors are limited by specific situations, such as protective ventilation, arrhythmia (e.g., atrial fibrillation), or vasopressor administration.

Studies on microcirculation during surgery have conflicting results. Some found maintained microcirculation,[15,16] whereas others found microvascular alterations.[17,18] This impact depends on the severity of the surgical procedure in terms of inflammation, blood loss, patient history, and macrovascular optimization. Postoperative alterations are also important to consider. Recently, Flick et al. [15] found that microcirculatory tissue perfusion is preserved during noncardiac surgery (120 elective non-cardiac surgery patients, major abdominal, orthopedic or trauma and minor urologic surgery) when macrocirculatory hemodynamics are maintained. On the other hand, in high-risk surgery, alterations of the microcirculation may persist postoperatively despite macrocirculatory optimization. [18,19] For example, Greenwood et al. [18] found persistent microvascular alterations in postoperative elective cardiac surgery requiring cardiopulmonary bypass, which was linked to organ failure. During major liver resection, Uz et al. [20] reported that a decrease in sublingual microvascular flow and in the proportion of perfused sublingual microvessels 24 hours after surgery was associated with glycocalyx degradation (Syndecan-1 levels as a parameter of glycocalyx degradation) and an increase in sublingual rolling leukocyte count despite macrovascular optimization. This underlines the fact that optimization of the macrocirculation is not always sufficient for intra- and postoperative microcirculatory optimization. Moreover, macrocirculatory optimization may differ depending on the surgery, the patient's history, and the team's practices.

Future studies need to validate protocols that either maintain macro- to microvascular coupling or detect uncoupling early. This is all the more true as we observe a modification of practices with a more liberal use of vasopressors at the expense of fluid administration during surgery, which can potentially cause organ damage and in particular that of the kidney.[21] There is a theoretical rationale for caution, as decreased fluids and increased vasopressors may actually decrease flow to tissues, but initial studies on more liberal vasopressors and microcirculation seem to be reassuring. For example, when Flick et al. used, during radical prostatectomy, a low-volume strategy associated with the administration of vasopressors until removal of prostate,[22] sublingual microcirculation was preserved. Furthermore, knowledge of the state of the microcirculation may lead to the discontinuation of macrovascular maximization. Indeed, if an already optimized microcirculation is targeted, it is possible that macrocirculatory maximization is useless or even potentially harmful due to excessive use of fluids and/or vasopressors.[23]

A Practical Approach to Integrating Microcirculation into Hemodynamic Management

The current state of evidence thus points to the possibility that macrocirculation optimization may not be sufficient during surgery. This is especially important in patients at risk of perioperative complications, such as during major abdominal surgery and trauma, where the dangers of inflammation, hemorrhagic shock, sepsis, and high vasopressor need are real. Future hemodynamic strategies in these patients should integrate both macrocirculatory and microcirculatory optimization to attempt to give clinicians the most comprehensive image of their patient's physiology and thus offer a clear path to treatment. Novel algorithms should be tested in prospective randomized-controlled trials of homogeneous populations at risk of perioperative morbidity. For the sake of clarity and to promote such studies, the following strategy is our expert opinion on a potentially useful approach to integrating microcirculation monitoring into goal-directed hemodynamic management. We suggest that any patient who requires continuous vasopressors be assessed for microcirculatory alterations. From a practical perspective, it is important to determine whether the patient is at risk of perioperative complications (i.e., either low to moderate risk and/or a high risk of complications). Determining that a patient is at high risk of hemodynamic instability before induction of anesthesia allows us to plan for difficulties and prepare more invasive monitoring techniques, such as invasive arterial blood pressure, pulse contour analysis, blood gas analysis, and so on.

Low- to Moderate-Risk Anesthesia

If the risk of perioperative complications is initially low, there is little benefit in invasive monitoring with arterial or central venous lines.[24] This limits the potential of fluid responsiveness assessment and removes the possibility to repeatedly measure arterial lactate unless a catheter is placed during the acute event. During low- to moderate-risk surgery, non-invasive monitoring is the norm. Fluid responsiveness can still be measured using tools such as the Pleth Variability Index (PVI; Masimo, Irvine, CA, USA), or the ClearSight monitor (Edwards Lifesciences, Irvine, CA, USA),[24] which provide important information of fluid administration needs. These monitors, however, have their limitations. PVI signal can decrease with increased vasopressor use, and both lose their capacities to predict fluid responsiveness in the presence of arrhythmia.[25] Furthermore, these tools are not ubiquitous to operating rooms. A more frequently available tool, but one that requires a certain level of subspeciality expertise, is ultrasound to assess the collapsibility of central veins (inferior vena cava, superior vena cava, or internal jugular vein).[26] If available, sublingual microcirculation examination may demonstrate improvement after a fluid bolus and thus participate in a goal-directed fluid strategy.[14] In parallel to non-invasive assessment of fluid responsiveness, tissue perfusion alterations can simultaneously be measured with the RER, which would be reassuring if normal.[8] Anesthesia depth should also be assessed, especially frontal electroencephalogram (EEG) with an analysis of burst suppression ratio, as burst suppression and hypotension when occurring concomitantly have been associated with increased mortality.[27] A single venous or arterial sample through the

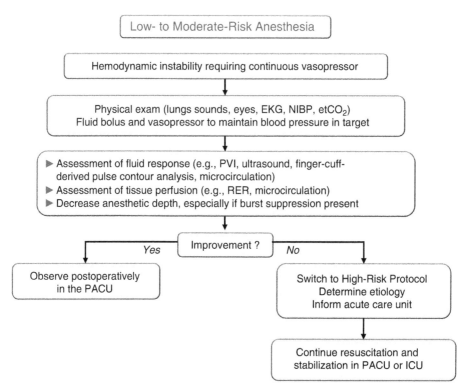

Figure 22.1 Proposed algorithm for assessing and treating hemodynamic instability in initially low- to moderate-risk patients monitored non-invasively. EKG, electrocardiogram; etCO$_2$, end-tidal carbon dioxide concentration; ICU, intensive care unit; NIBP, non-invasive blood pressure; PACU, post-anesthesia care unit.

radial artery or external jugular vein can also be of use, but should be limited, as multiple punctures can complicate future catheter placement. If the RER is abnormal, however, especially in the presence of persistently higher vasopressor need and concomitant surgical difficulties, arterial and central line placement with advanced macrovascular monitoring in conjunction with blood sampling and direct microcirculation assessment (e.g., sublingual microcirculation) are, in our view, justified (Fig. 22.1). We recommend moving to the high-risk protocol and determining the etiology of severe hemodynamic instability (hemorrhage, sepsis, anaphylaxis, embolus, metabolic disorders, pneumothorax, etc.).

High-Risk Anesthesia

If the risk of perioperative complications is considered high or a low- to moderate-risk patient develops considerable intraoperative challenges requiring continuous vasopressor infusion and an arterial line, clinicians should integrate both advanced macrovascular and direct microvascular monitoring (Fig. 22.2). Arterial lines allow both continuous blood pressure measurements and intermittent blood sampling (lactate, pH, bicarbonate, arterial CO$_2$ and O$_2$, and electrolytes). Many contemporary arterial blood pressure monitors display pulse pressure variation, which can more clearly determine if the patient is fluid responsive. Advanced hemodynamic monitors, such as the FloTrack (Edwards Lifesciences, Irvine, CA,

USA), give the additional ability to assess trends in stroke volume (and thus cardiac output), and, when coupled with a central line, will also continuously display peripheral vascular resistance.[28] Jugular and subclavian central venous catheters offer several other advantages to peripheral line placement, especially in high-risk patients. From a therapeutic perspective, these catheters allow rapid infusions of high concentrations of vasopressors directly into the superior vena cava, which become indispensable during hemodynamic instability. Central venous pressure, a static measurement, is a poor predictor of fluid responsiveness but continues to be extremely useful in the initial assessment of both the risk of right ventricular dysfunction and fluid overload, both of which can occur during hemodynamic instability.[29] In addition, central venous sampling can offer supplemental information on tissue perfusion by measuring surrogates such as Pv-aCO_2 gap and central venous hemoglobin saturation in oxygen ($ScvO_2$).[10] These measurements, in combination with arterial lactate, pH, and blood gases, can be used to determine whether an apparently optimized macrocirculation is mirrored by the patient's microcirculation. Although these surrogates can reflect poor microcirculation, their kinetics are either slow (as is the case of arterial lactate), or poorly understood (such as with RER and the Pv-aCO_2 gap). Furthermore, these markers can be limited by specificities in the patient's physiology. For example, Pv-aCO_2-gap and SvO_2 have been shown to be poor predictors of complications during liver transplantation.[9] This may be due to the increased cardiac output intrinsic to liver failure, which can cause these surrogates to be falsely reassuring. Lactate has become standard care in evaluating shock, but it decreases slowly after treatment, and tissue hypoxia is only one of the multiple causes of hyperlactatemia.[4,5] When there is a clear suspicion of poor tissue perfusion, confirmation through direct analysis of microcirculation (e.g., sublingual microcirculation) offers several advantages. Most importantly, it is a real-time analysis of the perfusion of capillaries, and the sublingual approach offers the clear benefit of being easily accessible in the vast majority of anesthetized patients, with the exception of head and neck surgery. As it offers real-time analysis of the patient's capillaries, it may thus reflect more quickly the patient's response to therapies.[30] Another essential component to optimization in the persistence of severe hemodynamic instability is cardiac ultrasound, which can assess left and right ventricular function, assess causes of shock, estimate pulmonary artery and left ventricular pressures, and estimate stroke volume. However, transesophageal cardiac ultrasound poses the disadvantage of limiting access to the sublingual capillaries for microcirculatory analysis.

When to Measure Microcirculation with the Hand-Held Vital Microscope

There are several potential moments to integrate the HVM into the goal-directed hemodynamic strategy. We recommend an early implementation even in low-risk patients suffering from acute hemodynamic instability, as it can quickly and non-invasively offer both a real-time image of the patient's current tissue perfusion and non-invasively guide fluid infusions.[14] Information from this analysis should be recorded and used as a baseline comparison for future interventions. In cases of greater severity that require more invasive monitoring and therapies, a sublingual microcirculation assessment can then be used to assess response to treatments and determine whether targets are adequate (see Fig. 22.2).[30] For example, if a personalized blood pressure is reached using both fluid boluses and a norepinephrine drip of 0.1 $\mu g\,kg^{-1}\,min^{-1}$, but the microcirculatory parameters indicate poor perfusion, clinicians may decide to lower the norepinephrine infusion and administer fluids or blood products in the hopes of optimizing flow while maintaining adequate perfusion pressure.

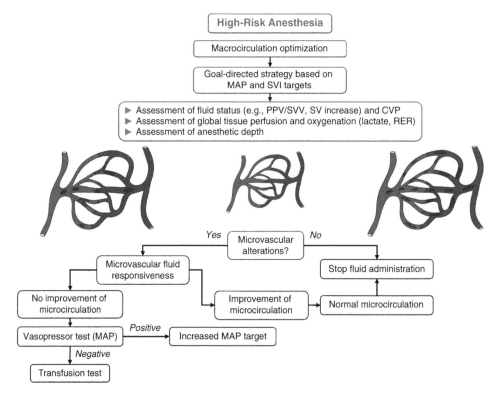

Figure 22.2 Proposed algorithm for assessing and treating hemodynamic instability in high-risk patients requiring invasive monitoring. CVP, central venous pressure; MAP, mean arterial pressure; PPV, pulse pressure variation; SV, stroke volume; SVI, stroke volume index; SVV. stroke volume variation; RER, respiratory exchange ratio. A black and white version of this figure will appear in some formats. For the color version, please refer to the plate section.

Conclusion

Hemodynamic therapy aims to optimize oxygen delivery to consumption ratio. Contemporary protocols overwhelmingly target improvements in macrocircular parameters, but uncoupling between macrocirculation and microcirculation can occur during surgery. Several tools exist for assessing tissue perfusion, and sublingual microcirculation is of particular interest as it offers a real-time non-invasive perspective of red blood cell flow through the capillaries. Future studies should focus on integrating this tool into goal-directed hemodynamic therapy strategies.

References

1. Shoemaker WC, Appel PL, Kram HB, Waxman K, Lee TS. Prospective trial of supranormal values of survivors as therapeutic goals in high-risk surgical patients. *Chest*. 1988;**94**(6):1176–86.

2. Pearse RM, Harrison DA, MacDonald N, et al. Effect of a perioperative, cardiac output-guided hemodynamic therapy algorithm on outcomes following major gastrointestinal surgery: a randomized clinical trial and systematic review. *JAMA*. 2014;**311**(21):2181–90.

3. Mythen MG, Webb AR. Perioperative plasma volume expansion reduces the incidence of gut mucosal hypoperfusion during cardiac surgery. *Arch Surg.* 1995;**130**(4):423–9.

4. Vincent JL, De Backer D. Circulatory shock. *N Engl J Med.* 2013;**369** (18):1726–34.

5. Kraut JA, Madias NE. Lactic acidosis. *N Engl J Med.* 2014;**371**(24):2309–19.

6. Regnier MA, Raux M, Le Manach Y, et al. Prognostic significance of blood lactate and lactate clearance in trauma patients. *Anesthesiology.* 2012;**117** (6):1276–88.

7. Bar S, Grenez C, Nguyen M, et al. Predicting postoperative complications with the respiratory exchange ratio after high-risk noncardiac surgery: a prospective cohort study. *Eur J Anaesthesiol.* 2020;**37** (11):1050–17.

8. Karam L, Desebbe O, Coeckelenbergh S, et al. Assessing the discriminative ability of the respiratory exchange ratio to detect hyperlactatemia during intermediate-to-high risk abdominal surgery. *BMC Anesthesiol.* 2022;**22**(1):211.

9. Coeckelenbergh S, Desebbe O, Carrier FM, et al. Intraoperative measurement of the respiratory exchange ratio predicts postoperative complications after liver transplantation. *BMC Anesthesiol.* 2022;**22** (1):405.

10. Ltaief Z, Schneider AG, Liaudet L. Pathophysiology and clinical implications of the veno-arterial PCO(2) gap. *Crit Care.* 2021;**25**(1):318.

11. Robin E, Futier E, Pires O, et al. Central venous-to-arterial carbon dioxide difference as a prognostic tool in high-risk surgical patients. *Crit Care.* 2015;**19**(1):227.

12. Verdant C, De Backer D. How monitoring of the microcirculation may help us at the bedside. *Curr Opin Crit Care.* 2005;**11** (3):240–4.

13. Ince C, Boerma EC, Cecconi M, et al. Second consensus on the assessment of sublingual microcirculation in critically ill patients: results from a task force of the European Society of Intensive Care Medicine. *Intensive Care Med.* 2018;**44** (3):281–99.

14. Bouattour K, Teboul JL, Varin L, Vicaut E, Duranteau J. Preload dependence is associated with reduced sublingual microcirculation during major abdominal surgery. *Anesthesiology.* 2019;**130** (4):541–9.

15. Flick M, Schreiber TH, Montomoli J, et al. Microcirculatory tissue perfusion during general anaesthesia and noncardiac surgery: an observational study using incident dark field imaging with automated video analysis. *Eur J Anaesthesiol.* 2022;**39** (7):582–90.

16. Bansch P, Flisberg P, Bentzer P. Changes in the sublingual microcirculation during major abdominal surgery and post-operative morbidity. *Acta Anaesthesiol. Scand.* 2014;**58**(1):89–97.

17. De Backer D, Dubois MJ, Schmartz D, et al. Microcirculatory alterations in cardiac surgery: effects of cardiopulmonary bypass and anesthesia. *Ann Thorac Surg;* 2009;**88**(5):1396–1403.

18. Greenwood JC, Jang DH, Spelde AE, et al. Low microcirculatory perfused vessel density and high heterogeneity are associated with increased intensity and duration of lactic acidosis after cardiac surgery with cardiopulmonary bypass. *Shock.* 2021;**56**(2):245–54.

19. den Os MM, van den Brom CE, van Leeuwen ALI, Dekker NAM. Microcirculatory perfusion disturbances following cardiopulmonary bypass: a systematic review. *Crit Care,* 2020;**24**(1):218.

20. Uz Z, Ince C, Shen L, Ergin B, van Gulik TM. Real-time observation of microcirculatory leukocytes in patients undergoing major liver resection. *Sci Rep.* 2021;**11**(1):4563.

21. Chiu C, Fong N, Lazzareschi D, et al. Fluids, vasopressors, and acute kidney injury after major abdominal surgery between 2015 and 2019: a multicentre retrospective analysis. *Br J Anaesth.* 2022;**129**(3):317–26.

22. Flick M, Briesenick L, Peine S, et al. The effect of moderate intraoperative blood loss and norepinephrine therapy on sublingual microcirculatory perfusion in patients having open radical prostatectomy: an observational study. *Eur J Anaesthesiol.* 2021;**38**(5):459–67.

23. Pottecher J, Deruddre S, Teboul JL, et al. Both passive leg raising and intravascular volume expansion improve sublingual microcirculatory perfusion in severe sepsis and septic shock patients. *Intensive Care Med.* 2010;**36**(11):1867–74.

24. Coeckelenbergh S, Delaporte A, Ghoundiwal D, et al. Pleth Variability Index versus pulse pressure variation for intraoperative goal-directed fluid therapy in patients undergoing low-to-moderate risk abdominal surgery: a randomized controlled trial. *BMC Anesthesiol.* 2019;**19**(1):34.

25. Coeckelenbergh S, Zaouter C, Alexander B, et al. Automated systems for perioperative goal-directed hemodynamic therapy. *J Anesth.* 2020;**34**(1):104–14.

26. Jozwiak M, Monnet X, Teboul JL. Prediction of fluid responsiveness in ventilated patients. *Ann Transl Med.* 2018;**6**(18):352.

27. Willingham M, Ben Abdallah A, Gradwohl S, et al. Association between intraoperative electroencephalographic suppression and postoperative mortality. *Br J Anaesth.* 2014;**113**(6):1001–8.

28. Grensemann J. Cardiac output monitoring by pulse contour analysis, the technical basics of less-invasive techniques. *Front Med (Lausanne).* 2018;**5**:64.

29. De Backer D, Vincent JL. Should we measure the central venous pressure to guide fluid management? Ten answers to 10 questions. *Crit Care.* 2018;**22**(1):43.

30. Tarazona V, Harrois, A, Duranteau, J. Monitoring of the sublingual microcirculation at the bedside: yes, it is possible and useful. In JL Vincent (ed.), *Annual Update in Intensive Care and Emergency Medicine 2020.* Cham: Springer; 2020: 235–44.

Chapter 23

Predictive Analytics and Artificial Intelligence

Jack E. Brooker and Kamal Maheshwari

Predictive analytics are a set of investigative tools that utilize existing data to predict future events. Artificial intelligence is a field of computer science dedicated to the development of systems and methods or smart machines which can mimic human intelligence. Many philosophers have warned against prediction of the future: *Prediction is hard, especially about the future.* However, the availability of large, near real-time datasets in medicine and advances in machine learning and artificial intelligence are challenging this prevailing wisdom.

In anesthesia and critical care, optimal hemodynamic management is critical for better patient outcomes.[1,2] Near universal heart rate, blood pressure, electrocardiogram, and pulse oximetry monitoring influence clinical interventions like fluid, vasopressor, or inotrope administration. In many cases, advanced hemodynamic monitoring is utilized in, for example, cardiac output-based goal-directed therapy.[2] Additionally, laboratory information such as blood electrolytes and lactate and radiologic information from chest radiograms can provide key insights into the hemodynamic state and specific interventions. The advances in monitoring and treatment have reduced intraoperative mortality by 99% compared with a century ago. However, morbidity and mortality in the early postoperative period remain common, with myocardial and renal injury being a leading cause.[3,4] Perfusion abnormalities are an intrinsic part of the ischemic insult on these organs in the perioperative phase. To further improve hemodynamic management, the focus has shifted to harnessing the information of real-time physiological monitoring data to guide clinical decisions.

Optimal Organ Perfusion

Tissue perfusion itself is dependent on a range of local and global factors, of which optimal blood pressure and cardiac output are key.[5] Preoperative factors such as fasting, gastrointestinal losses after bowel prep, losses to the interstitium in inflammatory states, and bleeding due to trauma are all common reasons for hypovolemia. Intraoperative effects from anesthesia such as vasodilation and cardiac depression, surgical bleeding, and lung insufflation affecting venous return may all be reasons for intraoperative hypotension. Postoperatively, continued bleeding, losses to the interstitium in the context of inflammation, or poor oral intake can all lead to protracted periods of hypovolemia and low blood pressure (BP). Losses due to bleeding require hemostasis for definitive control, and excessive blood loss requires transfusion for volume replacement. However, optimal fluid administration is critical because both restrictive and liberal fluid administration can lead to complications.[6]

A goal-directed approach may be adopted that relies on more invasive monitoring and working towards predetermined endpoints in these observed parameters. An example is intra-arterial waveform tracing measuring pulse-pressure variation or systolic waveform variation and estimating changes in these in response to fluid challenges. Other approaches include Doppler to assess stroke volume. As the name implies, goal-directed fluid management assigns pre-specified criteria to the above hemodynamic parameters to drive decision making (e.g., fluid boluses continue to be given if there are pulse-pressure variations of 10–15% implying responsiveness, whilst variations less than 10% mean fluid boluses are withheld to avoid hypervolemia).[2]

Current Gaps in Hemodynamic Management

Goal-directed fluid management is based on fluid responsive assessment and, recently, even the definition of fluid responsiveness has been debated.[7] Blood pressure itself is critically important to tissue perfusion as discussed above, not simply flow. Since both BP and flow are important to maintaining perfusion, it could be argued that goal-directed fluid therapy should categorize response based on 1) pressure and flow response, 2) pressure response only, 3) flow response only, 4) no response. Evidence does suggest that patients with goal-directed fluid therapy driven by pressure response do well irrespective of their flow responsiveness, with cardiac output a surrogate marker for the latter.[5] Within cardiology, cardiac power (mean arterial pressure × cardiac output/451) is believed to be predictive of outcomes in heart failure, and a similar metric drawing on both pressure and flow may be identified within perioperative fluid management. Further studies are required to assess the relative importance of flow and pressure response in goal-directed fluid management.

More broadly though, the current management of hypotension is based on reactive decisions, administering fluid or vasopressors after the hypotensive event has occurred. Since it is widely believed that periods of a minute or greater with a mean arterial pressure (MAP) <65 mmHg is deleterious to the brain, heart, kidney, and other organ systems, it follows that predicting a hypotensive event and proactively intervening should help to prevent morbidity and mortality in patients.[8]

Artificial Intelligence

Role Predictive Analytics and Artificial Intelligence

Artificial Intelligence (AI) at its most fundamental level is the construction of computer programs that can replicate human intellect. Within AI there are several major subdivisions: machine learning, deep learning, and natural language processing. Machine learning may be supervised or unsupervised and seeks patterns in high volumes of data to form predictions or make classifications. Deep learning is a more sophisticated form of machine learning that requires at least three layers of neural networks, removes the need for structured data, and is capable of automated feature extraction, removing the need for human pre-programming. Natural language processing is another subset of machine learning, which, as the name suggests, focuses on the computer's ability to understand the written and spoken word and make intelligent decisions based on that. With the huge amount of information held on electronic medical records, there is a near limitless source of data input available.

Predictive analytics, utilizing many data inputs, can play a huge role in augmenting clinician decision-making (Fig. 23.1). Predictive analytics is an important component of perioperative intelligence, where the focus is on identifying high-risk patients, early detection of complications, and timely treatment.[9] For example, multiple algorithms are available to predict readmission and mortality risks such as the Risk Stratification Index (RSI) and the National Surgical Quality Improvement Program (NSQIP).[2,10] AI can continually learn from patterns seen in huge datasets and predict specific outcomes.

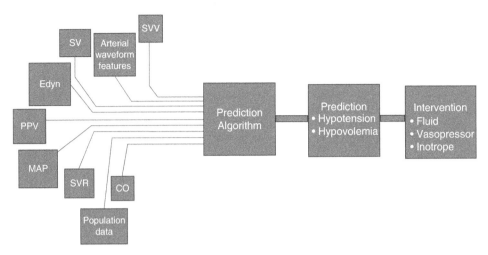

Figure 23.1 Illustration of the multiple inputs into a possible AI algorithm that integrates these, aiding the provider (or replacing them in a closed-loop system), resulting in an output (treatment). CO, cardiac output; Edyn, dynamic elastic moduli; MAP, mean arterial pressure; PPV, pulse pressure variation; SV, stroke volume; SVR, systemic vascular resistance; SVV, stroke volume variation.

Sensors allowing continuous vital sign monitoring provide an alternative source of contemporaneous data from which AI can conceivably learn to guide accurate prediction formation. Perioperative hypotension is an obvious target for this since extended periods of intraoperative and postoperative hypotension are clearly correlated with poor outcomes including mortality. Earlier prediction of hypotension would facilitate preventive measures including fluid administration, improving outcomes for patients. Acute kidney injury (AKI) is a common occurrence after surgery, likely due to hypotension and periods of inadequate perfusion. Machine learning based on various physiological data inputs including urine output, intra-abdominal pressure and core temperature accurately predicted the onset of AKI 24 minutes prior to the first objective evidence of kidney injury, a vital window that facilitates physician intervention.[11]

Example Solutions

A. Assisted Fluid Management Software

Assisted fluid management (AFM) software exists to automate the process of fluid bolus administration as part of a goal-directed fluid regimen.[12] Goal-directed regimens follow algorithms, which are frequently complex, with the end goal of maintaining predetermined hemodynamic parameters (usually a stroke volume variation of <12%).[13] As a consequence, adherence to algorithms is often poor, with under 30% of administered boluses achieving the desired alteration in stroke volume.[14] AFM typically utilizes invasive arterial pressure monitoring in the intraoperative phase to assess volume status and makes recommendations to the anesthesiology provider as to when they should consider administering fluid boluses. We undertook a large, prospective study enrolling at nine centers in the USA. Subjects were adults undergoing major non-cardiac surgery with American Society of Anesthesiology (ASA) status of class III or greater ($n = 330$) and were all assigned to a single study arm comprising fluid management by the Assisted Fluid Management Software (Edwards Lifesciences, Irvine, CA, USA). The endpoint of the study was the proportion of AFM-prompted boluses that achieved the desired hemodynamic response, compared with both the published rate of 30% in provider-directed boluses and the provider-directed boluses administered within the study when overriding the AFM prompts. The results were striking; of the provider-directed boluses in the study, the desired stroke volume (SV) response was only achieved in 41%, compared with 66% of the AFM-directed boluses.[12] AFM is very new and so little additional literature has been published about its safety and efficacy. Further trials will be required to establish superiority in postoperative outcomes before widespread adoption is likely within the field of anesthesiology.

B. Hypotension Prediction Index

The hypotension prediction index (HPI) is an algorithm developed through machine learning that is intended to better predict periods of hypotension (defined as MAP <65 mmHg for 1 minute or more). The algorithm processes the arterial waveform to extract relevant features, and these features are then mapped to obtain predictions. Input features in the HPI algorithm were numerous, including arterial pressure waveform time, amplitude, area, and slope features; FloTrac algorithm features; CO-Trek features; complexity features; Baroreflex features; variability features; and others.[15]

The algorithm performed well, based on a primary outcome of predicting periods of MAP <65 mmHg for at least 1 minute's duration, with sensitivity and specificity of 88% (85% to 90%) and 87% (85% to 90%), respectively, 15 minutes before a hypotensive event, calculated from receiver-operating characteristic curves with thresholds that minimized the difference between sensitivity and specificity.[15]

Maheshwari and colleagues evaluated the algorithm in adult patients over 45 years of age with ASA class III or above undergoing moderate- to high-risk non-cardiac surgery. They enrolled 214 eligible subjects and randomly assigned them to the HPI guidance group or a control group. Initial analysis found that the time-weighted average MAP below 65 mmHg was no different between the guided groups versus the unguided control group. However, post hoc analysis that restricted analysis to those events where guided providers actually intervened did demonstrate less hypotension than controls.[8] This suggests that an intervention is necessary after HPI alert to reduce hypotension. Similarly, Wijnberge and colleagues, in the HYPE trial of 68 non-cardiac surgical patients, reported significant reduction in hypotension with the use of HPI software.[16] Conversely, in a sub study of the HYPE trial, Schenk and colleagues assessed the HPI in postoperative patient in the postanesthetic care unit (PACU). Randomizing 60 adults undergoing non-cardiac surgery to either the HPI or control, they found that HPI made no difference to the median duration of postoperative hypotension.[17] Moving forward, clinical trials like SMART BP are focused on further evaluating the outcome benefits of hypotension prediction software.

A limitation to the algorithm, as demonstrated by Hatib and colleagues,[15] is that it relies on invasive arterial waveform data. Only a small fraction of patients undergoing major non-cardiac surgery requires arterial line monitoring, which limits its applicability in the real world. An obvious question is how well non-invasive monitors work with the HPI algorithm and whether data input from this source can be used to effectively predict periods of MAP < 65 mmHg. In a prospective study of 320 adult patients over 45 years of age undergoing moderate- to high-risk non-cardiac surgery, the algorithm predicted hypotension, with 0.86 sensitivity and specificity at 5 minutes in advance, 0.83 sensitivity and specificity at 10 minutes in advance, and 0.75 sensitivity and specificity at 15 minutes in advance of a hypotensive event.[18] It seems clear, therefore, that predictive software can be used with invasive and non-invasive arterial pressure monitoring.

Lee and colleagues tested a multichannel model comprising arterial pressure waveform, electrocardiography, photoplethysmography, and capnography and they compared this with single channel models (Table 23.1). The study also comprised invasive and non-invasive approaches. The former used both arterial waveform as a single channel and a multichannel approach, whilst the latter used photoplethysmography as a single channel approach and a multichannel approach (excepting arterial pressure). A hybrid model was also employed in which single systolic and diastolic BP points were provided to the non-invasive model. The classification was binary: a hypotensive event (MAP<65 mmHg for >1 minute) or a non-hypotensive event (MAP >65 mm Hg stable for >20 min) occurring after 5, 10, and 15 minutes. Using a multichannel approach had a greater accuracy of predicting hypotensive events in the 3301 patients included in the study.[19]

Closed-Loop Systems

An alternative to predictive models is a closed-loop system, which constantly monitors physiological parameters and applies boluses of fluid or vasopressors to maintain MAP within a narrow predetermined window (Table 23.2). Unlike open-loop systems where the provider has some degree of involvement, such as overriding the automated system or declining to comply with its prompts, the closed-loop cuts this step out and responds itself. A number of trials have been run, albeit with limited samples, which suggests that outcomes may be improved with the closed-loop (CL) approach. Reinhart and colleagues assessed CL in patients undergoing major hepatobiliary or abdominal surgery, matching them to patients with conventional fluid management, and found that heart rate trended lower for the CL patients who also spent less time in preload-independent states, possibly implying improved overall fluid management.[20] Joosten and colleagues assessed CL system for fluid management in patients undergoing major abdominal surgery ($n = 208$) and paired them with a historical cohort of equal size receiving conventional fluid management. Primary outcomes were intraoperative fluid balance, and secondary outcomes included a composite of major (e.g., acute coronary syndrome or arrhythmia, pulmonary embolism, bowel and surgical anastomotic leak, fistulae, or peritoneal effusions) and minor complications (paralytic ileus, superficial wound infection, urinary infection, postoperative nausea or vomiting, and confusion). Patients in the CL cohort had a significantly lower net fluid balance and lower major and minor complication rates as well as a lower hospital length of stay.[21]

The same CL system has been applied with vasopressors, though fewer studies have been conducted. Rinehart and colleagues performed a simulation comparing a closed-loop model with an unmanaged control in both stable and variable underlying blood pressure scenarios. The a priori target was 95% of time spent within target range, with the CL managed cases ($n = 250$) spending considerably more time in range with a higher mean MAP than the unmanaged cases ($n = 250$).[22] CL bolus versus continuous infusion has been assessed in spinal anesthesia with promising results, the authors reporting that CL management of phenylephrine provided superior consistency in BP compared with infusion though clinical outcomes such as cardiac output, nausea, and vomiting, and neonatal outcomes were not significantly different.[23] In septic patients ($n = 19$) closed-loop norepinephrine has been tested using conventional infusion as a control ($n = 20$). The CL-treated patients spent less time in sepsis and required less overall norepinephrine; however, other outcomes such as 28-day mortality and intensive care unit (ICU) length of stay were not significantly different.[24]

Table 23.1 Hypotension prediction evidence. Summary of articles reporting hypotension prediction index software, which aim to inform the anesthesiology provider who then makes the decision to administer fluid or not.

Authors	Study population	Study design	Main outcomes
Maheshwari et al., 2021 [18]	Non-cardiac surgery (n = 320)	Randomized trial	HPI of 80–89 using non-invasive arterial monitoring gave a median of 6 min notice before MAP <0.65 mmHg
Lee et al., 2021 [19]	Non-cardiac surgery (n = 3301)	Retrospective observational	Multichannel prediction shows greater accuracy than single input for AFM
Schenk et al., 2021 [17]	Non-cardiac surgery (n = 60)	Randomized trial	Total median duration of hypotension in PACU not different in HPI arm. Percentage time spent with MAP <65 mmHg less in AFM arm
Maheshwari et al., 2020 [8]	Non-cardiac surgery (n = 214)	Randomized trial	HPI with invasive arterial waveform analysis did not result in lower time-weighted average MAP <65 mmHg. Post hoc analysis restricted to clinician intervention per HPI prompting did show lower less hypotension
Wijnberge et al., 2020 [16]	Non-cardiac surgery (n = 68)	Randomized trial	Total median duration of hypotension in AFM group significantly less than control. Average time spent with MAP <65 mmHg significantly less with AFM group
Hatib et al., 2018 [15]	Non-cardiac surgery (n = 204)	Prospective cohort	Hypotension prediction algorithm using arterial waveform data from 1334 previous patients able to predict hypotension with 87% specificity and 88% sensitivity 15 minutes before an event in a prospective cohort of patients

AFM, assisted fluid management; HPI, hypotension prediction index; MAP, mean arterial pressure; PACU, postanesthetic care unit.

Table 23.2 Closed-loop hemodynamic management evidence. Summary of published work relating to closed-loop systems which both predict hemodynamic changes and make decision to administer fluid bolus.

Authors	Study population	Study design	Main outcomes
Joosten et al., 2019 [25]	Abdominal surgery (lap-assisted) (n = 40)	Randomized trial	Cardiac output and stroke volume variations similar, remained in target range > 90% of the study time
Joosten et al., 2018 [21]	Abdominal surgery (n = 208)	Cohort study with matched prospective and retrospective groups	Lower net fluid balance in CL group Major and minor complications composites lower in CL group Hospital LOS lower in CL group
Lilot et al., 2018 [26]	Abdominal surgery (n = 46)	Randomized trial	Greater increase CI in CL group, no other significant hemodynamic differences
Reinhart et al., 2015 [20]	Abdominal surgery (n = 40)	Matched cohorts	CL group spent more time in preload-independent state, trended to lower HR but difference non-significant
Reinhart et al., 2011 [27]	Simulated patient events (hemorrhage)	Simulated patients	Mean stroke volume, arterial pressure, CO, and final CO higher in the CL group than practitioners group

CI, Cardiac Index; CL, closed loop; CO, cardiac output; HR, heart rate; LOS, length of stay.

Future Considerations

Currently, the vast majority of interest in the role of predictive analytics and AI in fluid management concerns the intraoperative phase. Although this is crucial, the relatively unsupervised postoperative phase comprises a much greater risk for dehydration, poor fluid balance, and periods of hypotension. The same is true of non-surgical ICU patients, who spend extended periods sedated or unconscious on invasive ventilation and who are reliant on non-oral fluid replacement. Limited human resources and monitoring at the bedside further restrict our ability to deploy appropriate fluid or hemodynamic management algorithms. A natural role for entirely automated fluid management systems based on machine learning and advanced invasive or non-invasive monitoring seems to be the future, especially with increasing attention paid to both cost and quality. Extensive work focused on clinical validation would be required to demonstrate efficacy and safety and to achieve significant buy-in from patients, clinicians, and administrators.

Conclusion

In surgical and critically ill patients, optimal methods of fluid management are widely debated. However, it is clear that prolonged periods of hypotension and imprecise fluid management lead to increased morbidity and mortality. Current standard monitoring practices provide good but incomplete information, which, along with subjective clinical interpretation, inevitably lead to differences in clinical practice. Advanced hemodynamic data and predictive analytics are a welcome addition in hemodynamic management. The role of predictive analytics and artificial intelligence in blood pressure and fluid management is only likely to grow in the future, but we should rigorously test and validate the solutions in clinical trials before widespread adoption in practice.

References

1. Brandstrup B. Fluid therapy for the surgical patient. *Best Pract Res Clin Anaesthesiol.* 2006 Jun;**20**(2):265–83.

2. Miller TE, Myles PS. Perioperative fluid therapy for major surgery. *Anesthesiology.* 2019 May;**130**(5):825–32.

3. Li G, Warner M, Lang BH, Huang L, Sun LS. Epidemiology of anesthesia-related mortality in the United States, 1999–2005. *Anesthesiology.* 2009 Apr;**110**(4):759–65.

4. Spence J, LeManach Y, Chan MTV, et al. Association between complications and death within 30 days after noncardiac surgery. *CMAJ.* 2019 Jul 29;**191**(30):E830–7.

5. Maheshwari K, Pu X, Rivas E, et al. Association between intraoperative mean arterial pressure and postoperative complications is independent of cardiac index in patients undergoing noncardiac surgery. *Br J Anaesth.* 2021 Sep 1;**127**(3): e102–4.

6. Myles PS, Bellomo R, Corcoran T, et al. Restrictive versus liberal fluid therapy for major abdominal surgery. *N Engl J Med.* 2018 Jun 14;**378**(24):2263–74.

7. Maheshwari K, Saugel B. Defining fluid responsiveness: flow response vs. pressure response. *J Clin Anesth.* 2022 Aug 1;**79**:110667.

8. Maheshwari K, Shimada T, Yang D, et al. Hypotension prediction index for prevention of hypotension during moderate- to high-risk noncardiac surgery. *Anesthesiology.* 2020 Dec 1;**133**(6):1214–22.

9. Maheshwari K, Cywinski JB, Papay F, Khanna AK, Mathur P. Artificial intelligence for perioperative medicine: perioperative intelligence. *Anesth Analg.* 2023 Feb 24;**136**(4):637–45.

10. Harris AHS. Path from predictive analytics to improved patient outcomes: a framework to guide use, implementation, and

evaluation of accurate surgical predictive models. *Ann Surg.* 2017 Mar 1;**265**(3):461.

11. Prabhakar A, Stanton K, Burnett D, et al. Combining urine output and intra-abdominal pressures predict acute kidney injury early critical care medicine. *Crit Care Med.* 2021;**49**(1):567.

12. Maheshwari K, Malhotra G, Bao X, et al. Assisted fluid management software guidance for intraoperative fluid administration. *Anesthesiology.* 2021 Aug 1;**135**(2):273–83.

13. Benes J, Giglio M, Brienza N, Michard F. The effects of goal-directed fluid therapy based on dynamic parameters on post-surgical outcome: a meta-analysis of randomized controlled trials. *Crit Care.* 2014 Oct 28;**18**(5):584.

14. MacDonald N, Ahmad T, Mohr O, et al. Dynamic preload markers to predict fluid responsiveness during and after major gastrointestinal surgery: an observational substudy of the OPTIMISE Trial. *Br J Anaesth.* 2015 Apr;**114**(4):598–604.

15. Hatib F, Jian Z, Buddi S, et al. Machine-learning algorithm to predict hypotension based on high-fidelity arterial pressure waveform analysis. *Anesthesiology.* 2018 Oct;**129**(4):663–74.

16. Wijnberge M, Geerts BF, Hol L, et al. Effect of a machine learning-derived early warning system for intraoperative hypotension vs standard care on depth and duration of intraoperative hypotension during elective noncardiac surgery: the HYPE Randomized Clinical Trial. *JAMA.* 2020 Mar 17;**323**(11):1052–60.

17. Schenk J, Wijnberge M, Maaskant JM, et al. Effect of Hypotension Prediction Index-guided intraoperative haemodynamic care on depth and duration of postoperative hypotension: a sub-study of the Hypotension Prediction Trial. *Br J Anaesth.* 2021 Nov;**127**(5):681–8.

18. Maheshwari K, Buddi S, Jian Z, et al. Performance of the Hypotension Prediction Index with non-invasive arterial pressure waveforms in non-cardiac surgical patients. *J Clin Monit Comput.* 2021 Feb;**35**(1):71–8.

19. Lee S, Lee HC, Chu YS, et al. Deep learning models for the prediction of intraoperative hypotension. *Br J Anaesth.* 2021 Apr;**126**(4):808–17.

20. Rinehart J, Lilot M, Lee C, et al. Closed-loop assisted versus manual goal-directed fluid therapy during high-risk abdominal surgery: a case-control study with propensity matching. *Crit Care.* 2015 Mar 19;**19**:94.

21. Joosten A, Coeckelenbergh S, Delaporte A, et al. Implementation of closed-loop-assisted intra-operative goal-directed fluid therapy during major abdominal surgery: a case-control study with propensity matching. *Eur J Anaesthesiol.* 2018 Sep;**35**(9):650–8.

22. Rinehart J, Ma M, Calderon MD, Cannesson M. Feasibility of automated titration of vasopressor infusions using a novel closed-loop controller. *J Clin Monit Comput.* 2018 Feb;**32**(1):5–11.

23. Ngan Kee WD, Khaw KS, Tam YH, Ng FF, Lee SW. Performance of a closed-loop feedback computer-controlled infusion system for maintaining blood pressure during spinal anaesthesia for caesarean section: a randomized controlled comparison of norepinephrine versus phenylephrine. *J Clin Monit Comput.* 2017 Jun;**31**(3):617–23.

24. Merouani M, Guignard B, Vincent F, et al. Norepinephrine weaning in septic shock patients by closed loop control based on fuzzy logic. *Crit Care.* 2008 Dec;**12**(6):R155.

25. Joosten A, Raj Lawrence S, Colesnicenco A, et al. Personalized versus protocolized fluid management using noninvasive hemodynamic monitoring (Clearsight System) in patients undergoing moderate-risk abdominal surgery. *Anesth Analg.* 2019 Jul;**129**(1):e8–12.

26. Lilot M, Bellon A, Gueugnon M, et al. Comparison of cardiac output optimization with an automated closed-loop goal-directed fluid therapy versus non standardized manual fluid administration during elective abdominal surgery: first prospective randomized controlled trial. *J Clin Monit Comput.* 2018 Dec;**32**(6):993–1003.

27. Rinehart J, Alexander B, Manach YL, et al. Evaluation of a novel closed-loop fluid-administration system based on dynamic predictors of fluid responsiveness: an in silico simulation study. *Crit Care.* 2011 Nov 23;**15**(6):R278.

Clinical Decision Support and Closed-Loop Systems for Goal-Directed Hemodynamic Therapy

Sean Coeckelenbergh, Joseph Rinehart, Maxime Cannesson and Alexandre Joosten

Introduction

In 2001, the National Institutes of Health identified variance in healthcare practices and its inequalities as an underlying challenge of modern medicine. Clinical decision support systems (CDSS) and closed-loop (CL) systems have provided solutions by standardizing clinical care to improve patient management and outcome. Decreasing variability and improving compliance to goal-directed hemodynamic therapy (GDHT) have been at the heart these CDSS and CL systems innovations.

There are primarily two classes of decision support – active and passive. Passive decision support requires direct interaction from the provider for it to function. Document templates and medication dosing ranges are examples of passive decision support. Active decision support (e.g., graphical displays and alarms), on the other hand, interacts with providers to alert them of some event or otherwise present information. Both types have a role in clinical care, but active CDSS is actually more difficult to properly integrate into practice due to important design considerations and implementation challenges.

Decision Support – Design

Design plays a fundamental role in decision support efficacy. For applications like document templates, design may simply mean the elements that are included or excluded from the template. For active real-time decision support systems, design refers to the entire implementation of the decision support, including graphical elements, decision trees, and user interaction. All must be carefully planned for optimal use.[1] There are entire fields of study devoted to human factors and good design for usability, and these principles play an essential role in how clinical decision support tools are received and used.[2]

The key characteristics that make medical information useful to practitioners are relevance, validity, and accessibility.[3] Other factors that contribute, however, are clinical context of the information and acceptability.[4] Context of the information is important because even if information is relevant, valid, and easily accessible, if it does not guide decision making in a meaningful way (e.g., whether or not to apply treatment, or the odds of developing a disease), it is useless. For example, a rule set that identifies a disease with 80% accuracy is not useful if the 20% of misidentified patients will have bad outcomes that could have been prevented with low-risk treatment. It makes more sense to give everyone at risk the treatment until a better diagnostic rule set is found. Acceptability plays a role in advice that may be accurate, but will be ignored for medico-legal or financial reasons. A good example is CDSS that help triage patients in the emergency room. If the medico-legal risk of a missed diagnosis is sufficiently high, then all patients will receive treatment despite advice that it is not indicated.

Another key element of good CDSS is providing relevant information at the right time. Having a patient allergy list and body weight available when entering medication orders is obviously relevant. A popup alert during cardiopulmonary bypass reminding a care provider that the current patient is due for colonoscopy screening is obviously irrelevant and may even be dangerous if it distracts the provider from essential tasks. Evidence to date shows that the more specific and appropriate the advice a diagnostic system can give, the more clinicians will accept it. Low specificity and relevance quickly result in system fatigue and dismissal of the advice.[5]

Decision Support – Clinical Impact

Studies have examined the impact of CDSS and have found that regardless of whether commercially developed or locally developed, they are effective in improving process measures: hospital guidelines are followed more frequently and recommended treatments prescribed more often. There is very sparse evidence for clinical outcome improvements, workload benefits, economic impacts, or efficiency gains.[6,7] This may be due more to difficulty in designing and executing studies that focus on these factors as opposed to a lack of actual effect, but unfortunately many studies that attempted to examine these factors were equivocal.[8,9] For example, specific CDSS were able to show a reduction in variance in order sets in the neonatal intensive care unit (NICU), an improvement in blood utilization based on recommended guidelines, and a reduction in length of time in the emergency department.[10–12] A study designed to look at the impact on clinical outcomes in the intensive care unit (ICU), however, did not show any significant gains.[13]

While optimal patient outcomes with the most efficient possible use of resources is the ultimate goal of process improvement in healthcare, the existing evidence base alone is more than enough justification for implementation of CDSS in many situations. The proven ability of CDSS to reduce variability in practice is a laudable and necessary first step in any process improvement pathway, for as long as practice is "provider dependent" there is no true underlying "process" that can be improved upon. Standardization must therefore precede efforts aimed at improving patient outcomes. Another benefit of CDSS and CL systems is that they enable non-expert users to achieve expert-grade clinical performance. For example, Sondergaard et al. developed a computerized clinical decision support system making recommendations to novices regarding goal-directed fluid therapy and found a high concordance between the recommendations of the system and the actions of expert anesthesiologists. As such, this study is a good example of an "exportable expert" that could be used by practitioners with minimal training to obtain near equivalent quality GDHT to the experts.[14]

Decision Support – Challenges

Despite the safety and standardization gains that CDSS can provide, there are several challenges to overcome. A good design and high compliance are essential for optimal impact of CDSS. In addition, hospitals and health systems require a supportive infrastructure before CDSS can be implemented.[15] If there is no standardization of codification of data with CDSS, data sharing and cooperation across systems become very difficult. As an example, different companies design monitors and clinical systems and each presents information differently. Different colors mean different things on different systems, information such as patient name and ID may be located in various places on displays, and even alarms and alerts vary. Instead of having to learn a standard convention, providers must learn the nuances of every device, and this can lead to errors. Common standards and design elements (fonts, units, color schemes, lists, etc.) across an institution's systems comprise one factor that could substantially improve usability but may be difficult to achieve in practice. One such effort to provide standardization was undertaken by the National Health Service in the United Kingdom and Microsoft. The goal of this initiative is to provide a common appearance to similar information across health applications, allowing users to rapidly identify the information they need. Improving human-user interfaces is one of the most important challenges facing CDSS development. At the very least, interface design choices should be tested and refined by the intended users of the system. Good graphical displays can improve accuracy and reduce decision making time while increasing adherence to established protocols. Indeed, usability testing for medical devices is a requirement by the US Food and Drug Administration, though the rigor of testing is often left to the discretion of the device developer.

Another non-trivial factor is that physicians may perceive that advice and guidelines coming from CDSS infringe on their professional autonomy. In some regards, they are right: the CDSS are often recommending a pathway that the physician *should* follow as opposed to following his or her "gut" or personal algorithm. This is an incomplete view, however. CDSS recommend an algorithm in an effort to standardize care and reduce variability between providers and events. This does not mean the provider must *always* follow the advice of the CDSS, however; it just means that deviations from recommended care should be *justified*. As an example, a clinical pathway may recommend beta-blockers as a first-choice therapy for patients with hypertension. In a patient with severe asthma, however, a beta-blocker may not be the best first choice. If the CDSS does not account for this, a provider would be completely justified in prescribing a different class of agents. As no CDSS can possibly account for all of the potential scenarios, clinical providers are still required to use their own judgment in application of the tool. In fact, one potential new risk introduced by the CDSS is automation bias – a tendency to *over*-rely on the information provided by the system.[16] As evidence has shown that the way information is presented to physicians plays a key role in how decision support is accepted and what physician attitudes are towards the systems,[17] careful design and testing are warranted before clinical implementation.

Finally, time restraints linked to event reporting and subsequent notification to providers may be a limiting factor in CDSS design.[18] In fact, interruptions and the disruption of workflow they bring are a major potential drawback of active decision support systems. Interruptions have variable influences (sometimes positive, sometimes negative) on workflow [19] and often lead to reduction of time and attention to clinical tasks, and interrupted tasks may not be returned to a significant proportion of the time.[20]

Closed-Loop Systems: Automating Diagnosis and Therapy

A control unit, which measures some variable in a system and then intervenes in the same system based on the measurement, is a closed loop (Fig. 24.1). Simple common examples are household air conditioners and automobile cruise control. A sophisticated example is airline

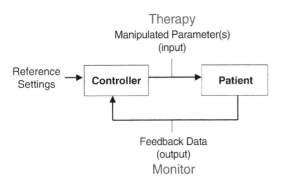

Therapy
Manipulated Parameter(s)
(input)

Reference Settings → **Controller** → **Patient**

Feedback Data
(output)
Monitor

Figure 24.1 Basic closed-loop scheme. A controller takes some form of measurement from a system; it then uses that measurement to direct some form of intervention on the system. A simple example is home air conditioning: the system is the house, the measurement is the thermometer reading, and the intervention is heating or cooling by the unit.

autopilot. Despite their ubiquity in engineering and life in general, their use has been heavily restricted in clinical practice, at least from the clinician's standpoint. The lag between the potential applications and implementation in medicine is largely due to regulatory factors, the complicated nature of biological systems, inaccuracies in measurement methodologies, and physician acceptance.[21] Nevertheless, the stability and consistency afforded by well-designed closed loops makes them potentially powerful tools for improving patient care while reducing costs,[22] and they are beginning to find use in clinical care. The best known medical example is probably the "artificial pancreas" – an automated insulin pump that matches insulin level to glucose level and can maintain tight control with minimal patient interaction. The limiting factor in developing these systems to date has primarily been the quality of the insulin sensor, but otherwise the control algorithms themselves have been studied by a variety of groups in both simulation and clinical settings.[23–25] Pacemakers, of course, are closed-loop devices, many of which have sophisticated respiratory rate and atrial tracking algorithms which attempt to optimize heart rate to physiological demand.

Decision Support for Goal-Directed Hemodynamic Therapy

CDSS for hemodynamic and fluid management has greatly evolved over the past decade, both in the intraoperative and critical care environments. One of the best known CDSS models in current use is probably the Rivers protocol for sepsis.[26] Following this pathway resulted in a 30% reduction in mortality in critically ill ED patients presenting with sepsis. Subsequently, a variety of studies looking at similar protocols in surgical and intensive care patients showed benefits ranging from improved outcomes to shorter length of stay.[27,28] In addition to recommendations for fluid administration, the Rivers protocol also includes inotropic and vasoactive agents. CDSS for pharmacological agents like these are not really found outside of more comprehensive management protocols because of the risks of under-resuscitation if a vasopressor is started instead of proper volume replacement therapy.

Since the development of the Rivers sepsis protocol, CDSS tools have been developed for other specific scenarios including massive transfusion and battlefield trauma.[29] One study looking at fluid resuscitation following severe burns in ICU patients showed a reduction in crystalloid volumes while simultaneously keeping patients within urinary output targets a higher percentage of the time.[30] Another study on trauma patients showed that a real-time CDSS resulted in improved protocol compliance and reduced errors and morbidity when applied during the first 30 minutes of trauma resuscitation.[31] CDSS have also been shown to help providers maintain a higher MAP in an ICU setting versus a standard alarm-based

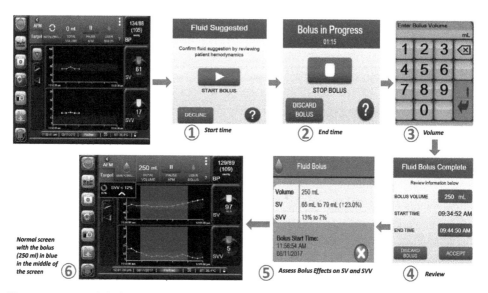

Figure 24.2 Assisted Fluid Management interface. SV, stroke volume; SVV, stroke volume variation. A black and white version of this figure will appear in some formats. For the color version, please refer to the plate section.

monitor.[32] The recently commercialized Assisted Fluid Management system (AFM) (Edwards Lifesciences) is a novel tool that assesses the patient's fluid responsiveness and suggests fluid infusions. Clinicians have been shown to better optimize hemodynamics with this system, when compared with manual goal-directed fluid therapy.[33–35] It is likely that hemodynamic management will become more heavily guided by CDSS like this in the coming years, especially given the impressive results that many of these studies have reported on outcomes. Figure 24.2 shows AFM steps.

Closed-Loop Hemodynamic and Fluid Therapy

CL systems offer enormous potential in optimizing blood pressure and fluid management. The general idea behind their use in perioperative GDHT is to automate CDSS. In other words, the system follows a recommended protocol to decrease variability and itself administers the treatment. This approach adds an essential benefit: increased protocol compliance. Initial studies began four decades ago and focused primarily on blood pressure management. Fluids, however, have also been a field of considerable interest over the past decades. Advances in preload assessment using pulse-contour technology and heart–lung interaction have given reliable targets for closed-loop systems.

Closed-Loop Fluid Therapy

Closed-loop control of fluid administration was first reported in the 1980s with the use of a computer-controlled intravenous (IV) fluid infusion pump directed by urine output in burn patients.[36] Additional studies targeting urine output and even postoperative auto-transfusion followed.[37] The latest and most innovative phase in closed-loop fluid administration only appeared recently with the use of indicators of fluid responsiveness, such as stroke volume variation and percentage increase in stroke volume following a fluid bolus.

Along with automation of propofol infusions for anesthesia and insulin infusion for glucose control, fluid resuscitation has been one of the major medical closed-loop research topics this decade.

One of two prime areas of focus has been closed-loop control in burn and shock resuscitation.[38,39] A variety of feedback signals have been used to direct infusion rates, including blood pressure and near infrared spectroscopy, and as with other closed-loop applications, these systems show improved consistency and stability of the controlled variable. Shock and burn resuscitation patients are ideal for closed-loop control, as the fluid needs in these patients can be considerable and may vary significantly as the pathophysiology evolves. A closed-loop system can maintain constant vigilance, administering fluid when needed and reducing infusions when patients stabilize.

The other area of active research is intraoperative fluid administration. A great deal of work has shown that various goal-directed fluid therapy approaches can improve patient outcomes and reduce hospital length of stay.[40,41] These protocols, however, can be time consuming to implement and require a constant high level of vigilance by the care provider, which may distract from other essential tasks. Automation of goal-directed fluid therapy with a closed-loop system can ease implementation and standardize performance on these protocols. Researchers at the University of California, Irvine developed an innovative system for automating fluid therapy, which has completed validation in engineering,[42] simulation,[43] animal studies,[44] and human studies.[40,45–47] This system was thoroughly evaluated and shown to safely administer fluids (Fig. 24.3). The interface allows both closed-loop and decision support options and functions with both semi-invasive and non-invasive pulse-contour analysis technologies.[45–47] Figure 24.4 shows important steps in the development of this closed-loop system. Two layers make up the controller. One allows it to predict fluid responsiveness based on previous population data (the "model" layer)

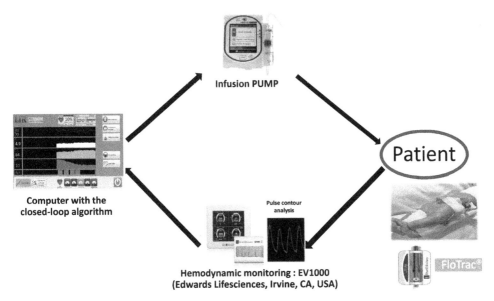

Infusion PUMP

Patient

Computer with the closed-loop algorithm

Pulse contour analysis

Hemodynamic monitoring : EV1000 (Edwards Lifesciences, Irvine, CA, USA)

FloTrac®

Figure 24.3 Closed-loop system for goal-directed fluid therapy. A black and white version of this figure will appear in some formats. For the color version, please refer to the plate section.

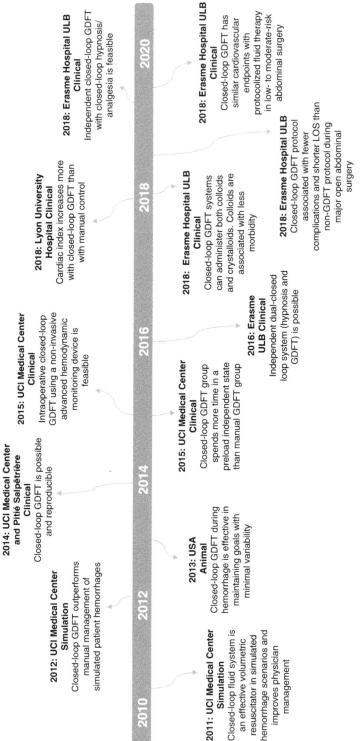

Figure 24.4 Evolution of closed-loop goal-directed fluid therapy (GDFT) over time. LOS, length of stay.

while the other, a learning component, evaluates bolus-based error after fluid administration (the "adaptive" layer). The adaptive layer, which modifies fluid infusion thresholds based on the patient's individual response, individualizes fluid therapy. This system maintains patients in preload independent state more consistently than manual goal-directed fluid therapy and was associated with improved outcome, when compared with fluid therapy based on a static parameters of fluid responsiveness.[40]

Closed-Loop Vasopressor Therapy

Intraoperative hypotension is linked to increased patient morbidity and mortality [48–50] and reversal often requires more than just fluids. Vasopressors are indispensable in perioperative medicine, as they can quickly improve hemodynamics. Strong variations in blood pressure may also be harmful, and a high systolic blood pressure variability is associated with increased perioperative renal failure and mortality. Effective blood pressure management should consistently maintain an individualized blood pressure threshold with minimal variability. When an individualized vasopressor strategy that aimed to maintain blood pressure within 10% of the patient's baseline was used, it significantly reduced postoperative organ dysfunction.[51] As many factors impact hemodynamic response during surgery, maintaining a precise and stable blood pressure value requires frequent and repetitive interventions. The challenge of vasopressor titration is a clinically relevant problem, and a recent observational study indicated that norepinephrine infusions in the ICU and operating rooms are around 50% of treatment time outside of predetermined target ranges.[52] This illustrates the need for improvement and decision support or even closed-loop systems may be the solution.[53,54]

Closed-loop blood pressure research for hemodynamic control began in the 1970s. Initial interest focused on blood pressure control, with research into heart rate control during rehabilitation and computer-controlled nitroprusside infusions for hypertension. Nitroprusside was initially the most heavily investigated vasoactive agent, probably because its short duration of action makes it easy to titrate. Additional studies were published through the 1980s and 1990s, all of which showed tighter and more consistent control with the closed-loop system.[55–59] Other studies have been published looking at blood pressure control in critical care settings using vasopressors to support blood pressure,[60–66] treat circulatory shock,[67] or in one case, study efficiency of weaning from vasopressors.[68] During obstetric care for caesarean section, Ngan Kee et al. developed a phenylephrine closed-loop system guided noninvasively with oscillometrically derived systolic blood.[69–71] This extensively tested system, in comparison to manually titrated phenylephrine, provides better blood pressure control for hypotension associated with spinal anesthesia. [69] The University of California, Irvine / University Libre de Bruxelles team has tested another controller in simulation studies [70,71] and an animal model and showed excellent performance metrics (i.e., target within ±5 mmHg for 98 ± 1% (mean ± SD) of the treatment time).[72] Even more recently, they published a proof of concept study that showed that this system minimized perioperative hypotension in patients undergoing moderate- or high-risk surgery.[73–75] The same team has also demonstrated the superiority of the closed-loop vasopressor therapy to decrease perioperative hypotension compared with manual control. [35,76,77]

Despite more than 40 years of research into closed-loop controllers for direct management of infusion of vasoactive agents, to date no system has been widely accepted or commercialized. The reasons for this are probably myriad, but one of the chief difficulties is ensuring patient safety with agents that are supporting life and have a very narrow safety margin with severe consequences of overdose. These features do not make closed-loop control of vasoactive agents impossible or even impractical –after all, we let computers manage commercial flights all the time and they have an incredible safety record – but the overall design, safety, and regulatory challenges have not been worth the potential commercial benefit to date. These factors may be changing, however, as cost pressure on the healthcare system is driving insurers and regulators to seek consistent outcomes.

Conclusion

Decision support and closed-loop systems are still finding their place in hemodynamic and fluid management. Given the increasing attention being paid to disparities in outcomes and care decisions across providers and institutions, it is likely that the coming years will see an increase in development and use of tools like these to standardize healthcare delivery.

References

1. Horsky J, Schiff GD, Johnston D, et al. Interface design principles for usable decision support: a targeted review of best practices for clinical prescribing interventions. *J Biomed Inform*. 2012;**45**(6):1202–16.

2. Enticott JC, Jeffcott S, Ibrahim JE, et al. A review on decision support for massive transfusion: understanding human factors to support the implementation of complex interventions in trauma. *Transfusion*. 2012;**52**(12):2692–705.

3. Shaughnessy AF, Slawson DC, Bennett JH. Becoming an information master: a guidebook to the medical information jungle. *J Fam Pract*. 1994;**39**(5):489–99.

4. Ahmadian L, van Engen-Verheul M, Bakhshi-Raiez F, et al. The role of standardized data and terminological systems in computerized clinical decision support systems: literature review and survey. *Int J Med Inform*. 2011;**80**(2):81–93.

5. Jaspers MW, Smeulers M, Vermeulen H, Peute LW. Effects of clinical decision-support systems on practitioner performance and patient outcomes: a synthesis of high-quality systematic review findings. *J Am Med Inform Assoc*. 2011;**18**(3):327–34.

6. Bright TJ, Wong A, Dhurjati R, et al. Effect of clinical decision-support systems: a systematic review. *Ann Intern Med*. 2012;**157**(1):29–43.

7. Wolfstadt JI, Gurwitz JH, Field TS, et al. The effect of computerized physician order entry with clinical decision support on the rates of adverse drug events: a systematic review. *J Gen Intern Med*. 2008;**23**(4):451–8.

8. Sahota N, Lloyd R, Ramakrishna A, et al. Computerized clinical decision support systems for acute care management: a decision-maker-researcher partnership systematic review of effects on process of care and patient outcomes. *Implement Sci*. 2011;**6**:91.

9. Eslami S, Abu-Hanna A, de Jonge E, de Keizer NF. Tight glycemic control and computerized decision-support systems: a systematic review. *Intensive Care Med*. 2009;**35**(9):1505–17.

10. Taylor JA, Loan LA, Kamara J, Blackburn S, Whitney D. Medication administration variances before and after implementation of computerized physician order entry in a neonatal intensive care unit. *Pediatrics*. 2008;**121**(1):123–8.

11. Adams ES, Longhurst CA, Pageler N, et al. Computerized physician order entry with decision support decreases blood transfusions in children. *Pediatrics*. 2011;**127**(5):e1112–19.

12. Spalding SC, Mayer PH, Ginde AA, Lowenstein SR, Yaron M. Impact of computerized physician order entry on ED patient length of stay. *Am J Emerg Med*. 2011;**29**(2):207–11.

13. Al-Dorzi HM, Tamim HM, Cherfan A, et al. Impact of computerized physician order entry (CPOE) system on the outcome of critically ill adult patients: a before-after study. *BMC Med Inform Decis Mak*. 2011;**11**:71.

14. Sondergaard S, Wall P, Cocks K, Parkin WG, Leaning MS. High concordance between expert anaesthetists' actions and advice of decision support system in achieving oxygen delivery targets in high-risk surgery patients. *Br J Anaesth*. 2012;**108**(6):966–72.

15. Gamble KH. Wired for CPOE. CIOs are finding that computerized physician order entry starts with a solid infrastructure. *Healthc Inform*. 2009;**25**(13):30–2.

16. Goddard K, Roudsari A, Wyatt JC. Automation bias – a hidden issue for clinical decision support system use. *Stud Health Technol Inform*. 2011;**164**:17–22.

17. Jung M, Hoerbst A, Hackl WO, et al. Attitude of physicians towards automatic alerting in computerized physician order entry systems. A comparative international survey. *Methods Inf Med*. 2013;**52**(2):99–108.

18. Epstein RH, Dexter F, Ehrenfeld JM, Sandberg WS. Implications of event entry latency on anesthesia information management decision support systems. *Anesth Analg*. 2009;**108**(3):941–7.

19. Li SY, Magrabi F, Coiera E. A systematic review of the psychological literature on interruption and its patient safety implications. *J Am Med Inform Assoc*. 2012;**19**(1):6–12.

20. Westbrook JI, Coiera E, Dunsmuir WT, et al. The impact of interruptions on clinical task completion. *Qual Saf Health Care*. 2010;**19**(4):284–9.

21. Rinehart J, Liu N, Alexander B, Cannesson M. Review article: closed-loop systems in anesthesia: is there a potential for closed-loop fluid management and hemodynamic optimization? *Anesth Analg*. 2012;**114**(1):130–43.

22. Dumont GA, Ansermino JM. Closed-loop control of anesthesia: a primer for anesthesiologists. *Anesth Analg*. 2013;**117**(5):1130–8.

23. Abbes IB, Richard PY, Lefebvre MA, Guilhem I, Poirier JY. A closed-loop artificial pancreas using a proportional integral derivative with double phase lead controller based on a new nonlinear model of glucose metabolism. *J Diabetes Sci Technol*. 2013;**7**(3):699–707.

24. Dauber A, Corcia L, Safer J, et al. Closed-loop insulin therapy improves glycemic control in children aged <7 years: a randomized controlled trial. *Diabetes Care*. 2013;**36**(2):222–7.

25. Elleri D, Allen JM, Kumareswaran K, et al. Closed-loop basal insulin delivery over 36 hours in adolescents with type 1 diabetes: randomized clinical trial. *Diabetes Care*. 2013;**36**(4):838–44.

26. Rivers E, Nguyen B, Havstad S, et al. Early goal-directed therapy in the treatment of severe sepsis and septic shock. *N Engl J Med*. 2001;**345**(19):1368–77.

27. Hamilton MA, Cecconi M, Rhodes A. A systematic review and meta-analysis on the use of preemptive hemodynamic intervention to improve postoperative outcomes in moderate and high-risk surgical patients. *Anesth Analg*. 2011;**112**(6):1392–1402.

28. Pearse R, Dawson D, Fawcett J, et al. Early goal-directed therapy after major surgery reduces complications and duration of hospital stay. A randomised, controlled trial [ISRCTN38797445]. *Crit Care*. 2005;**9**(6):R687-693.

29. Salinas J, Nguyen R, Darrah MI, et al. Advanced monitoring and decision support for battlefield critical care environment. *US Army Med Dep J*. 2011:73–81.

30. Salinas J, Chung KK, Mann EA, et al. Computerized decision support system improves fluid resuscitation following severe burns: an original study. *Crit Care Med*. 2011;**39**(9):2031–8.

31. Fitzgerald M, Cameron P, Mackenzie C, et al. Trauma resuscitation errors and computer-assisted decision support. *Arch Surg.* 2011;**146**(2):218–25.

32. Giuliano KK, Jahrsdoerfer M, Case J, Drew T, Raber G. The role of clinical decision support tools to reduce blood pressure variability in critically ill patients receiving vasopressor support. *Comput Inform Nurs.* 2012;**30**(4):204–9.

33. Joosten A, Hafiane R, Pustetto M, et al. Practical impact of a decision support for goal-directed fluid therapy on protocol adherence: a clinical implementation study in patients undergoing major abdominal surgery. *J Clin Monit Comput.* 2019;**33**(1):15–24.

34. Maheshwari K, Malhotra G, Bao X, et al. Assisted fluid management software guidance for intraoperative fluid administration. *Anesthesiology.* 2021;**135**(2):273–83.

35. Joosten A, Rinehart J, Van der Linden P, et al. Computer-assisted individualized hemodynamic management reduces intraoperative hypotension in intermediate- and high-risk surgery: a randomized controlled trial. *Anesthesiology.* 2021;**135**(2):258–72.

36. Bowman RJ, Westenskow DR. A microcomputer-based fluid infusion system for the resuscitation of burn patients. *IEEE Trans Biomed Eng.* 1981;**28**(6):475–9.

37. Blankenship HB, Wallace FD, Pacifico AD. Clinical application of closed-loop postoperative autotransfusion. *Med Prog Technol.* 1990;**16**(1–2):89–93.

38. Chaisson NF, Kirschner RA, Deyo DJ, et al. Near-infrared spectroscopy-guided closed-loop resuscitation of hemorrhage. *J Trauma.* 2003;**54**(5 Suppl):S183–92.

39. Hoskins SL, Elgjo GI, Lu J, et al. Closed-loop resuscitation of burn shock. *J Burn Care Res.* 2006;**27**(3):377–85.

40. Joosten A, Coeckelenbergh S, Delaporte A, et al. Implementation of closed-loop-assisted intra-operative goal-directed fluid therapy during major abdominal surgery: a case-control study with propensy matching. *Eur J Anaesthesiol.* 2018;**35**(9):650–8.

41. Messina A, Robba C, Calabrò L, et al. Association between perioperative fluid administration and postoperative outcomes: a 20-year systematic review and a meta-analysis of randomized goal-directed trials in major visceral/noncardiac surgery. *Crit Care.* 2021;**25**(1):43.

42. Rinehart J, Alexander B, Le Manach Y, et al. Evaluation of a novel closed-loop fluid-administration system based on dynamic predictors of fluid responsiveness: an in silico simulation study. *Crit Care.* 2011;**15**(6):R278.

43. Rinehart J, Chung E, Canales C, Cannesson M. Intraoperative stroke volume optimization using stroke volume, arterial pressure, and heart rate: closed-loop (learning intravenous resuscitator) versus anesthesiologists. *J Cardiothorac Vasc Anesth.* 2012;**26**(5):933–9.

44. Rinehart J, Lee C, Canales C, et al. Closed-loop fluid administration compared to anesthesiologist management for hemodynamic optimization and resuscitation during surgery: an in vivo study. *Anesth Analg.* 2013;**117**(5):1119–29.

45. Rinehart J, Lilot M, Lee C, et al. Closed-loop assisted versus manual goal-directed fluid therapy during high-risk abdominal surgery: a case-control study with propensity matching. *Crit Care.* 2015;**19**(1):94.

46. Joosten A, Huynh T, Suehiro K, et al. Goal-directed fluid therapy with closed-loop assistance during moderate risk surgery using noninvasive cardiac output monitoring: a pilot study. *Br J Anaesth.* 2015;**114**(6):886–92.

47. Lilot M, Bellon A, Gueugnon M, et al. Comparison of cardiac output optimization with an automated closed-loop goal-directed fluid therapy versus non standardized manual fluid administration during elective abdominal surgery: first prospective randomized controlled trial. *J Clin Monit Comput.* 2018;**32**(6):993–1003.

48. Gregory A, Stapelfeldt WH, Khanna AK, et al. Intraoperative hypotension is associated with adverse clinical outcomes after noncardiac surgery. *Anesth Analg.* 2021;**132**(6):1654–65.

49. Joosten A, Lucidi V, Ickx B, et al. Intraoperative hypotension during liver transplant surgery is associated with postoperative acute kidney injury: a historical cohort study. *BMC Anesthesiol.* 2021;**21**(1):12.

50. de la Hoz MA, Rangasamy V, Bastos AB, et al. Intraoperative hypotension and acute kidney injury, stroke, and mortality during and outside cardiopulmonary bypass: a retrospective observational cohort study. *Anesthesiology.* 2022;**136**(6):927–39.

51. Futier E, Lefrant JY, Guinot PG, et al. Effect of individualized vs standard blood pressure management strategies on postoperative organ dysfunction among high-risk patients undergoing major surgery: a randomized clinical trial. *JAMA.* 2017;**318**(14):1346–57.

52. Rinehart J, Ma M, Calderon MD, et al. Blood pressure variability in surgical and intensive care patients: is there a potential for closed-loop vasopressor administration? *Anaesth Crit Care Pain Med.* 2019;**38**(1):69–71.

53. Michard F, Liu N, Kurz A. The future of intraoperative blood pressure management. *J Clin Monit Comput.* 2018;**32**(1):1–4.

54. Joosten A, Rinehart J. Part of the steamroller and not part of the road: better blood pressure management through automation. *Anesth Analg.* 2017;**125** (1):20–2.

55. Petre JH, Cosgrove DM, Estafanous FG. Closed loop computerized control of sodium nitroprusside. *Trans Am Soc Artif Intern Organs.* 1983;**29**:501–5.

56. Rosenfeldt FL, Chang V, Grigg M, et al. A closed loop microprocessor controller for treatment of hypertension after cardiac surgery. *Anaesth Intensive Care.* 1986;**14** (2):158–62.

57. Reid JA, Kenny GN. Evaluation of closed-loop control of arterial pressure after cardiopulmonary bypass. *Br J Anaesth.* 1987;**59**(2):247–55.

58. Bednarski P, Siclari F, Voigt A, Demertzis S, Lau G. Use of a computerized closed-loop sodium nitroprusside titration system for antihypertensive treatment after open heart surgery. *Crit Care Med.* 1990;**18** (10):1061–5.

59. Mackenzie AF, Colvin JR, Kenny GN, Bisset WI. Closed loop control of arterial hypertension following intracranial surgery using sodium nitroprusside. A comparison of intra-operative halothane or isoflurane. *Anaesthesia.* 1993;**48**(3):202–4.

60. Mason DG, Packer JS, Cade JF, McDonald RD. Closed-loop management of blood pressure in critically ill patients. *Australas Phys Eng Sci Med.* 1985; **8** (4):164–7.

61. Colvin JR, Kenny GN. Development and evaluation of a dual-pump microcomputer-based closed-loop arterial pressure control system. *Int J Clin Monit Comput.* 1989;**6**(1):31–5.

62. Murchie CJ, Kenny GN. Comparison among manual, computer-assisted, and closed-loop control of blood pressure after cardiac surgery. *J Cardiothorac Anesth.* 1989;**3**(1):16–19.

63. McKinley S, Cade JF, Siganporia R, et al. Clinical evaluation of closed-loop control of blood pressure in seriously ill patients. *Crit Care Med.* 1991; **19**(2):166–70.

64. Martin JF. Closed-loop control of arterial pressure during cardiac surgery. *J Clin Monit.* 1992;**8**(3):252–5.

65. Nafz B, Persson PB, Ehmke H, Kirchheim HR. A servo-control system for open- and closed-loop blood pressure regulation. *Am J Physiol.* 1992;**262**(2 Pt 2): F320–5.

66. Potter DR, Moyle JT, Lester RJ, Ware RJ. Closed loop control of vasoactive drug infusion. A preliminary report. *Anaesthesia* .1984;**39**(7):670–7.

67. Mason DG, Packer JS, Cade JF, Siganporia RJ. Closed-loop management of circulatory shock. *Australas Phys Eng Sci Med.* 1988;**11**(4):133–42.

68. Merouani M, Guignard B, Vincent F, et al. Norepinephrine weaning in septic shock patients by closed loop control based on fuzzy logic. *Crit Care*. 2008;**12**(6):R155.

69. Ngan Kee WD, Tam YH, Khaw KS, Ng FF, Lee SWY. Closed-loop feedback computer-controlled phenylephrine for maintenance of blood pressure during spinal anesthesia for cesarean delivery: a randomized trial comparing automated boluses versus infusion. *Anesth Analg*. 2017;**125**(1):117–23.

70. Ngan Kee WD, Khaw KS, Ng FF, Tam YH. Randomized comparison of closed-loop feedback computer-controlled with manual-controlled infusion of phenylephrine for maintaining arterial pressure during spinal anaesthesia for caesarean delivery. *Br J Anaesth*. 2013;**110**(1):59–65.

71. Ngan Kee WD, Tam YH, Khaw KS, et al. Closed-loop feedback computer-controlled infusion of phenylephrine for maintaining blood pressure during spinal anaesthesia for caesarean section: a preliminary descriptive study. *Anaesthesia*. 2007;**62**(12):1251–6.

72. Joosten A, Delaporte A, Alexander B, et al. Automated titration of vasopressor infusion using a closed-loop controller: in vivo feasibility study using a swine model. *Anesthesiology*. 2019;**130**(3):394–403.

73. Joosten A, Alexander B, Duranteau J, et al. Feasibility of closed-loop titration of norepinephrine infusion in patients undergoing moderate- and high-risk surgery. *Br J Anaesth*. 2019;**123**(4):430.

74. Joosten A, Coeckelenbergh S, Alexander B, Cannesson M, Rinehart J. Feasibility of computer-assisted vasopressor infusion using continuous non-invasive blood pressure monitoring in high-risk patients undergoing renal transplant surgery. *Anaesth Crit Care Pain Med*. 2020;**39**(5):623–4.

75. Rinehart J, Cannesson M, Weeraman S, et al. Closed-loop control of vasopressor administration in patients undergoing cardiac revascularization surgery. *J Cardiothorac Vasc Anesth*. 2020;**34**(11):3081–5.

76. Joosten A, Chirnoaga D, Van der Linden P, et al. Automated closed-loop versus manually controlled norepinephrine infusion in patients undergoing intermediate- to high-risk abdominal surgery: a randomised controlled trial. *Br J Anaesth*. 2021;**126**(1):210–18.

77. Desebbe O, Rinehart J, Van der Linden P, et al. Control of postoperative hypotension using a closed-loop system for norepinephrine infusion in patients after cardiac surgery: a randomized trial. *Anesth Analg*. 2022;**134**(5):964–73.

25

Postoperative Surveillance: The Rise of Wireless Sensors, Pocket Ultrasound Devices and AI-Enabled Tools

Frédéric Michard

Introduction

Around 17% of patients undergoing non-ambulatory surgery develop at least one postoperative complication, and 1–2% ultimately die within 30 days following the procedure.[1] Given the global volume of surgeries, it represents over 4 million postoperative deaths every year, that is, more than the number of deaths related to malaria, tuberculosis, and HIV combined.[2]

Many retrospective observational studies have reported a significant association between perioperative hypotension and postoperative morbidity and mortality. Until recently, most studies focused on intraoperative hypotension, which is very common, in particular during anesthesia induction. During surgery, blood pressure is closely monitored (every 3–5 min, when not continuously) so that hypotensive events are quickly detected and usually last only a few minutes. In contrast, once patients have been admitted on surgical wards, blood pressure spot-checks are typically done every 4 to 8 hours. In this context, hypotensive events may be overlooked for hours. In the control group (5001 patients undergoing non-cardiac surgery) of the POISE-2 study,[3] the median cumulative duration of hypotension exceeded 8 hours on surgical wards whereas it was only 15 minutes during surgery (Fig. 25.1). In addition, hypotension on the wards was associated with a 183%

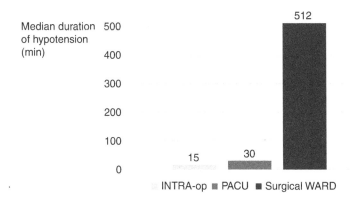

Figure 25.1 Median duration of hypotension during and after surgery in the control group (5001 patients undergoing non-cardiac surgery) of the POISE 2 trial. The median cumulative duration of hypotension exceeded 8 h on surgical wards, whereas it was only 15 min during surgery. Therefore, initiatives to improve patient safety should focus on the early detection and treatment of hypotensive events on the wards. INTRA-op, intraoperative; PACU, postanesthesia care unit. A black and white version of this figure will appear in some formats. For the color version, please refer to the plate section.

increase (odds ratio 2.83) in myocardial injury and death.[4] Therefore, preventing hours of hypotension after surgery may have a much bigger impact on patient outcome than preventing minutes of hypotension during surgery.[5]

The implementation of continuous blood pressure monitoring systems beyond the postanesthesia care unit (PACU) would enable the detection of hypotensive events without any delay.[6] Once hypotension is detected, point of care ultrasound devices may enable a quick assessment of cardiac function that would help to make rational therapeutic decisions.[7] In this chapter, I will first discuss new methods designed to monitor blood pressure non-invasively and continuously on surgical wards. Then, I will describe several hardware and software innovations, including artificial intelligence-enabled tools, for point-of-care echocardiography. Finally, I will briefly discuss how machine learning algorithms may help predict clinical deterioration during the postoperative period.

Continuous, Non-Invasive, and Mobile Blood Pressure Monitoring

Volume clamp methods have been proposed to monitor blood pressure continuously and non-invasively during surgery and could, at least in theory, be used as well after surgery.[8] Patients wear a finger cuff that is inflated during each heart beat by an air pump to precisely counterbalance the intramural finger arterial pressure and prevent any increase in arterial blood volume during systole. Knowing the counterbalancing pressure enables an estimation of the finger arterial pressure. Then, a mathematical transfer function provides an estimation of the corresponding brachial arterial pressure.

Clinical validation studies of volume clamp methods have yielded conflicting results. A recent meta-analysis [9] showed that only one-third of published studies reported an accuracy and precision meeting international standards (bias <5 mmHg, standard deviation <8 mmHg). Volume clamp methods are not reliable when the peripheral perfusion is shut down, which is often the case in patients with circulatory shock. In addition, volume clamp methods are part of bulky monitoring systems that have not been designed to be used beyond the PACU and are not wireless. Alternative techniques have therefore been proposed for the continuous and mobile monitoring of blood pressure on surgical wards.[5] At least two of them, the pulse wave transit time and the pulse decomposition methods, have been approved for medical use in Europe and/or in the USA.

Pulse Wave Transit Time Methods

The pulse wave transit time (PWTT) or pulse arrival time is the time difference between a heart beat and the arrival of the corresponding pulse in peripheral arteries. The PWTT depends on stroke volume and vascular tone. Any decrease in stroke volume or in vascular tone is responsible for an increase in PWTT. In this respect, changes in PWTT are known to correlate with changes in blood pressure. Acute changes in PWTT have been used with success to track changes in blood pressure during anesthesia induction.[10] In ward patients, blood pressure changes can be detected continuously in patients wearing simultaneously skin electrodes to detect the R wave of the electrocardiogram (ECG) and a pulse oximeter to detect the peripheral pulse arrival. As of today, at least two systems (from Sotera Wireless, Carlsbad, CA, USA and Biobeat, Petah Tikva, Israel) have been approved for continuous blood pressure monitoring in ambulatory ward patients. The Sotera system combines skin electrodes to record the ECG and a classic transductive finger pulse oximeter, whereas the Biobeat system uses a single thoracic adhesive sensor to capture both the ECG and pulse oximetry (reflective method) signals. Validation studies remain scarce, but the implementation of such mobile monitoring systems has been shown to be associated with improved postoperative outcome.[11]

Pulse Decomposition Method

The pulse decomposition method enables the continuous recording of a blood pressure waveform wirelessly with a low-pressure finger cuff (40 mmHg), a piezo electric sensor, and a proprietary algorithm analyzing pulse wave morphology. This method is implemented in the VitalStream monitoring system (Caretaker Medical, Charlottesville, VA, USA). At least two clinical studies.[12,13] suggest that the pulse decomposition method is accurate and precise enough to monitor blood pressure during surgery and in stable intensive care unit (ICU) patients. Studies are now needed to assess its reliability in awake ward patients, but such studies are challenging to conduct because of the lack of reference continuous monitoring technique in ambulatory patients. In addition to blood pressure, the VitalStream system continuously monitors advanced hemodynamic variables including stroke volume and cardiac output. This may help to identify the root cause of hypotension (a decrease in blood flow or systemic vasodilation) and select the most appropriate treatment.

Future Methods Not Yet Approved for Medical Use

Many different sensors are currently under development and testing. They include graphene, piezo-electric, and ultrasound sensors that, when positioned next to the radial or carotid artery, enable the wireless recording of high-fidelity blood pressure waveforms. [14] Both applanation tonometry and the volume clamp method have been miniaturized and could play a part in the future of bracelets or finger rings, respectively.[5]

Recently, artificial intelligence (AI) has been proposed to estimate blood pressure changes from a pulse oximetry signal. Machine learning algorithms trained with a large number of pulse oximetry and invasive arterial pressure waveforms become capable of recognizing specific morphological patterns that are characteristics of changes in arterial pressure. In a recent clinical study,[15] acute changes in systolic and mean arterial pressure during anesthesia induction were accurately tracked from the mere analysis of a pulse oximetry waveform. In the future, machine learning algorithms may enable continuous blood pressure monitoring between two intermittent oscillometric measurements and the automatic triggering of brachial cuff measurements as soon as significant changes in blood pressure are suspected (Fig. 25.2).

Challenges to the Implementation of Wireless Blood Pressure Monitoring Systems on Surgical Wards

Once a monitoring system has been selected, it is crucial to ensure its implementation is not going to result in a significant increase in false alarms and nurse workload.[16] To do so, smart algorithms, including machine learning algorithms, may be needed to filter artifacts. [17] Alarm settings should consider individual heart rate and blood pressure values recorded during the preoperative visit (personalization of alarm limits). Increasing the

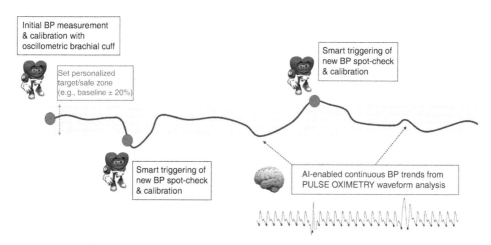

Figure 25.2 Principles of continuous blood pressure monitoring with a machine learning algorithm and a pulse oximeter. Assuming the oscillometric brachial cuff and the pulse oximeter are wireless, mobile and continuous monitoring of blood pressure may become a reality for patients at high risk of clinical deterioration on regular wards. BP, blood pressure. A black and white version of this figure will appear in some formats. For the color version, please refer to the plate section.

time between the detection of an abnormal blood pressure and the alarm (aka annunciation delay) may also help to reduce false alerts related to transient technical failure or movement artifacts.[6] Connectivity should be robust enough to prevent prolonged disruptions that could generate false alarms as well. Importantly, to enhance patient satisfaction and prevent sleep disorders, alarms should be banned from hospital rooms and received by caregivers on a central station, on their pager or smartphone, or in a dedicated command center.[16] Finally, processes must be put in place to ensure that the detection of hypotension is followed by a quick and appropriate response.[17] Indeed, if the lack of effective "afferent limb" has been advocated to explain disappointing results after the implementation of rapid response systems, the lack of "efferent limb" would likely be responsible for the same disappointment when using monitoring systems alone. These processes should be tailored to clinician habits and hospital organization but, in any case, must clearly define who should be informed (the nurse, the ward physician, or the rapid response team) and what should be done in case of hemodynamic deterioration. The key elements for a successful implementation of wireless wearable sensors on the wards are presented in Figure 25.3.

The Rise of Pocket Ultrasound Devices and Artificial Intelligence–Enabled Tools

Over the past decade, ultrasound devices became smaller, smarter, and affordable. Most cart-based point-of-care ultrasound (POCUS) systems are light and easy to move from one room to another. Some POCUS devices fit in the pocket, and several transducers can be connected to an electronic tablet or a smartphone, sometimes wirelessly.[18] As a result, POCUS devices may ultimately replace the stethoscope in the pocket of many clinicians, including those who are part of rapid response teams (RRT) or medical emergency teams (MET). In case of hemodynamic instability during the postoperative period, they enable a quick evaluation of cardiac anatomy and function.[7]

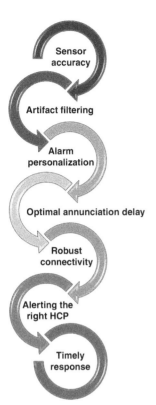

Figure 25.3 The implementation chain for wireless wearables on hospital wards. All links are indispensable for a successful implementation. HCP, healthcare professional. A black and white version of this figure will appear in some formats. For the color version, please refer to the plate section.

All pocket ultrasound devices are not created equal. Some enable a qualitative evaluation only. Interestingly, in case of RRT activation, a recent study [7] showed that a quick and qualitative evaluation of cardiac function with a pocket ultrasound device was associated with early therapeutic intervention and improved outcome in patients who developed hemodynamic instability.

Other ultrasound systems integrate pulsed Doppler and enable the quantification of the sub-aortic velocity time integral (VTI), a variable useful to guide therapy in patients with circulatory shock (Fig. 25.4). Most recent ultrasound devices come with software innovations, such as speckle tracking or machine learning algorithms. Speckle tracking or strain echocardiography enables the measurement of the global longitudinal strain (GLS) of the right and left ventricles. The GLS is a quantification of myocardial longitudinal shortening during systole.[19] GLS values are expressed as a negative percentage (shortening) and usually range between −20% and −30% for both ventricles. Less negative values (e.g., −15%) indicate a decrease in longitudinal shortening. The GLS is automatically calculated by modern echocardiographic software from a single cardiac view. In this respect, the estimation of GLS has been shown to be quicker and less operator-dependent than the estimation of classic echo-Doppler indices of systolic function.[20]

Machine learning algorithms have been developed to facilitate and automate the measurement of several key echocardiographic variables such as ventricular volumes, left

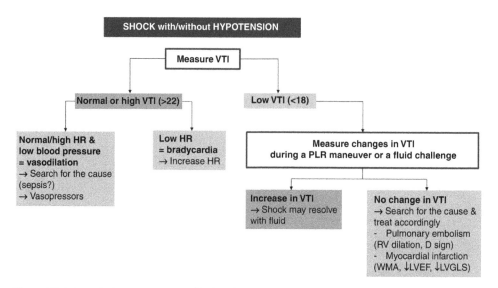

Figure 25.4 A simple decision tree to quickly identify the determinants of acute circulatory failure. The sub-aortic velocity time integral (VTI) is now easy to measure with a point-of-care ultrasound (POCUS) device and a machine learning algorithm.

HR, heart rate; LVEF, left ventricular ejection fraction; LVGLS, left ventricular global longitudinal strain; PLR, passive leg raising; RV, right ventricular; WMA, wall motion abnormalities.

ventricular ejection fraction (LVEF), and sub-aortic VTI. Most clinical validation studies published so far have been done in ambulatory cardiac patients.[21] However, a few recent studies done in critically ill patients yielded promising results, in particular for beginners in echocardiography (typically ICU residents). A neural network algorithm has been designed to provide real time LVEF measurements. To do so, the algorithm automatically detects the apical four-chamber view, endocardial left ventricular (LV) borders and end-diastolic/ systolic times from mitral valve motion. Then, it calculates LV volumes and LVEF. A recent clinical study done in 95 critically ill patients reported an excellent specificity (>95%) to detect LV dysfunction in critically ill patients.[22] Interestingly, in this study, the reproducibility of LVEF measurements was better when novices were using the machine learning algorithm than when experts in echocardiography were performing the measurements manually. Another machine learning algorithm, trained to automatically recognize the apical five-chamber view and the left ventricular outflow tract (Fig. 25.5), has been shown to be useful to estimate the sub-aortic VTI with a low percentage error.[23] This AI-enabled tool may therefore assist trainees in quickly identifying the underlying mechanisms of circulatory shock (see Fig. 25.4).

Prediction of Clinical Deterioration Using Machine Learning Algorithms

Early warning scores have been proposed to detect and quantify clinical deterioration on hospital wards. They are based on the aggregation of several vital signs into a single variable. They are better predictors of serious adverse events than any individual vital sign.

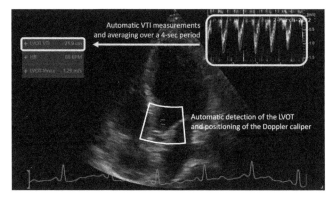

Figure 25.5 Example of machine learning algorithm for the automatic measurement of the sub-aortic velocity time integral (VTI).
First, the algorithm detects the five-chamber apical view and the left ventricular outflow tract (LVOT). A colored trapezoid around the LVOT indicates the quality of the ultrasound image and Doppler signal (green when optimal, yellow when fair, red when not acceptable). There is no need to position the caliper manually in the LVOT.
Then, the algorithm automatically measures and averages VTI over a 4-sec period. A black and white version of this figure will appear in some formats. For the color version, please refer to the plate section.

In hospital wards, they are increasingly used to trigger nurse intervention and to define the optimal timing for the next spot-check. Thanks to the development of connectivity and electronic medical record systems, early warning scores can now be automatically calculated.[6] When automated early warning systems are combined with paging functionality, they enable the immediate communication of clinical deterioration to a responsible nurse or physician. The use of automated early warning systems has been associated with improved outcomes in several large prospective studies.[24] Continuous monitoring of vital signs, including blood pressure, would give the opportunity to "refresh" early warning scores in the electronic medical record system on a very frequent basis (e.g., every 5 min) and has therefore potential to further improve their clinical value.

More sophisticated approaches, based on machine learning algorithms, can integrate multiple variables (in theory, all data contained in the electronic medical record system) and consider their trends over time and complex relationships, in order to better predict clinical trajectories.[6] The electronic Cardiac Arrest Risk Triage (eCART) and the Hospital wide Alerting Via Electronic Noticeboard (HAVEN) scores are examples of machine learning–derived fusion of age, vital signs, and laboratory data collected from electronic medical records. They have been shown to better predict cardiac arrest, ICU transfer, and death than classical early warning scores.[25] They may be useful to select patients who should be monitored more closely with mobile and wireless monitoring solutions.

Conclusion

Because of the low nurse-to-patient ratio on surgical wards and the intermittent nature of blood pressure spot-checks, there is increasing evidence that hemodynamic deterioration may be overlooked for hours. Several non-obtrusive systems have recently been developed to monitor blood pressure continuously and non-invasively. They may help to relieve nurses from time-consuming and repetitive tasks and to detect clinical deterioration earlier, decrease the number of RRT interventions, ICU admissions, cardiac arrests, and deaths. From a sensor standpoint, wireless wearables are emerging as the ideal solution for monitoring on the wards because they are patient friendly and they enable early mobilization, which is a key element of enhanced recovery programs. Clinical studies are needed to clarify what are the best strategies to effectively respond to early deterioration alerts. Such strategies may include the quick assessment of cardiac function with a POCUS device. Future trials will also have to investigate what is the impact on key outcome variables such as ICU admission and hospital length of stay, and which patients may benefit the most from mobile monitoring and ultrasound innovations.

References

1. International Surgical Outcomes Study Group. Global patient outcomes after elective surgery: prospective cohort study in 27 low-, middle-, and high-income countries. *Br J Anaesth.* 2016;**117**:601–9.

2. Nepogodiev D, Martin J, Biccard J, et al. Global burden of postoperative death. *Lancet.* 2019;**393**:401.

3. Devereaux PJ, Sessler DI, Leslie K, et al. Clonidine in patients undergoing non-cardiac surgery. *N Engl J Med.* 2014;**370**:1504–13.

4. Sessler DI, Meyhoff CS, Zimmerman NM, et al. Period-dependent associations between hypotension during and for 4 days after noncardiac surgery and a composite of myocardial infarction and death: a substudy of the POISE-2 trial. *Anesthesiology.* 2018;**128**:317–27.

5. Michard F, Scheeren TWL, Saugel B. A glimpse into the future of postoperative arterial blood pressure monitoring. *Br J Anaesth.* 2020;**125**:113–15.

6. Michard F, Kalkman C. Rethinking patient surveillance on hospital wards. *Anesthesiology.* 2021;**135**:531–40.

7. Zieleskiewicz L, Lopez A, Hraiech S, et al. Bedside POCUS during ward emergencies is associated with improved diagnosis and outcome: an observational, prospective, controlled study. *Crit Care.* 2021;**25**:34.

8. Michard F, Sessler DI, Saugel B. Non-invasive arterial pressure monitoring revisited. *Intensive Care Med.* 2018;**44**:2213–15.

9. Saugel B, Hoppe P, Nicklas JY, et al. Continuous non invasive pulse wave analysis using finger cuff technologies for arterial blood pressure monitoring in perioperative and intensive care medicine: a systematic review and meta-analysis. *Br J Anaesth.* 2020;**125**:25–37.

10. Kim SH, Song JG, Park JH, et al. Beat-to-beat tracking of systolic blood pressure using noninvasive pulse transit time during anesthesia induction in hypertensive patients. *Anesth Analg.* 2013;**116**:94–100.

11. Eddahchouri Y, Peelen RV, Koeneman M, et al. Effect of continuous wireless vital sign monitoring on unplanned ICU admissions and rapid response team calls: a before-and-after study. *Br J Anaesth.* 2022;**128**:857–63.

12. Gratz I, Deal E, Spitz F, et al. Continuous non-invasive finger cuff Caretaker comparable to invasive intra-arterial pressure in patients undergoing major abdominal surgery. *BMC Anesthesiol.* 2017;**17**:48.

13. Kwon Y, Stafford PL, Enfield K, et al. Continuous noninvasive monitoring of beat-by-beat blood pressure and heart rate using Caretaker compared with invasive arterial catheter in the intensive care unit. *J Cardiothorac Vasc Anesth.* 2022;**36**:2012–21.

14. Michard F. Hemodynamic monitoring in the era of digital health. *Ann Intensive Care.* 2016;**6**:15.

15. Ghamri Y, Proença M, Hofmann G, et al. Automated pulse oximeter waveform analysis to track changes in blood pressure

during anesthesia induction: a proof-of-concept study. *Anesth Analg.* 2020;**130**:1222–33.

16. Michard F, Thiele RH, Saugel B, et al. Wireless wearables for postoperative surveillance on surgical wards: a survey of 1158 anesthesiologists in Western Europe and in the USA. *BJA Open.* 2022;**1**:100002.

17. Michard F, Bellomo R, Taenzer A. The rise of ward monitoring: opportunities and challenges for critical care specialists. *Intensive Care Med.* 2019;**45**:671–73.

18. Le MPT, Voigt L, Nathanson R, et al. Comparison of four handheld point of care ultrasound devices by expert users. *Ultrasound J.* 2022;**14**:27.

19. Gonzalez F, Gomes R, Bacariza J, Michard F. Could strain echocardiography help to assess systolic function in critically ill COVID-19 patients? *J Clin Monit Comput.* 2021;**35**:1229–34.

20. Karlsen S, Dahlslett T, Grenne B, et al. Global longitudinal strain is a more reproducible measure of left ventricular function than ejection fraction regardless of echocardiographic training. *Cardiovasc Ultrasound.* 2019;**17**:18.

21. Nabi W, Bansal A, Xu B. Applications of artificial intelligence and machine learning approaches in echocardiography. *Echocardiography.* 2021;**38**:982–92.

22. Varudo R, Gonzalez FA, Leote J, et al. Machine learning for the real time assessment of left ventricular ejection fraction in critically ill patients: a bedside evaluation by novices and experts in echocardiography. *Crit Care.* 2022;**26**:386.

23. Gonzalez FA, Varudo R, Leote J, et al. Automation of sub-aortic velocity time integral measurements by transthoracic echocardiography: clinical evaluation of an artificial intelligence-enabled tool in critically ill patients. *Br J Anesth.* 2022;**129**: e116–e119.

24. Escobar GJ, Liu VX, Schuler A, et al. Automated identification of adults at risk for in-hospital deterioration. *N Engl J Med.* 2020;**383**:1951–60.

25. Pimentel MAF, Redfern OC, Malycha J, et al. Detecting deteriorating patients in hospital: development and validation of a novel scoring system. *Am J Respir Crit Care Med.* 2021;**204**:44–52.

Chapter 26

Can Perfusion Index Be Useful for Fluid and Hemodynamic Management?

Maxime Coutrot, Emmanuel Dudoignon, Benjamin Deniau and François Dépret

Introduction

In the 1970s, following previous works, pulse oximetry was developed using red and infrared lights transmission through tissues.[1]

Recently, there has been heightened interest in non-invasive monitoring of macrohemodynamic and microcirculation, particularly within anesthesia, perioperative and critical care. Photoplethysmography (PPG) signal, which was historically only used to monitor oxygen saturation, now offers itself as an interesting tool in hemodynamic monitoring.

PPG is a non-invasive tool that is cheap, fast and simple to use. However, the interpretation of PPG data can be challenging. Due to an initial lack of knowledge and through the misunderstanding of its determinants, the technique of hemodynamic monitoring utilizing PPG signal was not used effectively. However, analysis of PPG signal has benefitted from regained interest in the past years; its usefulness has been highlighted by several works in anesthesia and perioperative and critical care.[2–4]

Among the different components of PPG signal, perfusion index (PI), which represents the proportion of the pulsatile part of PPG, has been widely studied and presents a promising tool for physicians. A good understanding of the principles of PPG and PI determinants, as well as the knowledge of their limits, is therefore essential to optimize correct use and performance. Physical principles and the physiological determinants of PI will be explained thereafter in this chapter.

This chapter also covers the physiological and technical aspects of PPG and PI that clinicians need to understand, and presents the clinical usefulness of PI in the operating theater and in perioperative and critical care.

Measurement of Perfusion Index: Technical Aspects

Principles of Photoplethysmography

The basic principle of conventional PPG is based on indirect measurement of tissue volume variations, using absorbance variations of light beams through this tissue or by reflection properties of the light in the tissue. The oximeter probe generates incident red and ultra-red light beams, whose transmitted or reflected intensities by the tissues are transformed into electrical currents by a photodetector (Fig. 26.1).

Usually, red light (660 nm) and infrared light (940 nm) are used for PPG. Those are mainly absorbed by deoxyhemoglobin and oxyhemoglobin, respectively. The PPG curve represents infrared light absorption variations. However, some PPG devices use one or often more than two wavelengths.

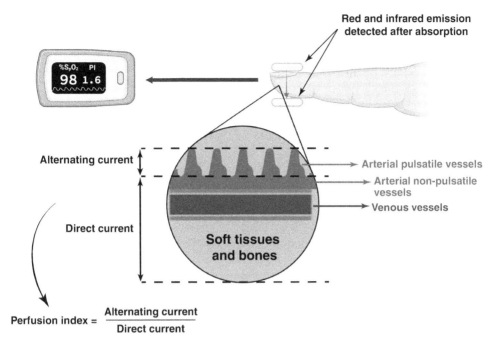

Figure 26.1 Principles of photoplethysmography and PI calculation. A black and white version of this figure will appear in some formats. For the color version, please refer to the plate section.

Perfusion Index Components: Alternating Current (AC) and Direct Current (DC)

Light absorption varies across the cardiac cycle. The absorption is maximal during the systole, because it reflects the dilation of vessels under systolic pressure, that is, the increase of arterial blood volume under the light source. The signal received by the photodetector is then decomposed into pulsatile and non-pulsatile signals. Pulsatile variation in light absorption during systole is commonly referred to as alternating current (AC). AC represents variations of absorbance or reflectance of the incident light beams due to pulsatile vessels under arterial pressure variations, that is, the sum of the variations of the diameters of pulsatile vessels through which the light beams pass. Therefore, AC represents an indirect measure of arterial volume change during the cardiac cycle, but not a flow measurement in those vessels.

The PPG curve displayed on actual monitors represents AC, derived from the infrared light signal, after signal processing. Restitution of AC requires computer processing (via computer filters) of the raw signal received by the photodetector to reduce signal artifacts. These manufacturer-dependent algorithms can significantly deform the PPG curve; each impacting the data in different ways.

In contrast, continuous absorption is referred to as direct current (DC), from which AC varies. DC corresponds to light absorption from other tissues, such as non-pulsatile capillaries and venous vessels, skin, soft tissues and bones. DC is not displayed in current practice on a usual oximeter's monitors.

PI Calculation: AC/DC

PI represents the ratio of pulsatile light absorption on continuous light absorption, that is, the ratio AC/DC (Fig. 26.1). PI, often referred to as "peripheral PI," was initially used as a quality signal indicator for pulse oximetry. However, PI represents the local blood volume variation during systole and varies according to systemic and local hemodynamic status. Hence, PI can be used for non-invasive hemodynamic monitoring.

Determinants of Perfusion Index: Physiological and Pathophysiological Aspects

Physiological Value of PI

In healthy awake volunteers, mean PI values (± standard deviation) measured at the finger were in two studies 2.2% ± 2.0 and 3.5% ± 2.4.[5,6] This means that AC represents only around 2–3% of DC, and that the blood volume under the sensor increases by around 2–3% at each heart beat. However, the ranges of PI normal values in healthy volunteers are wide (from <1% to >10%), and it is difficult to propose a reliable normal value of this parameter.

Determinants of PI are numerous and complex. When measured in a peripheral site, both AC and DC and their ratio are the results of systemic and local factors, which are discussed below, and summarized in Table 26.1.

Determinants of Direct Current (DC)

PI represents the ratio AC/DC. Thus, any variation of DC will result in a variation of PI. Soft tissues or venous compression (e.g., by a finger clip) may decrease DC and increase PI. Likewise, congestion due to global fluid overload would have the opposite consequences. Changes in DC due to limb position and induced changes of venous filling would also affect PI value: increase in DC if the limb is in declive (venous congestion) and its opposite, proclive.[3] DC is also not constant, and small variations are observed due to variations in venous return and sympathetic tone in spontaneously breathing patients, or under those mechanical ventilation. Similarly, DC may also change if vascular tone changes, as under action of vasoactive drugs (i.e., decrease of DC while vascular tone increases).[7]

Determinants of Alternating Current (AC)

Some authors have described PI as a surrogate of vascular tone only. Lima et al. showed that PI was correlated with central to toe temperature gradient – an accurate surrogate of vascular tone.[5] Indeed, PI rapidly increases after local vasodilation induced by plexus or epidural anesthesia, measured in the blocked area. PI was also strongly influenced by changes of vascular tone under action of vasopressors in patients under general anesthesia (i.e., decrease in PI secondary to norepinephrine infusion).[8]

Several recent studies suggested that stroke volume (SV) is another important determinant of PI. PI was correlated with superior vena cava flow and cardiac output in infants. [9–11] Low flow could be associated with increased vascular tone, but such data are not presented in these works. Van Genderen et al. exposed healthy volunteers to a lower body negative pressure.[12] They observed a rapid decrease in median PI (from 2.2% to 1.3%), while SV decreased, and skin temperature difference between forearm and fingertip did not

Table 26.1 Determinants of Perfusion Index and artifacts

Systemic factors	Local factors
Factors influencing AC	
• Volemia and venous return[*]	• Obliterative arteriopathy
• Diastolic function and inotropism[*]	• Position of the limb in relation to the heart
• Valvulopathy[*]	• Vascular compression
• Vascular tone[*] (sympathetic, parasympathetic and nonadrenergic/ noncholinergic tones)	• Local temperature exposure
• Arterial stiffness[*]	• Local arterial compliance
• Vasoactive and cardiac medications[*]	• Local vascular tone
Factors influencing DC	
• Vascular tone[*] (notably venous tone)	• Position of the limb
• Volemia[*]	• Body position
	• Vascular compression
	• Soft tissues compression
	• Local vascular tone
Artifacts that may influence AC and DC	
• External light	• Tissues and vascular extrinsic compressions
• Nail polish	• Probe and/or patient movements

Numerous intrinsic or extrinsic factors influence AC and/or DC, and therefore their ratio, i.e., Perfusion Index. The main determinants are stroke volume and vascular tone, themselves influenced by many factors. Determinants of stroke volume (*) all may influence AC and PI. Volemia, external temperature, stress, nociception, medications (e.g., norepinephrine, vasodilatator effect of anesthetic drugs) are determinants of vascular tone and therefore of Perfusion Index.
[*] Determinants of stroke volume
AC, alternating current; DC, direct current

increase significantly. Lack of significant variation in skin temperature gradient between forearm and fingertip may be explained by the reduced scale of the study (the study population comprised 25 males) or because of temperature change inertia. This suggested that PI was not only influenced by local vascular tone but also by SV itself. Another study performed in healthy volunteers showed PI variations induced by body positioning modifications (e.g., Trendelenburg, 45-degree, supine).[13] The highest values of PI were observed in Trendelenburg position (7.8 ± 3.8%). Conversely, PI was the lowest in the sitting position (4.5 ± 2.5%), suggesting a positive relationship between PI and SV. This has been confirmed in a work showing that variation of PI was highly correlated to variation of SV ($r = 0.9$), and mean arterial pressure (MAP) ($r = 0.9$) during head up and down tilt test in patients under general anesthesia with low basal sympathetic tone or reactivity to position-induced hypovolemia.[14] Additionally, other recent works found significant correlation of cardiac index and PI variations after passive leg raising and fluid challenge.[15–17] These works

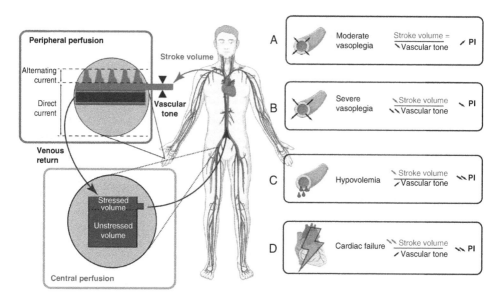

Figure 26.2 Determinants of perfusion index (PI) and typical clinical situations. A black and white version of this figure will appear in some formats. For the color version, please refer to the plate section.

confirmed the major influence of SV on PI and the complexity of PI variations interpretation, especially in septic shock.[18]

The respective influence of vascular tone and SV variations in vasoplegia are shown in Figure 26.2, cases A and B. Figure 26.2, case A, represents moderate vasoplegia (e.g., intraoperative hypotension secondary to anesthetic drugs). In this case, the increase of PI (from 5% to 10%) would mainly be the consequence of a fall in arterial vascular tone (secondary to vasodilation induced by anesthetic drugs) without substantial SV variations.[5,7,8] In severe vasoplegia (Fig. 26.2, case B), such as under general anesthesia with an overdose of anesthetics leading to a significant decrease in stressed volume, venous return and thus in SV, or in surgical bleeding, PI decreases secondarily compared with Figure 26.2, case A, despite a low arterial vascular tone. In this case, SV would be the predominant determinant, leading to a PI secondary decrease, that is, "hiding" the effect of the decrease of vascular tone on PI. [12–14,16] However, data are lacking to quantify the respective contributions of vascular tone and stroke volume in PI values and interpret its variations in such clinical situations.

Conversely, as illustrated in the Figure 26.2, case C, in the case of hypovolemia with preserved baroreceptors activation, SV will decrease and vascular tone increase. Both variations of SV and vascular tone will contribute to a decrease in AC. In such conditions, a decrease in DC secondary to the activation of the sympathetic system also participates in the drop of PI, suggesting that the decrease in AC is predominant over the decrease in DC. [7,12,13] Another comparable situation characterized by a low SV and potential increased vascular tone is cardiac failure, where both also contribute to the fall of AC, DC and PI values (Fig. 26.2, case D). In this situation, PI would be typically extremely low PI (<0.5%). After inotropic drugs, an increase in SV would lead to a greater PI value.[7]

Local Conditions

As PI measurement assesses local perfusion, its value varies according to the measurement site, even for sites within a few centimeters of each other. Thus, PI is highly influenced by systemic macrohemodynamic status as well as local conditions, since local vascular tone is mainly influenced by thermoregulation and non-thermoregulatory stimuli (e.g., nociception, exercise).[19,20] As an example, in one study PPG waveform variations were substantially different between ear and finger after cold exposure.[21] Regional anesthesia also illustrates the influence of local conditions: the increase in PI measured in the blocked area after regional anesthesia shows a decrease in local vascular tone associated with an increase in local blood flow and volume at each heart beat in the blocked region. Both the decrease in vascular tone and the increase in local blood flow and volume are contributing to the rise of AC and PI values. As for other variations of vascular tone, it is expected that DC also increases in the blocked area, although this has not been studied. In this situation, PI is a tool for local but not central hemodynamic monitoring. Likewise, many local conditions must be taken into account to interpret PI value: local compression (soft tissues, veins and/or arteries), outside temperature variations, positions of the limbs or severe arterial abnormalities such as obliterating arteriopathy. In the conditions mentioned above, peripheral PI rather reflects local conditions than the central hemodynamic status.[11,22] However, no difference was found in basal PI in volunteers with or without vascular disease (hypertension and diabetes mellitus). On the contrary, macrohemodynamic status (i.e., cardiac index) can influence PI value depending on the measurement site. In infants, PI tends to be higher at the right hand compared with the foot for low cardiac output, and inversely for high cardiac output.[9] All these elements suggest the importance of regional perfusion variation secondary to changes of sympathetic response and central hemodynamic status on local PI value.

Sources of Errors and Variations of PPG Signal and PI Value

Clinicians must be aware of the frequent sources of known errors in the measurement of PI. Any extrinsic compression of soft tissues and/or vascular bed can affect AC and/or DC and so the value of PI and/or its variations.[3] A common example is the digital compression by the clamping of PPG. The ear and finger PPG sensors are usually fitted with a clip, which avoids venous stasis and its influence on DC and thus on PI. Without a clip, forehead PPG waveform, that is, AC signal, has been described as significantly affected by a strong venous signal. Therefore, venous compression by a clip may result in a more reliable arterial waveform.[23] However, the use of an external pressure on the forehead probe with a dedicated headband in order to suppress the impact of venous pulsation may also result in a more reliable PPG waveform. Other classical sources of errors or factors that may influence PPG waveform, such as nail polish, obesity, age, gender, ambient lights changes, course artifacts of movement of the probe, or the patient, have been pointed out.[22]

PI and Fluid Therapy

PI, Fluid Responsiveness and Fluid Removal

PI variations were assessed during passive leg raising (PLR) for prediction of fluid responsiveness in intensive care unit (ICU) patients, most of them under mechanical ventilation. [15] An increase of PI > 9% induced by PLR predicted an increase of cardiac index > 10% induced by PLR with a sensitivity of 91%, a specificity of 79% and an area under the receiver operating characteristics curve (AUC) of 0.89. Another study also showed that PI variations during end-expiratory occlusion test could predict positive PLR.[16] However, the cut-off value of relative PI increase during end-expiratory occlusion test was very low (2.5%), compared with the PI values displayed today in most monitors with most often only one decimal place, and with respect to spontaneous variations in PI. The ratio PI before weaning trial/PI during weaning trial was also studied in a trial of mechanically ventilated patients during spontaneous breathing to predict weaning failure.[24] During the spontaneous breathing trial, the lack of increase in PI was associated with trial failure. This suggests than when PI increases during a spontaneous breathing trial, patients may be on the initial vertical part of the Frank–Starling curve, that is, fluid responders, and thus at lower risk of weaning-induced pulmonary edema. Following the same pathophysiology, PI and its variations during renal replacement therapy were studied to predict arterial hypotension. A PI value ≤ 0.82% at the beginning of renal replacement therapy predicts arterial hypotension during ultrafiltration with an AUC of 0.8. A decrease in PI during fluid removal was also predictive of arterial hypotension.[25] As for neuraxial anesthesia, low PI could be associated with high vascular tone and/or low SV, and thus predictive of arterial hypotension due in part to hypovolemia induced by fluid removal. However, these data should be confirmed in larger cohorts.

PI Respiratory Variations for Prediction of Fluid Responsiveness

The variability of PI is low during steady-state conditions under deep general anesthesia, because general anesthesia reduces the oscillatory components of the perfusion signal related to sympathetic, myogenic activity and the component modulated by the endothelium. Therefore, in this situation PI variations are mainly due to SV variations. PI respiratory variations, measured by the Pleth Variability Index (PVI), have been widely studied in mechanically ventilated patients for the prediction of fluid responsiveness, notably in the operating room. The physiological concept is based on tracking PI variations as a surrogate of SV variations (or pulse pressure) induced by positive pressure ventilation. The respiratory variations of PI, then, could have nearly the same accuracy in predicting fluid responsiveness as pulse pressure variation.

A recent meta-analysis highlighted the wide range of PVI cut-off values (from 7% to 20%), depending on the studied population and ventilation settings (e.g., ICU, tidal volume, positive end-expiratory pressure) to predict fluid responsiveness.[26] Furthermore, PVI is also (as it is derived from PI) largely influenced by the measurement site and seems to be more accurate in predicting fluid responsiveness when measured in the forehead, where it is less influenced by vasomotor tone, than the finger and earlobe.[27] Although a study showed that PVI-guided intraoperative fluid management was associated with reduced volume of fluid infused and reduced lactate levels, a perioperative management based on PVI (compared with standard management) was not associated with shorter duration of hospitalization.[28,29] Therefore, further studies are needed to assess whether using PVI for hemodynamic management in the operating room is useful in improving prognosis of these patients.

Clinical Usefulness of PI during Anesthesia for Hemodynamic Monitoring

PI has been studied in the operating theater for patients under regional or general anesthesia in different clinical settings.

Usefulness of PI for Hemodynamic Management under Neuraxial Anesthesia

After spinal-epidural anesthesia for Caesarean delivery, basal PI measured at the finger is correlated with a decrease in systolic arterial pressure (SAP) ($r = 0.66$).[30] Baseline PI is also better correlated with SAP or MAP decrease than baseline heart rate, SAP or MAP. A PI value ≥ 3.5% before spinal anesthesia is a risk factor for anesthesia-induced arterial hypotension.[31] A high PI value at baseline suggests a low basal vascular tone. Therefore, the decrease in sympathetic tone induced by spinal epidural in patients with already low basal sympathetic tone is more likely to induce a decrease in the stressed volume, resulting in a decrease of venous return and SV. Thus, PI can easily detect low sympathetic tone in parturient patients at high risk of arterial hypotension induced by the sympatholysis induced by neuraxial anesthesia.

Usefulness of PI for Hemodynamic Management during General Anesthesia

The value of PI for detection of arterial hypotension during general anesthesia has been shown. During induction of anesthesia, PI variations are inversely correlated with MAP variations.[8] An increase of 51% or more from baseline PI can detect a decrease of MAP of ≥20%. Conversely, during the maintenance of general anesthesia, in patients who underwent head-up and head-down tilt, PI variations are positively correlated to MAP variations. [14] Head-up tilt induces a decrease in SV, correlated to MAP decrease, suggesting no significant variations in vascular tone during this maneuver and resulting in a drop in PI. In contrast, induction of anesthesia is associated with a severe drop in vascular tone. The two relationships between PI and MAP show that PI should be considered as the balance between SV and vascular tone, as schematically described in Figure 26.2. Then, a rapid variation of PI represents an alarm signal that should warn and force the clinician to quickly check the occurrence of an arterial hypotension in patients under general anesthesia monitored with intermittent cuff blood pressure measurement. The kinetics of PI variation may also help clinicians to identify the mechanism of arterial hypotension and manage these situations quickly and accurately: an increase in PI suggests excessive vasodilation (e.g., relative to excessive depth of anesthesia), while a secondary decrease in PI in a patient deeply anesthetized may reveal SV decrease (hypovolemia and/or cardiac dysfunction).

Prognostic Value of PI in the Operating Room

Intraoperative PI is associated with severe postoperative complications and death. Lower values of PI are associated with worst outcomes in a time dependent manner, even after adjustment for confounding variables.[32] The association between PI with the postoperative complications is higher in patients with MAP > 65 mmHg than in patients with MAP ≤ 65 mmHg.

However, the impact of PI use in hemodynamic management during anesthesia on clinical outcomes remains to be assessed in randomized-controlled trials.

Perspectives

PPG having long been used for oximetry only, renewed interest and increasing use of PI (notably in anesthesia) have been observed recently. However, some important issues remain to be dealt with (Fig. 26.3).

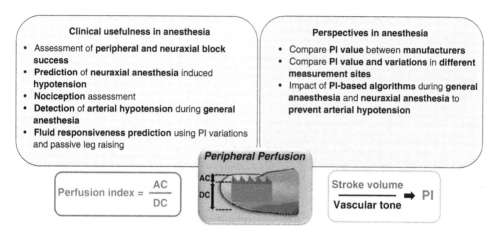

Figure 26.3 Summary of clinical usefulness and perspectives of perfusion index (PI) use in anesthesia. A black and white version of this figure will appear in some formats. For the color version, please refer to the plate section.

Technical Aspects

First, certain technical aspects need to be assessed, as the measured values of PI between manufacturers have never been evaluated and could vary significantly. Algorithms and filters used by manufacturers to process the signal could be sources of distortion of the PPG signal, and therefore influence PI performances in various clinical settings. Furthermore, these differences between monitors could also impact the absolute value of PI and could lead to misinterpretations of values. Therefore, the adequate cut-off value could be different between manufacturers. For such reasons, studies assessing PI should always indicate which PPG device has been used.

Impact of PI Use in Hemodynamic Management during Anesthesia

Should the data indicate the usefulness of PI for hemodynamic monitoring, it remains to be explored whether its application would improve the prognosis of patients undergoing surgery. To date, no comprehensive studies have been conducted. One notable study reported the use of an algorithm integrating PI and pulse pressure variation to guide fluid administration and the use of vasopressors (i.e., in the case of an arterial hypotension event, fluids should be administered if the PI value remains steady during the 15 min previous to the arterial hypotension; conversely, the increase of the PI value should lead to the use of vasopressors). The use of this algorithm was associated with a significant lower duration of arterial hypotension (7.7 ± 5.0 min vs. 17.1 ± 10.6 min) and lower intraoperative fluid administration (4.3 ± 1.3 ml/kg/hr vs. 7.2 ± 3.3 ml/kg/hr).[33] However, this study suffers from several limitations. For example, there was no algorithm in the control group, and the use of an algorithm itself may have favored an early use of vasopressors rather than fluid challenge. We could assume that another algorithm using other variables without PI may have similar effects.

PI value before neuraxial anesthesia predicts arterial hypotension.[30,31] Similarly, variations of PI allow real-time detection of arterial hypotension during the induction of general anesthesia.[8] Nevertheless, the impact of PI use in these fields remains to be explored. Indeed, algorithms using PI for early use of vasopressors should be evaluated to prevent arterial hypotension following neuraxial anesthesia or induction of general anesthesia.

Assessment and Impact of Mucosal PI Measurement

In addition to measurements in external sites (limbs, forehead, etc.), PPG signal and PI have been studied in urinary and digestive mucosa.[34–36]

Urethral PI (uPI) was the most studied. Using the IKORUS UP® probe (Vygon) during major abdominal surgery, signal quality was almost always good or excellent. Urethral PI was strongly and positively correlated with SV for 45% of measurement time, positively correlated with MAP for 47% of measurement time, but negatively correlated with MAP for 18% of measurement time.[35] As previously described, the dissociation of correlation between PI and MAP results from the balance between local vascular tone and SV. The MAP threshold for which the correlation reverses varies from one individual to another.[36]

These data strongly suggest that mucosal PI could also be useful in tailoring vasopressors and fluids in order to improve microcirculation and tissue perfusion, particularly once macrohemodynamic targets are achieved. Although uPI has already been studied during abdominal surgery, none of this work was designed to assess the impact of its use on the prognosis of the patient.[37,38]

Conclusion

PI derived from the PPG signal is already measured by most devices. PI is at the crossroads between central and peripheral perfusion, and appears to be a useful, non-invasive supplementary tool for hemodynamic monitoring in perioperative care for clinicians. It is essential to know its determinants in order to interpret its potential variations. Further study is required to determine whether the use of PI in resuscitation algorithms improves patient outcomes.

Glossary of Terms

PPG: photoplethysmography
PI: perfusion index
PVI: Pleth Variability Index
AC: alternating current
DC: direct current
SV: stroke volume
MAP: mean arterial pressure
ICU: intensive care unit
PLR: passive leg raising
CI: confidence interval
uPI: urethral perfusion index

References

1. Aoyagi T. Pulse oximetry: its invention, theory, and future. *J Anesth*. 2003 Nov 1;**17**(4):259–66.

2. Alian AA, Shelley KH. Photoplethysmography. *Best Pract Res Clin Anaesthesiol*. 2014 Dec;**28**(4):395–406.

3. Reisner A, Shaltis PA, McCombie D, Asada HH. Utility of the photoplethysmogram in circulatory monitoring. *Anesthesiology*. 2008 May;**108**(5):950–8.

4. Elgendi M. Optimal signal quality index for photoplethysmogram signals. *Bioengineering*. 2016 Sep 22;**3**(4):21.

5. Lima AP, Beelen P, Bakker J. Use of a peripheral perfusion index derived from the pulse oximetry signal as a noninvasive indicator of perfusion. *Critl Care Med.* 2002;**30**(6):1210–13.

6. Keller G, Cassar E, Desebbe O, Lehot JJ, Cannesson M. Ability of Pleth Variability Index to detect hemodynamic changes induced by passive leg raising in spontaneously breathing volunteers. *Crit Care.* 2008;**12**(2):R37.

7. Jeong I, Jun S, Um D, Oh J, Yoon H. Non-invasive estimation of systolic blood pressure and diastolic blood pressure using photoplethysmograph components. *Yonsei Med J.* 2010;**51**(3):345.

8. Coutrot M, Joachim J, Dépret F, et al. Noninvasive continuous detection of arterial hypotension during induction of anaesthesia using a photoplethysmographic signal: proof of concept. *Br J Anaesth.* 2019 May;**122**(5):605–12.

9. Corsini I, Cecchi A, Coviello C, Dani C. Perfusion index and left ventricular output correlation in healthy term infants. *Eur J Pediatr.* 2017 Aug;**176**(8):1013–18.

10. Janaillac M, Beausoleil TP, Barrington KJ et al. Correlations between near-infrared spectroscopy, perfusion index, and cardiac outputs in extremely preterm infants in the first 72 h of life. *Eur J Pediatr.* 2018 Apr;**177**(4):541–50.

11. Takahashi S, Kakiuchi S, Nanba Y, et al. The perfusion index derived from a pulse oximeter for predicting low superior vena cava flow in very low birth weight infants. *J Perinatol.* 2010;**30**(4):265–9.

12. Van Genderen ME, Bartels SA, Lima A, et al. Peripheral perfusion index as an early predictor for central hypovolemia in awake healthy volunteers. *Anesth Analg.* 2013 Feb;**116**(2):351–6.

13. Tapar H, Karaman S, Dogru S, et al. The effect of patient positions on perfusion index. *BMC Anesthesiol.* 2018 Dec;**18**(1):111.

14. Højlund J, Agerskov M, Clemmesen CG, Hvolris LE, Foss NB. The peripheral perfusion index tracks systemic haemodynamics during general anaesthesia. *J Clin Monit Comput.* 2020 Dec;**34**(6):1177–84.

15. Beurton A, Teboul JL, Gavelli F, et al. The effects of passive leg raising may be detected by the plethysmographic oxygen saturation signal in critically ill patients. *Crit Care.* 2019 Dec;**23**(1):19.

16. Beurton A, Gavelli F, Teboul JL, De Vita N, Monnet X. Changes in the plethysmographic perfusion index during an end-expiratory occlusion detect a positive passive leg raising test. *Crit Care Med.* 2021 Feb;**49**(2):e151–60.

17. Lian H, Wang X, Zhang Q, Zhang H, Liu D. Changes in perfusion can detect changes in the cardiac index in patients with septic shock. *J Int Med Res.* 2020 Aug;**48**(8):030006052093167.

18. He HW, Liu WL, Zhou X, Long Y, Liu DW. Effect of mean arterial pressure change by norepinephrine on peripheral perfusion index in septic shock patients after early resuscitation. *Chin Med J (Engl).* 2020 Sep 20;**133**(18):2146–52.

19. Charkoudian N. Mechanisms and modifiers of reflex induced cutaneous vasodilation and vasoconstriction in humans. *J Appl Physiol.* 2010 Oct;**109**(4):1221–8.

20. Hodges GJ, Johnson JM. Adrenergic control of the human cutaneous circulation. *Appl Physiol Nutr Metab.* 2009 Oct;**34**(5):829–39.

21. Awad AA, Ghobashy MA, Ouda W, et al. Different responses of ear and finger pulse oximeter wave form to cold pressor test. *Anesth Analg.* 2001 Jun;**92**(6):1483–6.

22. Fine J, Branan KL, Rodriguez AJ, et al. Sources of inaccuracy in photoplethysmography for continuous cardiovascular monitoring. *Biosensors.* 2021 Apr 16;**11**(4):126.

23. Shelley KH, Tamai D, Jablonka D, et al. The effect of venous pulsation on the forehead pulse oximeter wave form as a possible source of error in Spo2 calculation. *Anesth Analg.* 2005 Mar;**100**(3):743–7.

24. Lotfy A, Hasanin A, Rashad M, et al. Peripheral perfusion index as a predictor of failed weaning from mechanical ventilation. *J Clin Monit Comput.* 2021 Apr;35(2):405–12.

25. Klijn E, Groeneveld ABJ, van Genderen ME, et al. Peripheral perfusion index predicts hypotension during fluid withdrawal by continuous veno-venous hemofiltration in critically ill patients. *Blood Purif.* 2015;40(1):92–8.

26. Liu T, Xu C, Wang M, Niu Z, Qi D. Reliability of Pleth Variability Index in predicting preload responsiveness of mechanically ventilated patients under various conditions: a systematic review and meta-analysis. *BMC Anesthesiol.* 2019 Dec;19(1):67.

27. Desgranges FP, Desebbe O, Ghazouani A, et al. Influence of the site of measurement on the ability of plethysmographic variability index to predict fluid responsiveness. *Br J Anaesth.* 2011 Sep;107(3):329–35.

28. Fischer MO, Lemoine S, Tavernier B, et al. Individualized fluid management using the Pleth Variability Index: a randomized clinical trial. *Anesthesiology.* 2020;133 (1):31–40.

29. Forget P, Lois F, de Kock M. Goal-directed fluid management based on the pulse oximeter–derived Pleth variability index reduces lactate levels and improves fluid management. *Anesth Analg.* 2010 Oct;111 (4):910–14.

30. Toyama S, Kakumoto M, Morioka M, et al. Perfusion index derived from a pulse oximeter can predict the incidence of hypotension during spinal anaesthesia for Caesarean delivery. *Br J of Anaesth.* 2013 Aug 1;111(2):235–41.

31. Duggappa D, Lokesh M, Dixit A, et al. Perfusion index as a predictor of hypotension following spinal anaesthesia in lower segment caesarean section. *Indian J Anaesth.* 2017;61(8):649.

32. Agerskov M, Thusholdt ANW, Holm-Sørensen H, et al. Association of the intraoperative peripheral perfusion index with postoperative morbidity and mortality in acute surgical patients: a retrospective observational multicentre cohort study. *Br J Anaesth.* 2021 Sep;127 (3):396–404.

33. Godai K, Matsunaga A, Kanmura Y. The effects of hemodynamic management using the trend of the perfusion index and pulse pressure variation on tissue perfusion: a randomized pilot study. *JA Clin Rep.* 2019 Dec;5(1):72.

34. Kyriacou PA. Pulse oximetry in the oesophagus. *Physiol Meas.* 2006 Jan 1;27 (1):R1–35.

35. Dépret F, Leone M, Duclos G, et al. Monitoring tissue perfusion: a pilot clinical feasibility and safety study of a urethral photoplethysmography-derived perfusion device in high-risk patients. *J Clin Monit Comput.* 2020 Oct;34 (5):961–9.

36. Cardinali M, Magnin M, Bonnet-Garin JM, et al. A new photoplethysmographic device for continuous assessment of urethral mucosa perfusion: evaluation in a porcine model. *J Clin Monit Comput.* 2021 May;35 (3):585–98.

37. Chirnoaga D, Coeckelenbergh S, Ickx B, et al. Impact of conventional vs. goal-directed fluid therapy on urethral tissue perfusion in patients undergoing liver surgery: a pilot randomised controlled trial. *Eur J Anaesthesiol.* 2022 Apr 1;39 (4):324–32.

38. Joosten A, Chirnoaga D, Van der Linden P, et al. Automated closed-loop versus manually controlled norepinephrine infusion in patients undergoing intermediate- to high-risk abdominal surgery: a randomised controlled trial. *Br J Anaesth.* 2021 Jan;126 (1):210–8.

Index